OVERCOMING YEAST INFECTIONS

A Ten-Step Program of
Medical Care and Self-Help
for Candidiasis

Marjorie Crandall, Ph.D.

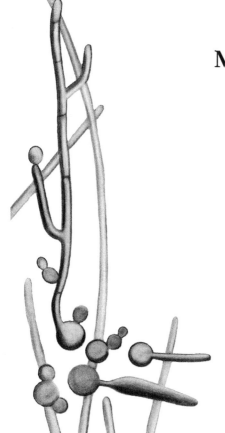

Yeast Consulting Services
YCS Press
P.O. Box 11157
Torrance CA 90510

Cover: Yeasts are oval cells that grow by forming buds. Under starvation conditions, yeast cells form filaments called *pseudohyphae* that lack cross walls. In the presence of serum, Candida albicans yeast cells form *germ tubes* that are true hyphae with cross walls.

Requests for such permissions should be addressed to:
YCS Press
P.O. Box 11157
Torrance CA 90510, USA

For single copies or bulk orders, contact author at:
yeastconsulting.com
Telephone: 1-310-375-1073
Email: DrCrandall@aol.com

Library of Congress Cataloging-in-Publication Data
Name: Crandall, Marjorie (Ann), 1940-
Title: Overcoming Yeast Infections: A Ten-Step Program of Medical Care and Self-Help for Candidiasis / Marjorie Crandall, Ph.D.

979-8-9864890-0-1 (paperback)
979-8-9864890-1-8 (eBook)

Library of Congress Control Number: 2022911963

First Edition

Printed in the United States of America

Dedication

To Morris Cohen, Ph.D., whose friendship and support made this book possible.

Acknowledgments

Special thanks to C. Orian Truss, M.D., and William G. Crook, M.D., whose 1983 books helped me regain my former good health, and opened up a new area of study—chronic candidiasis.

I am indebted to the thousands of Candida sufferers who have shared their personal experiences with me about the difficulties they faced trying to obtain proper medical care for chronic yeast infections from their physicians.

I obtained the knowledge I needed to self-publish this book from membership in the Authors Guild, Independent Writers of Southern California, and Publishers Association of Los Angeles.

Thanks to the following persons for help with this book:

- Susan Jamele drew the graphic of yeasts and hyphae on the book cover.
- Deanna Hockett drew the graphic of my logo for Yeast Consulting Services and YCS Press.
- Bob Cook, at Business Printing and Imaging, prepared Figure 1, Figure 2, and the circular graphic indicating YEAST INFECTIONS prohibited.
- David Wogahn, at AuthorImprints, designed this paperback and the ebook *Overcoming Yeast Infections.*

Disclaimer

The suggestions in this book are designed to help otherwise healthy, immunocompetent people overcome superficial yeast infections and yeast allergies. You must be under the supervision of a medical doctor or other licensed health care professional to receive the medical tests and therapies described herein. Before self-treating with natural remedies, obtain diagnostic testing. Since every patient is different, you need a treatment program based on your test results, and individual susceptibility factors. Your response to antiyeast treatment is influenced by your other health conditions, and how closely you follow your personalized healing plan. Therefore, the information in this book must not be viewed as a prescription for anyone. The author disclaims any and all liability for any adverse reactions you might experience while following this ten-step program. If you have a problem while following this program, consult your physician immediately.

Contents

Part II: A Ten-Step Program of Medical Care and Self-Help for Candida Infections and Candida Allergy 87

List of Tables and Figures

Part III: Literature Cited 217

Why I Wrote This Book

My Story

I AM A CANDIDA RESEARCHER AND FORMER CANDIDA PATIENT. My unique insights into yeast-related problems have been gained from my decades-long battle against Candida infections and my academic research on candidiasis.

Initially, I struggled against the idea of going public with my medical history in this book, but finally decided to tell my story to help other people avoid similar problems.

My yeast infections started during my twenties. Soon after I was married in 1960, I developed "honeymoon cystitis." This bacterial infection of the bladder often develops in women after vaginal intercourse. None of my doctors told me that the diaphragm I used for birth control predisposes women to develop bladder infections due to the physical trauma to the bladder during intercourse. Neither did my doctors tell me that spermicidal jelly used with the diaphragm causes chemical irritation of the vaginal mucosa, which predisposes women to develop vaginal yeast infections.

Adding insult to injury, none of my doctors told me that the antibiotic prescribed for my bladder infection makes women susceptible to vaginal yeast infections. Neither did they offer prophylactic antifungals to prevent recurrences. The antibiotic-induced vaginal yeast infections caused urethral inflammation and swelling that prevented me from emptying my bladder completely. Urine left in the bladder allowed bacteria to grow and produce another episode of cystitis, followed by another episode of vaginitis, leading to a self-perpetuating cycle of cure and relapse. These bacterial and yeast infections could suddenly appear overnight and fulminate into highly symptomatic episodes that required immediate treatment.

Self-Perpetuating Cycle

I still remember my despair at not being able to see my doctor right away when I felt that old familiar itching and burning again. When I called for a doctor's appointment, the receptionist would always say, "Is next week okay?" Each time, I had to explain that I could not tolerate the symptoms and needed immediate treatment.

During my thirties, my episodes of yeast vaginitis became more and more frequent. I was trapped in a whirlpool of yeast vaginitis alternating with bacterial cystitis that dragged me down physically and mentally. I was willing to do anything to get relief from my chronic vulvar and urethral pain. I endured many urological procedures including a cystoscopy with removal of polyps from my bladder, filling my bladder with silver nitrate, painful urethral dilations with a long rod (I call this urethral rape), and worst of all—surgical removal of the Skene glands surrounding the urethra. Called the Richardson Operation, this surgery was supposed to remove the reservoir of infection in my periurethral Skene glands causing recurrent cystitis. The bad news is that all these procedures failed to cure my recurrent bladder infections and produced additional problems.

At that time in my life, I thought physicians knew everything about their specialty, and I agreed to whatever they suggested. It never occurred to me to question my doctor's recommendations. There was no discussion about the risks and benefits of this surgery, no informed consent, no second opinion. I trusted my urologist and anticipated that this surgery would solve all my urogenital problems. Well, I was wrong!

Immediately after the surgery, I developed another bladder infection, and was back in the urologist's office! After being treated with antibiotics—again, I developed another vaginal yeast infection—again. My urogenital inflammation became even worse, and my self-perpetuating cycle of alternating vaginitis and cystitis continued unabated.

Not only that, after the Richardson operation, my urethra was wide open, exposing the internal mucosal lining of my urethra to chemical irritants, or to friction during intercourse. This made me even more susceptible to bladder infections because bacteria were more easily pushed up my urethra during sex. Furthermore, certain sexual positions became painful or impossible, and I started to leak urine whenever I sneezed or coughed. The bad news continues: I am not the only unfortunate victim of this ill-designed, experimental surgery. The only good news is that urologists no longer perform the Richardson operation, which never received official board certification.

Take home message: Do not agree to the removal of any urogenital tissue without a valid medical reason such as cancer, and always get a second opinion. Uncomplicated infections and inflammation should be treated with medications and lifestyle changes—not surgery!

After more antibiotic and antifungal treatments, my condition evolved into chronic vulvar pain and inflammation, which is now called vulvodynia. To make a very long story very short, once my gynecologist realized that I could correctly recognize symptoms of yeast vaginitis, he prescribed a refillable prescription for clotrimazole vaginal inserts. (These inserts were less irritating than vaginal antifungal creams, which also contain alcohols and detergents. Unfortunately, clotrimazole vaginal inserts are no longer available.)

Having antifungal medication on hand greatly improved the quality of my life because I could obtain prompt treatment without having to wait for a doctor's appointment. Since none of my physicians had a permanent solution for preventing my long-standing yeast problems, I became obsessed with learning everything I could about Candida infections.

My Quest for a Cure

So, in 1978, I switched the focus of my university-based laboratory work from basic research on yeast genetics to studying the medically important yeast, *Candida albicans*. I started by reviewing the research literature on candidiasis. My Eureka moment came one day while I reading medical journals in the library and I came across one study showing that yeast infections don't just occur on the surface of skin and mucous membranes, but yeasts also invade underlying tissues, and grow inside epithelial cells!

This fact led me to realize why yeast infections tend to recur after standard antifungal therapy and resolution of symptoms. The answer is that after short-term antifungal treatment, some yeasts remain inside tissue cells in a hibernating or latent condition. Even though these intracellular yeasts are not actively growing, they continuously release antigens into tissues thereby causing immune reactions that produce inflammation. Thus, after your first yeast infection, you are in a different state. The yeasts remaining inside your subsurface tissues can start growing again the next time you are exposed to a predisposing risk factor.

I also learned from my review of the scientific and medical literature on candidiasis that there are dozens of risk factors that make people susceptible to Candida infections. Before I became aware of all these predisposing conditions, I discovered a new risk factor each time I had another vaginal yeast infection. My personal risk factors were antibiotics for cystitis, use of spermicides with the diaphragm, personal hygiene products, estrogen-based contraceptive pills, swimming in chlorinated pools, becoming pregnant, and wearing pantyhose. These risk factors were cumulative, and worsened my yeast condition.

Progressive Yeast Disease

Initial episodes of yeast vaginitis become recurrent, and then chronic. Subsequently, I also developed oral thrush and chronic intestinal candidiasis. As time went by, I developed associated diseases including allergy, idiopathic (Id) reactions, inflammation, autoimmunity, and endocrine disorders. With this clinical condition, I became a textbook case of autoimmune polyendocrinopathy immune dysregulation candidiasis hypersensitivity (APICH):

- My autoimmune diseases include endometriosis and multiple sclerosis.
- My endocrine disorders include hypothyroidism, premature ovarian failure, and type II diabetes.
- My immune dysregulation is deduced from my 40-year battle with candidiasis.
- My hypersensitivities include allergies to Candida and many other substances, multiple food intolerances, chemical sensitivities, and medication-induced photosensitivity.

In 1980, I accepted a research faculty appointment, at the Associate Professor level, in the Division of Infectious Diseases, at Harbor-UCLA Medical Center, in Torrance, California. There I continued my federally funded research on Candida, published papers, and networked with colleagues studying candidiasis at other institutions.

I learned that in 1983, two pivotal books for the general public were published independently by community-based physicians: *The Missing Diagnosis* by C. Orian Truss, M.D., and *The Yeast Connection* by William G. Crook, M.D. Both described a syndrome caused by chronic intestinal candidiasis that offered me the first ray of hope for escaping from my Candida quagmire.

Following the publication of these two books, several research laboratories developed blood tests that measured levels of anti-Candida antibodies, Candida antigens, and Candida immune complexes for diagnosing chronic intestinal candidiasis.

I asked my primary care physician to order the test for anti-Candida antibody levels. When the results came back higher than normal, I asked for a prescription for Nizoral (oral ketoconazole). Diflucan was not yet available. (At that time, I was unaware of the importance of taking oral nystatin powder at the same time as a systemic antifungal for intestinal candidiasis.) I took Nizoral for about nine months, stopping occasionally to recover from side effects, and gradually my oral, intestinal and vaginal yeast infection symptoms subsided.

At the same time, I asked my allergist to test me for allergy to Candida and other substances. My scratch tests were positive for many allergens including Candida. So, I started long-term allergy shots containing all my allergens including Candida. Finally, I was on the road to recovery. But antifungal therapy and immunotherapy do not produce overnight cures.

There were many bumps along the road to my recovery. I relapsed whenever I was exposed to a new risk factor. To prevent recurrences, I had to avoid vaginal contact with all chemicals, use an antifungal concurrently whenever I took antibiotics, and treat each new yeast infection promptly in order to nip it in the bud!

My Candida Crusade

While still dealing with my personal yeast problems, I continued pursuing academic research on Candida. In 1986, I was interviewed about my research at Harbor-UCLA Medical Center in Torrance, California, by Linda Marsa, a freelance journalist. Her article, "The Infection Women Don't Talk About," was published in *Parade Magazine* on August 17, 1986. That morning, my phone started ringing, and it hasn't stopped since.

People who had read Marsa's article called or wrote me because they could not obtain proper medical care for chronic or recurrent candidiasis from their personal physicians. After receiving so many distressing inquiries, I embarked upon a crusade to correct the confusion in this field. I began writing evidence-based guidelines for the diagnosis, treatment, and prevention of oral, vaginal, and intestinal candidiasis.

Initially, I wrote a one-page handout that I distributed at my Grand Rounds lectures to physicians in the Divisions of Infectious Diseases and Allergy and Immunology at Harbor-UCLA Medical Center. By the time I retired from academia in 1988, I had read thousands of medical journal articles on the causes and cures of candidiasis, networked extensively with scientists and physicians who were studying and/or treating yeast-related disorders, and I had been invited to give lectures at several Candida conferences.

At this point, I realized that I knew more about yeast infections than most doctors, and that Candida sufferers needed accurate information about their yeast conditions. So, I switched the focus of my career from laboratory studies of Candida, to writing about candidiasis for the general public. To achieve this goal, I founded my business firm, Yeast Consulting Services, in Torrance, California, in 1988.

My Mission

The mission of Yeast Consulting Services is to help people overcome yeast infections. I counsel people on the telephone, discuss their symptoms and medical history, review their Candida test results and medical conditions, answer their questions, and make recommendations. I have also given lectures to support groups, offered expert witness testimony, and consulted for industrial firms on research and development of new antifungals and diagnostics.

As part of my mission to improve medical care for people with candidiasis, I wrote letters to medical organizations, researchers, and self-help groups, and published articles in medical journals and online. Here are some of my outreach efforts.

In 1988, I sent a letter to many members of the Infectious Diseases Society of America urging them not to adopt the draft IDSA guidelines for the yeast connection written by Edwards (1988b).

In 1989, I published a short booklet entitled, *How to Prevent Yeast Infections.* Over the following years, the helpful tips in my booklet grew into a detailed *Candida Information Packet* with supporting references.

In 1990, when the sale of vaginal antifungals over-the-counter was being decided by a panel of experts at the Food and Drug Administration (FDA), I wrote them a letter in support of their proposal. The FDA approved OTC sale of antifungal treatments for vaginal yeast infections in 1991, thereby improving the lives of many women by making prompt treatment available.

In 1991 and 2004, I wrote letters to journal editors, objecting to their negative—and incorrect—articles denying the existence of the candidiasis hypersensitivity syndrome.

In 1996, I founded my website, www.yeastconsulting.com, to sell my *Candida Information Packet* and telephone consultations.

In 2008, I sent letters to Paul Fidel, his coauthors, and their Institutional Review Board at Louisiana State University, objecting to their 2004 *Infection and Immunity* study. These researchers inserted living Candida cells into women's vaginas and, afterwards, one-third of the women subjects developed vulvovaginal candidiasis. I warned patients, if you are asked to participate in such an objectionable research protocol, just say "No!"

Also, in 2008, I published an article on www.empowher.com explaining that if Candida vulvovaginitis is not treated long enough with a sufficient dosage of an antifungal, women are left with residual Candida vulvitis (chronic atrophic erythematous candidiasis), which produces chronic vulvar pain (vulvodynia).

In 2021, my *Candida Information Packet* finally became this book. *Overcoming Yeast Infections* contains the most comprehensive scholarship available on superficial Candida infections.

My Qualifications for Writing This Book

Evidence-based information in this book is based on a synthesis of everything I have learned from all sources including:

- my personal experience with recurrent vaginal yeast infections and chronic oral and intestinal candidiasis since the 1960s
- my comprehensive review of the medical and scientific literature on candidiasis since 1980
- my experience counseling Candida patients since 1988
- my professional contacts and personal acquaintances with:
  - physicians who discovered the yeast syndrome and developed best practices for clinically diagnosing and treating chronic candidiasis in their 1983 books
  - researchers who developed and validated diagnostic tests and screening questionnaires for Candida infection
  - academic skeptics who denied the existence of the candidiasis hypersensitivity syndrome and the yeast connection to chronic disease

By taking charge of my health and learning everything I could about yeast-related conditions, I was able to overcome my long-standing problems with yeast infections. Now you too can benefit from what I have learned. By following the evidence-based guidelines in my ten-step program, you can overcome chronic candidiasis and prevent recurrences by obtaining appropriate medical care, make lifestyle changes to avoid risk factors, and obtain antifungal protection when some predisposing conditions are unavoidable. Form a partnership with your physician and offer her/him a copy of this book. They will find my evidence-based protocols valuable to other patients as well in their medical practices.

If my career efforts to help people overcome yeast infections are successful, then I will consider my Candida crusade to have been worthwhile.

My best wishes for a yeast-free future,

Marjorie Crandall, Ph.D.
Founder and Owner
Yeast Consulting Services
YCS Press
PO Box 11157
Torrance CA 90510
310-375-1073

www.yeastconsulting.com
drcrandall@aol.com
Helping Candida patients since 1988

PART I

Spectrum of Yeast Infections

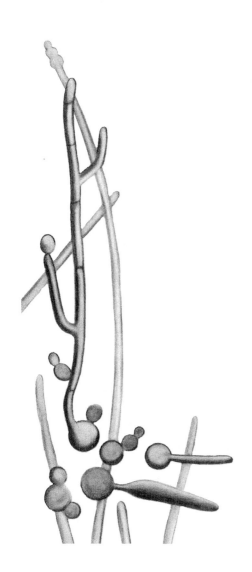

INTRODUCTION

"Your doctor said what!?"

WHEN YOU DESCRIBED YOUR WHOLE-BODY SYMPTOMS and said you thought they were yeast-related, did your doctor say something like this?

> *"The yeast connection is quackery!"*
>
> *"No studies have been done!"*
>
> *"Everyone has yeast in their intestine!"*
>
> *"It's all in your head!"*
>
> *"There's nothing more we can do for you!"*
>
> *"Learn to live with it!"*
>
> *"Stop taking antifungals, and let your body heal itself!"*

If your doctor made such uninformed, unsympathetic, and disrespectful comments, you are not alone. Candida sufferers routinely tell me they receive insulting dismissals of their symptoms, and want to know: *Why don't my physicians want to help me?*

The answer is that physicians in community practices have been influenced by skeptical academic physicians who wrote negative position statements denying the existence of a yeast connection to chronic illnesses (see Chapter 6. The Candida Controversy and the Hall of Shame).

Even though these negative papers by academic skeptics lacked scientific data and were based only on opinions, they influenced community-based physicians to deny patients medical care. Nowadays, most doctors refuse even to test patients for Candida—let alone treat them! This is tantamount to medical malpractice and condemns patients who have chronic yeast infections to needless suffering and disability.

Some adults with chronic Candida infections become so debilitated that they can no longer work or attend school. As a result, they lose their health insurance and must go on disability, live off their credit cards, and/or ask their parents or acquaintances for financial support and housing after having previously lived independently.

Children with chronic candidiasis cannot describe their discomfort. Instead, they misbehave or act out. When parents seek medical help for their child's presumed yeast infection, they are usually denied testing and treatment ironically by the same pediatrician who prescribed the antibiotics that caused the child's yeast infection in the first place!

Purpose of this Book

The purpose of this book is to educate patients about how to diagnose, treat and prevent chronic and recurrent candidiasis and yeast allergies.

Then, through Candida patients, to educate doctors about accurate scientific articles on yeast-related diseases published in medical journals. Doctors who claim that "the yeast connection does not exist" or "the candidiasis hypersensitivity syndrome is quackery" will learn how wrong these skeptical comments are, and how much suffering they have inflicted on Candida patients.

Overcoming Yeast Infections offers everything you need to know about conquering Candida infections and related yeast allergies. It is a guide through the confusing maze of myths, misinformation, misconceptions, misnomers, contradictory statements, controversies, and errors found on the internet, in popular books, and—yes—even in some academic publications!

Because there is so much nonsense written about yeast infections, you cannot believe everything you read. In your quest for a cure, keep in mind that science and medicine advance by confirming previous findings. When independent researcher groups report the same results and form a consensus, then you can believe it. That is why this book mainly cites controlled clinical studies that were published in medical and scientific journal articles. These are called primary sources of information and are the most reliable. To help you understand medical articles, scientific terms are defined the first time they are mentioned.

Overcoming Yeast Infections explains:

- how to recognize yeast-related symptoms
- what screening questionnaires and diagnostic laboratory tests for Candida have been validated in controlled clinical studies
- what treatments are proven effective for candidiasis and Candida allergy
- what risk factors cause yeast infections in susceptible people
- how to prevent candidiasis from recurring

To receive proper medical care for yeast infections, you must take charge of your health. Advocate for yourself. Discuss the information in this book with your doctor. Ask for tests and treatments that are tailor-made for your individual case.

Be assertive. Just say *"No!"* to any test, treatment, or procedure that sounds phony. If something seems hokey, it probably is! Unproven procedures offered by some alternative practitioners are named in this book.

Please be assured that yeast-related illnesses **can** be cured if you obtain effective medical care and make appropriate lifestyle changes. You should not have to endure symptoms of candidiasis for weeks or months—*or even years*—when definitive diagnostic tests, effective treatments, and preventive protocols are available. *You **can** conquer Candida!*

How to Get the Most from this Book

To get started right away on your healing plan, first read the Introduction and Chapter 1 to learn important background information. Then read the chapter that applies to your yeast condition, and fill in Tables 1, 3 and 4 in Part I. Then read the Overview of the Ten-Step Program in Part II.

Table 1. Summary of Your Medical History

Download this questionnaire from www.yeastconsulting.com, fill in your answers, print it out, and give a copy to your physician. Ask for the tests recommended in Steps 1 and 5 that are relevant for your yeast condition. If the results are positive for Candida infection and/or Candida allergy, ask for treatments recommended in Steps 2 and 5 that are appropriate for your case. Lend this book to your doctor or buy another copy for her or him.

Information you provide about your case will help your doctor make a preliminary evaluation of your yeast condition, and decide what diagnostic tests to order. After performing a physical examination and evaluating your medical history, risk factors for candidiasis, and diagnostic test results for Candida and other illnesses, your physician can arrive at a more accurate diagnosis of your condition.

1. Name, age, height, weight, and male or female:
2. Current signs and symptoms:
3. On a scale from 1 (lowest) to 10 (highest), fill in the number that best describes the degree of pain and discomfort you feel:
4. On a scale from 1 (lowest) to 10 (highest), fill in the number that indicates how much your yeast condition interferes with your work, relationships, and recreational activities:
5. When did your symptoms start?
6. History of yeast infections indicating your susceptibility to Candida:
7. Recent risk factors that predisposed you to develop a yeast infection:
8. Women:
   - What birth control method are you using?
   - When during your monthly menstrual cycle are your yeast symptoms the worst?
   - Or are you postmenopausal?
9. Men: Are you circumcised?
10. Medically diagnosed diseases:

11. List your results from tests for Candida infection and immune function using the following headings:

    Date, Doctor, Specimen, Test, Result and Normal Range, Interpretation
    - **Blood tests for:** Candida antibodies, Candida antigens, Candida immune complexes, and/or Candida DNA.
    - **Specimens collected:** stool (fecal) samples; swabs of vagina and/or rectum; scrapings of vulva, tongue, and/or skin.
    - **Procedures performed on specimens:** Microscopy, Candida culture, yeast species identification, and antifungal susceptibility testing.
    - **Urine test for:** yeast metabolites.
    - **Immune function tests for:** Candida allergy (RAST, scratch or prick tests, and/or intradermal testing); Candida anergy (delayed hypersensitivity and T lymphocyte function).

12. Any other abnormal medical test results:

13. Blood test results for: WBC count, liver function, diabetes, and HIV:

14. Any allergies? If yes, what ones? Candida, baker's yeast, molds, pollen, dander, foods, other?

15. What antifungals have you taken? Dose, treatment time, and response to therapy.

16. Current medications and supplements you are taking:

17. Are you taking oral probiotics containing the friendly bacteria Lactobacillus and Bifidobacterium?

18. Are you following the Candida diet? What foods do you eliminate from your diet? What happens if you eat those foods?

19. Questions about your case:

Your clinical signs and symptoms of Candida infection and Candida allergy are the justification you need for your doctor to order diagnostic tests (Steps 1 and 5). If your test results are positive, they justify antifungal therapy and immunotherapy (Steps 2 through 5). If you develop recurrences, you require preventive Steps 6 through 10.

I strongly urge you to stay with your own personal physician. She or he knows your history yeast infections and risk factors that cause recurrences. Lend your copy of *Overcoming Yeast Infections* to your physician, or buy a second copy and give it to her or him. Doctors will find this book a valuable reference manual containing evidence-based treatment protocols and citations of over 500 original research articles. It also contains practical advice and self-help programs for Candida patients to follow.

CHAPTER 1

Diseases Caused by Candida

CANDIDIASIS IS LIKE A CHAMELEON—its appearance changes under different conditions. Symptoms of yeast infections vary depending on the body site, virulence of the yeast strain, and strength of your immune system. The winner of this battle between host and pathogen is determined by factors explored in this chapter. We start with a description of what yeasts are, and infections they cause. Then explanations are given for how symptoms are caused by both Candida and the immune system.

What Yeasts Are

Yeasts are defined as single-celled fungi that reproduce by budding. They are so small you cannot see them without magnification under a microscope. That is why they are called *microorganisms*, or *microbes* for short. Candida yeast cells are round or oval-shaped, about 3 x 5 μm.

In the older literature, yeast cells were called *blastospores.* However, this term should not be used because *spore* means an environmentally resistant dormant cell with a hard cell wall that protects it from heat and chemicals. In contrast, growing (*vegetative*) yeast cells are not spores, and they are sensitive to high temperatures and chemicals.

The yeast species that causes most infections is *Candida albicans.* It grows as a single cell, and also elongates in serum and tissues into filaments called *hyphae, germ tubes,* or *mycelia.* This form has individual cells separated by cross walls (*septa*). When hyphae are transferred to growth medium, yeast cells bud off indicating that both forms are the same organism.

C. albicans is the only species that forms true hyphae or germ tubes with cross walls. All other pathogenic Candida species grow only as single yeast cells. When Candida cells are grown under starvation conditions in laboratory media lacking nutrients, they elongate forming false or *pseudo-hyphae* that lack cross walls.

How Yeasts Are Named

Plants, animals, and microorganisms are assigned two Latin names consisting of the *genus* and *species*. For the major pathogenic yeast, *Candida albicans*, the genus name is *Candida*, and the species name is *albicans*. Once the genus name has been mentioned in the text, it can be abbreviated (for example, *C. albicans*). Italics are used only when both the genus and species names are used together. When the genus name is used alone, it is not italicized (for example, Candida).

The correct pronunciation of Candida is "kan' di dah" with emphasis on the first syllable. The letter "i" is pronounced as in the word "did" (not as in the word "deed"). Please don't say "Candeeda!" That is the pronunciation for Candida, a woman's given name.

Where Yeasts Are Found

Yeasts are ubiquitous. They are present everywhere—in the air, soil, oceans, lakes, and streams, and on the surfaces of plants and animals. For example, the yeast *Saccharomyces cerevisiae* grows on the surfaces of grapes and ferments the sugar in grape juice forming wine. Candida yeast species are normally found on skin and mucous membranes of the mouth, intestine, and vagina in humans (Akiyama, 2000).

Because Candida yeasts obtain their nutrients from our tissues, they are called *commensals,* a Latin term which means eating at the same table. *Commensalism* is defined as a relationship between two organisms in which one organism benefits, and one is unaffected. In general, Candida is present on our body surfaces in small numbers and does us no harm. The presence of yeasts on tissue surfaces in the absence of disease is called *asymptomatic colonization.*

Babies become colonized with yeasts and bacteria from the mother's vagina as they travel down the birth canal. When newborns swallow, yeasts and bacteria spread from their mouth to their intestines. The microbes attach to the bowel wall and also grow on the contents of the *lumen,* the opening inside the intestine where the food and feces are located.

When the same yeasts and bacteria are repeatedly isolated from body surfaces on thousands of healthy people, they are considered part of the *normal flora* or *microbiome,* i.e., the resident microbial population. The normal intestinal bacterial flora is referred to as "friendly" because they help prevent infections by:

- producing antimicrobial substances
- competing for nutrients
- blocking attachment sites on body surfaces
- assisting with digestion
- detoxifying chemicals
- synthesizing vitamins

Probiotics supplements containing friendly bacteria are taken to help replace normal flora killed by antibiotics.

Yeast Species that Cause Infections

Dozens of yeasts have been isolated from people, but most are environmental yeasts that transiently contaminate body surfaces, but do not live there. The yeast species found most consistently in healthy people is *Candida albicans*. It normally colonizes skin and mucous membranes because the immune system tolerates its presence. In other words, Candida is not recognized as a pathogen (Jouault et al., 2009). This phenomenon is called *immune tolerance.*

Yet, *Candida albicans* is also a major pathogen (*etiological agent*) that causes infections. A yeast infection caused by any species of Candida is called *candidiasis*. Older names for Candida are Oidium and Monilia, and the infection used to be called *moniliasis*. Oidium is the "O" in the T.O.E. vaccine that was used to treat fungal infections before antifungal drugs became available. The other components of this fungal vaccine are Trichophyton and Epidermophyton.

Candida albicans accounts for 60% of the Candida species isolated from the mouth, intestine, vagina, and skin. Gentles and La Touche (1969) suggested that its predominance as a pathogen derives from its high incidence as a commensal. Most yeast infections are caused by *C. albicans* and most are susceptible to Diflucan.

Other pathogenic Candida species, such as *C. glabrata, C. krusei, C. parapsilosis,* and *C. tropicalis*, are present as commensals at lower frequencies and are often resistant to Diflucan. That's why in cases of chronic candidiasis recalcitrant to permanent cure, yeast cultures should be ordered, the species identified, and tested for antifungal susceptibility.

Harmless Flora or Dangerous Pathogen?

Candida is our constant companion, and occasional enemy. Commensal yeasts do not cause infections unless we are exposed to risk factors that lower our immunity or promote yeast growth. Then Candida takes advantage of the opportunity to overgrow. That is why Candida is called an *opportunistic pathogen.*

Exposure to Risk Factors

Susceptibility to yeast infections is determined by many different predisposing risk factors (explained in Step 6). *The number one cause of candidiasis is treatment with antibiotics.* Antibacterial drugs not only kill pathogenic bacteria, they also kill friendly bacteria in our body that keep yeast growth under control. Other medications that predispose people to develop yeast infections include corticosteroids that lower immunity; antacids that raise the stomach pH thereby promoting yeast growth; and drugs called sodium-glucose cotransporter-2 inhibitors for type 2 diabetes that cause genital yeast infections in men and women. Estrogen makes women more susceptible to vaginal yeast infections. Other causes of yeast infections include medical, hospital, physiological, disease, and transmission risk factors.

Number of Yeasts in Your Body

Yeasts are normally present in low numbers in healthy people. However, each time you are exposed to a predisposing condition, yeast numbers increase. Multiple risk factors have a cumulative effect. Once yeasts increase above a threshold or tipping point, a full-blown yeast infection will occur.

Virulence of Your Yeast Strain

Susceptibility to yeast infections is also determined by the degree of pathogenicity or *virulence* of your yeast strain. Virulence of *C. albicans* depends on its ability to produce digestive enzymes, evade WBC killing, and form hyphae that penetrate into underlying tissues.

Strength of Your Immune System

Candidiasis is like a "red flag" signaling decreased immunity. A little recognized factor that lowers your immunity is allergy to Candida (Step 5). Allergic reactions release chemical mediators (such as histamine, leukotrienes, and prostaglandin E2), which inhibit WBCs. You must identify your individual susceptibility to candidiasis before you can develop a preventive program.

Spectrum of Yeast Infections

Yeasts and fungi can infect any site in your body. Yeast infections on the surfaces of skin and mucous membranes are termed *superficial*. Such infections are referred to as *benign* because they are not life threatening. While superficial and benign are medical terms, sometimes patients misinterpret their meaning and think doctors are downplaying their symptoms.

Superficial yeast infections are common, easy to diagnose, and well documented in the medical literature. Candida yeasts commonly overgrow skin and mucous membranes because they reside there as part of the normal flora. In rare cases, when people have very low WBC counts, Candida infects the blood (*candidemia*), and spreads to the deep organs (liver, kidney, and spleen), causing *disseminated candidiasis*, a potentially fatal infection.

Over the last two decades, there has been a dramatic increase in the rate of superficial and disseminated fungal infections (Moosa et al., 2004). Paradoxically, the intensity of symptoms does not correlate with the seriousness of the yeast infection. A life-threatening yeast infection often has few or no symptoms, whereas yeast infections of the mouth, intestine, vagina, or penis can torment people night and day. Hence, in this book, *severe* is used to describe intense symptoms, whereas *serious* is used to describe life-threatening infections.

Between the extremes of superficial and disseminated candidiasis are many other yeast-related illnesses. These are arranged in order of seriousness in Table 2. Candida Continuum.

Table 2. Candida Continuum

Normal flora (Candida colonization) is present without symptoms.

↓

Superficial yeast infections (mucosal, cutaneous, and allergic) can be highly symptomatic.

↓

The yeast syndrome and Candida autoimmunity can be disabling.

↓

Chronic mucocutaneous candidiasis, chronic granulomatous disease, and candidemia can be life threatening.

↓

Disseminated candidiasis is often fatal.

Mucosal Candidiasis

Yeast infections on mucous membranes can be acute or chronic. The scientific names for these two types of yeast infection are *acute pseudomembranous candidiasis* and *chronic atrophic erythematous candidiasis*. To make the terminology easier, I call these two conditions the white form and the red form of yeast infection because of the color of the infected mucosal tissue.

The white form of mucosal yeast infection (called *acute pseudomembranous candidiasis)* is a full-blown, active, acute yeast infection. A swab of infected tissue yields a positive yeast culture and a positive microscope smear. White patches or lesions observed on infected mucosal tissue is dead tissue called false membranes (*pseudomembranes*). Here is how they are formed.

When yeasts infect mucosal tissues, they grow on the surface and also invade the deeper layers of tissue where they grow inside epithelial cells. There, yeasts release fermentation products and digestive enzymes that kill tissue cells. When mucosal epithelial tissue cells die, they turn white. White patches are not "visible colony-forming units of Candida on the mucosal surface" as claimed by van Burik and Magee (2001). You cannot see Candida cells because they are microscopic. The white lesions you see are clumps of dead mucosal epithelial tissue.

Examples of *acute pseudomembranous candidiasis* include the following yeast infections:

- *Thrush* or *oral candidiasis* is characterized by white patches on the tongue. When scraped off, the infected tissue underneath may bleed. Oral thrush is common in people who have been treated with antibiotics, corticosteroids, chemotherapy or radiation for cancer, and in infants and elderly people who have weak immune systems.
- *Geographic tongue* is a common condition in which tuft-like projections on the tongue, called *lingual papillae,* (some of which are associated with taste buds), are lost, leaving smooth, red areas. Sometimes, white patches develop first and migrate over the surface of the tongue. The name comes from the map-like appearance of the tongue like the earth's

continents on a globe. In some cases, fissures may also develop. Some people with geographic tongue may experience pain or burning when eating hot, acidic, or spicy foods.

- *Esophageal candidiasis* is identified by white patches in the throat and on the esophagus seen during endoscopy. It is common in people whose immune system is weakened by HIV infection or who have been treated intensively with antibiotics or corticosteroids. If you have Candida esophagitis, get tested for HIV as well as for diabetes and other predisposing conditions (listed in Step 6). If you have an unavoidable risk factor, obtain antifungal prophylaxis (described in Step 10).
- *Vulvovaginal candidiasis* is diagnosed by white lesions on the vaginal wall seen during colposcopy. This dead vaginal tissue peels or *sloughs* off forming a white clumpy or creamy vaginal discharge. Yeast vaginitis is common in women treated with antibiotics, corticosteroids, estrogen, or sodium-glucose cotransporter-2 inhibitor drugs for type 2 diabetes, and in pregnant women who have high levels of estrogen and cortisol.
- *Intestinal candidiasis* produces white lesions on the intestinal wall seen during sigmoidoscopy and colonoscopy. The false membrane sloughs off the intestinal wall and appears as white clumps or strings in feces. Intestinal candidiasis is caused by antibiotics, antacids, and corticosteroids.

The red form of yeast infection (called *chronic atrophic erythematous candidiasis*) is a chronic, inactive, or low-grade yeast infection. *Atrophic* means not feeding, not growing; *erythematous* means red, inflamed tissue. Yeasts reside inside mucosal tissue causing redness and burning, but because yeasts are inside epithelial cells, and not on the mucosal surface, swabs of the surface yield negative cultures and no yeasts are seen on microscope smears. Yet, dormant or *latent* Candida cells inside epithelial cells continuously release Candida antigens and digestive enzymes, which trigger inflammation. Inactive, nongrowing, intracellular yeast infections are difficult to cure because antifungals only kill yeasts that are actively growing.

Examples of *chronic atrophic erythematous candidiasis* include the following yeast infections:

- *Denture stomatitis* is characterized by red, burning gums in people with false teeth or poor dental hygiene (Webb et al., 1998). It also develops after antibiotic treatment, and is called "antibiotic sore mouth."
- *Oral, pharyngeal, and esophageal candidiasis* and *Candida gastroenteritis* cause redness and burning of tongue, buccal membranes, throat, the swallowing tube (*esophagus*) and stomach seen during endoscopy. It occurs in people with HIV infection (Dodd et al., 1991), and after antibiotic treatment.
- *Vulvodynia* or *vulvar vestibulitis* is characterized by residual redness and burning of the vulva or vestibule remaining after short-term antifungal treatment of yeast vaginitis.
- *Prostatodynia* or nonbacterial prostatitis remaining after antibiotic treatment might be an unrecognized example of inactive yeast infection.
- *Intestinal candidiasis* produces red lesions on the intestinal wall seen during sigmoidoscopy and colonoscopy, and is caused by antibiotics, antacids, corticosteroids, and sodium-glucose cotransporter-2 inhibitor drugs for type 2 diabetes.

Take home message: *Any red, inflamed tissue without an identifiable etiology is a candidate for the diagnosis of chronic atrophic erythematous candidiasis.*

Because the red or erythematous form of yeast infection is not generally recognized, it is underdiagnosed (Dodd et al., 1991). Short-term treatment with an antifungal agent may cure an active infection, but it is inefficient for eradicating latent yeasts inside tissue cells.

Cutaneous Candidiasis

Fungal infections of the skin are very common, affecting about 1.7 billion people worldwide (Havlickova et al., 2008). Colloquial names for fungal skin infections are *tinea* or *ringworm*. Lesions of ringworm tend to be circular, but are caused by a fungus—not a worm! Fungi that cause skin infections include Trichophyton, Epidermophyton, and Microsporum. Dandruff is caused by the fungus Malassezia (previously named Pityrosporum).

Nonspecific illnesses such as *dermatitis, psoriasis, eczema,* and *urticaria* can be caused by Candida or other fungal infections. They produce red, inflamed tissue called a *rash*, with itching and burning, red patches that are either flat (*macular*) or raised (*papular*), companion (*satellite*) lesions around the edges that can be red bumps, tiny water blisters, or flaky, scaly, white (dead) skin that peels off.

Cutaneous candidiasis usually occurs in warm moist body locations such as the genital and anal areas, and inside skin folds such as underarms, under breasts, and the *inguinal* area where the thigh meets the groin. Examples include "jock itch" in adults and diaper rash in babies and the elderly. Diaper rash is usually a mixed infection with fecal bacteria and yeasts. Other skin rashes can be due to chemical irritation, other infections, autoimmune diseases, or allergic reactions.

Allergic Candidiasis

Immune reactions to a pathogen produce symptoms typical of that infection (Waksman, 1979). For example, it is widely acknowledged that Candida infections provoke allergic responses, which are immune reactions. When Candida acts as both an infectious agent and an allergen, the disease is called *allergic candidiasis* or *candidiasis hypersensitivity*.

A classic example of a disease caused by allergy to Candida is *Candida asthma.* It is a chronic inflammatory condition of the lungs that causes difficulty in breathing. While asthma is usually caused by airborne allergens (such as pollen, dust mites, mold spores, and animal dander), it can also be caused by internal (*endogenous*) allergens such as Candida, which has overgrown the intestines.

Candida asthma is an example of an allergic reaction called an *idiopathic (Id) reaction.* According to Odds (1988; pp. 136, 231-2), an Id reaction is caused by an allergic reaction in a target organ to an infection at a distant site in the body. Another definition of Id reaction is a secondary inflammatory reaction that develops from a remotely localized immunological insult (Ilkit et al. (2012). Id reactions on skin caused by Candida are called *candidids* (Odds, 1979; p. 113). *Dermatophytids* are Id reactions on skin caused by fungi (Ilkit et al., 2012). Failure of the clinician to recognize Id reactions could result in an unwarranted early withdrawal of antifungal treatment (Sorey, 2009).

Allergic bronchopulmonary candidiasis is both a Candida infection in the lungs, and an allergy to Candida located in the lungs (Akiyama et al., 1984).

The Yeast Syndrome

Intestinal yeast overgrowths produce symptoms locally in the gut as well as systemically throughout the body. This group of symptoms has several names including *the yeast connection, the missing diagnosis,* and *the yeast syndrome* (after books by these titles). This disease is also called the *Candida-related complex, candidiasis hypersensitivity syndrome*, and *polysystem chronic candidiasis* by authors of scientific papers. An incorrect name for intestinal candidiasis often used on the internet is *"systemic yeast."*

"Systemic Yeast" is a misnomer!

Candida sufferers who could not get help for symptoms of the yeast syndrome often sought help from alternative practitioners. While these health care practitioners acknowledged the existence of the yeast syndrome, they used the misnomer "systemic yeast" to describe chronic intestinal candidiasis. People eagerly embraced this diagnosis because it accounted for their long-standing yeast symptoms in the gut and at other body sites. But patients who received this diagnosis became alarmed because they mistakenly thought that yeasts had spread throughout their body.

How did this inappropriate terminology arise? I tracked down its origin to pages 35 through 37 of Truss's 1983 book, *The Missing Diagnosis*. There, Truss incorrectly used the term *systemic candidiasis* to describe systemic symptoms caused by the release of toxic metabolites from Candida into infected intestinal mucosal tissues.

Later, the term, systemic candidiasis, was corrupted into "systemic yeast." This misnomer has been repeated so often in popular books, magazines, and on the internet that it has become common parlance. People suffering from chronic fatigue, gastrointestinal distress, and brain fog were diagnosed with "systemic yeast" by alternative practitioners, nutritionists, chiropractors, and herbalists—even by some medical doctors who should know better!

Take a lesson from this backstory. Never use the term *"systemic yeast"* when describing your symptoms to your doctor, or you will lose credibility. Physicians know that systemic candidiasis develops only in people who have extremely low white blood cell (WBC) counts after receiving chemotherapy or radiation for cancer, or organ transplants, or in people who have terminal acquired immune deficiency syndrome (AIDS).

When Candida patients consult with me and claim they have "systemic yeast," I explain that, *"The yeast syndrome is a real disease, but it is not a systemic infection. While some symptoms can be systemic, the yeast infection is localized in the intestinal tract. Intestinal yeast infections are not life threatening—they just make your life miserable!*

To obtain proper medical care, always use the correct terminology when asking for tests and treatments recommended in this book. The term used herein to describe the physical and mental symptoms caused by intestinal candidiasis is the yeast syndrome.

Chronic Mucocutaneous Candidiasis

CMCC refers to several syndromes caused by congenital abnormalities of T cell-mediated immunity (Kirkpatrick, 1989). These disorders predispose people to persistent or recurrent Candida and/or other infections, plus endocrine dysfunctions (such as hypoparathyroidism, adrenal insufficiency, hypogonadism, thyroid disease, and diabetes), and other disorders such as alopecia, vitiligo, malabsorption, and neoplasms (Merck Manual for Health Care Professionals).

Laypersons often mistakenly think CMCC refers to superficial candidiasis and the yeast syndrome. Even though both diseases share many clinical features, CMCC is a genetic disease that is usually identified in childhood when symptoms arise, whereas superficial candidiasis occurs in otherwise healthy people, and is usually caused by antibiotics.

Chronic Granulomatous Disease

CGD is a rare disorder (Segal et al., 2000) caused by an inherited (genetic) immune system disorder. The CGD patient's WBCs, called *neutrophils* or *granulocytes*, are unable to produce activated oxygen compounds. As a result, these defective WBCs cannot kill bacteria and fungi.

Candidemia

Continuing along the Candida continuum, the next disease is yeast infection of the bloodstream. *Candidemia* is of intermediate seriousness. It occurs in eight of every 100,000 persons per year (Centers for Disease Control, 2008). Hospitalized people are at high risk for developing candidemia if they have intravenous (IV) catheters, or very low WBC counts. Yeasts attach to IV catheters, and form biofilms. These contaminated IV catheters continuously seed the bloodstream with yeast cells. Also, at risk for candidemia are addicts who inject illegal drugs into their veins, and low-birth-weight babies whose immune systems are undeveloped.

Disseminated Yeast Infections

The most serious yeast infection occurs when yeasts enter the bloodstream and spread (*disseminate*) to the deep tissues and organs such as the liver, kidney and spleen. At these body sites, yeasts establish a potentially fatal yeast infection variously called *disseminated, systemic, deep, deep-seated, hematogenous, blood borne,* or *invasive candidiasis.* The term *systemic candidiasis* has fallen into disuse to avoid confusion with the misnomer "systemic yeast," which is used incorrectly to describe the yeast syndrome. The term *invasive candidiasis* should also be avoided because it can be confused with invasion of skin and mucous membranes by yeasts in superficial candidiasis.

Healthy people with normal WBC counts do not develop disseminated candidiasis because germs entering the circulatory system from the intestines are quickly killed by WBCs called *neutrophils* or *granulocytes* in blood.

Critically ill, hospitalized people with terminal AIDS, malignant neoplasms, or organ transplants often develop disseminated candidiasis after treatment with broad-spectrum antibacterial agents, corticosteroids, cancer chemotherapy, or anti-rejection medications (Pappas et al., 2009). These diseases and drugs decrease the number of neutrophils in the blood resulting in extremely low WBC counts (*neutropenia*). Then, Candida cells entering the bloodstream overwhelm the small number of WBCs and grow uncontrolled throughout the body.

To prevent serious yeast infections, standard hospital protocols emphasize best practices such as hand washing, sterile technique, universal precautions, replacing IV catheters on schedule, and administering prophylactic antifungals.

Expanding Spectrum

As our medical knowledge has increased, so has the number of illnesses attributed to Candida. To understand how different yeast-related diseases develop, we must examine the pathogenic mechanisms involved at both the cellular and molecular levels. So, next we examine how symptoms of yeast infections are produced by Candida as well as by our immune system.

How Candida Causes Symptoms

Candida disease activities include microbiological processes, enzymatic mechanisms, and putative toxins.

Microbiological Processes

Candida infectious processes include tissue invasion, intracellular protection, and latent yeast infection.

Tissue invasion: During active yeast infections of skin and mucous membranes, Candida yeast cells proliferate by budding, but *C. albicans* is the only yeast that produces hyphae. Both yeast cells and hyphae burrow into underlying tissues, and penetrate into epithelial cells (Filler and Sheppard, 2006). *C. albicans* invades tissues by degrading intercellular junctions using lytic enzymes, such as proteases and phospholipases (Zhu and Filler, 2010).

When biopsies from active vaginal yeast infections were sectioned and examined under the electron microscope, yeast cells and hyphae were seen invading tissues as shown below in Figure 1. Pathogenesis of Vaginal Candidiasis.

Figure 1.

PATHOGENESIS OF VAGINAL CANDIDIASIS

STRATIFIED VAGINAL EPITHELIUM

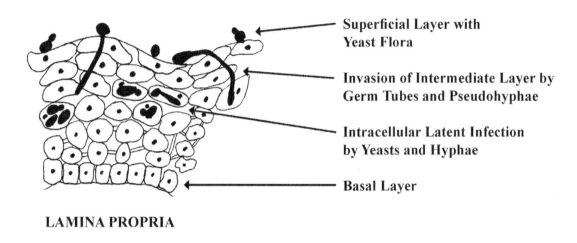

Superficial Layer with Yeast Flora

Invasion of Intermediate Layer by Germ Tubes and Pseudohyphae

Intracellular Latent Infection by Yeasts and Hyphae

Basal Layer

LAMINA PROPRIA

Figure 1 is a drawing that represents what is seen in electron micrographs published in Schnell and Voigt (1976), García-Tamayo et al. (1982), and Montes and Wilborn (1985). Yeasts and hyphae were seen inside vaginal epithelial cells by Schnell (1982a, b). Other scientists have made similar observations of yeasts inside epithelial cells from biopsies of oral and intestinal candidiasis.

Intracellular protection: Yeast cells inside tissue cells are protected from antifungal drugs and the immune system. Only low concentrations of antifungals can be attained inside host cells. This explains why antifungals are *fungistatic*, and only inhibit growth, but are not *fungicidal*, and do not kill yeasts. While yeasts can be killed in laboratory cultures by adding high concentrations of antifungals, such a high drug level in the body would kill the patient!

Thus, persistence of colonization and endogenous reinfection are explained by the fungistatic activity of antifungals (Vazquez et al., 1994). Yeasts inside epithelial cells also evade immune surveillance because WBCs and antibodies cannot enter host cells (García-Tamayo et al., 1982). Intracellular protection explains why yeast infections are so difficult to cure.

Latent intracellular yeast infection: After standard short-term antifungal treatment, symptoms of active yeast infections usually resolve, and swabs of tissue surfaces become negative for yeasts. But some yeast cells remain inside tissues in a nongrowing state. I coined the term *latent intracellular yeast infection* to describe this condition (Crandall, 1991a). *Latent* means hidden, dormant, or hibernating. Latent or persister cells are known in other microorganisms as well (Lewis, 2010).

After exposure to antifungals, yeasts stop growing, but remain alive. When antifungal therapy is discontinued, yeasts may start to grow again when the person is exposed to a risk factor for candidiasis. After a lag period, actively growing yeasts may then erupt into another full-blown yeast infection. The lag period before yeasts start growing again is called the *postantifungal effect* (Gunderson et al., 2000). Persistence of colonizing *C. albicans* occurred in five out of eight individuals for up to seven years despite intervals of antifungal therapy (Bartie et al., 2001). Thus, intracellular yeasts are a *reservoir of infection*. This condition explains why:

- Swabs of tissue surfaces yield negative yeast cultures, but tissue scrapings containing epithelial cells yield positive yeast cultures.
- Symptoms come back at the same body site after discontinuing antifungal therapy.
- Recurrences happen at higher rates than the rate of first-time yeast infections.
- Yeasts isolated from difficult-to-cure infections are usually sensitive to antifungals when tested in the laboratory. This means that persistence or latency is not due to antifungal resistance.

These results explain why standard short-term antifungal therapy (one day or three days) results in incomplete cures. Nongrowing yeasts remain inside tissue cells and continuously release Candida antigens, degradative enzymes, and metabolic products that trigger chronic inflammation and pain, i.e., the red (*erythematous*) form of yeast infection.

Take home message: Eradication of yeasts inside tissues requires longer treatment times, with both topical and systemic antifungals, at higher than standard doses, or with two or three antifungals used concurrently. After the intracellular infection is eradicated, it takes time for the inflammatory reactions to dampen down, and for tissues to repair the damage.

During the healing process, dead epithelial cells containing intracellular yeasts slough off tissue surfaces, and new tissue cells without intracellular yeasts grow up from the bottom (*basal*) layers. While tissue regeneration is occurring, antifungal treatment should be in place to make sure new cells do not become infected. Corticosteroid cream helps with the repair process by reducing inflammation, but only if used together with an antifungal. Once symptoms have resolved, daily antifungal treatment should be switched to weekly suppression to prevent recurrences.

Enzymatic Mechanisms

Another infectious process in Candida infection that results in symptoms is the release of degradative enzymes that allow yeast cells and hyphae to penetrate into tissues. *Enzymes* are protein molecules that catalyze biochemical reactions. Degradative enzymes break down large molecules into smaller constituents. Candida secretes these degradative enzymes:

- *Hemolysins* cause red blood cells (RBCs) to burst (*lyse*).
- *Phospholipase* breaks down fats in epithelial cell membranes.
- *Acidic proteinase* breaks down proteins in epithelial cell membranes.

These three enzymes are involved in pathogenesis as shown by the following observations. Higher amounts of phospholipase and proteinase are produced by Candida isolated from women with yeast vaginitis than by Candida isolated from healthy women (Kalkanci et al., 2012). *Candida albicans* acidic proteinase antigen is isolated from women with yeast vaginitis (Crandall et al., 1988). It functions optimally at pH 4.5, the same pH as in the healthy vagina during the child-bearing years. It is likely that during active yeast infections, phospholipase and acidic proteinase kill tissues forming the characteristic white pseudomembranous lesions. During inactive yeast infections, these enzymes cause inflammation, turning tissues red.

Putative Candida Toxins

Canditoxin: The mistaken idea that *Candida albicans* produces a toxin originated with a series of papers by Iwata and coinvestigators from 1967 to 1977 and 1978. Iwata reported on a *Canditoxin*, but refused to send the so-called Canditoxin-producing yeast strain to other scientists for verification. Other investigators were unable to repeat Iwata's results using different clinical isolates of *C. albicans* (Chattaway et al., 1971). Even though extracts of *C. albicans* were lethal in mice, a specific toxin could not be isolated or identified (Cutler et al. (1972). Therefore, it was concluded that *the toxic effects of Candida infections are most likely caused by immune reactions of the host, not by Candida activity* (Odds, 1988; pp. 264-6). Despite the fact that Iwata's reports were discredited by several groups of investigators, the myth about a Canditoxin became dogma on the internet and among alternative practitioners.

Adding to this confusion was the misinterpretation of a journal article published by Axelsen (1976) who identified 79 antibodies against Candida antigens. Some practitioners mistakenly interpreted this finding to mean that Candida produced 79 toxins.

Gliotoxin: Further confusion was caused by conflicting reports about an immunosuppressive toxin called *gliotoxin*. Shah et al. (1995) reported that *C. albicans* produced gliotoxin in vivo, but Kupfahl et al. (2007) and Kosalec et al. (2008) reported that Candida did not produce gliotoxin in vitro. Actually, all these reports may be correct because cofactors required for gliotoxin synthesis in the body may not be supplied in laboratory media. The clinical significance of these gliotoxin reports remains unknown.

Candidalysin: The first valid report of the isolation of a toxin from *C. albicans* was by Moyes et al. (2016). Candidalysin is a 31-amino acid α-helical peptide toxin that acts as a virulence factor during hyphal morphogenesis. Candidalysin promotes invasion and rupture (*lysis*) of epithelial cells during active infections of mucosal membranes. This cytolytic toxin also activates epithelial cells to produce an immune response. *C. albicans* strains lacking candidalysin do not damage epithelial cells and cannot infect mucosal tissues.

A few words to the wise: While Candidalysin is called a toxin by Moyes and coinvestigators, it does not fit the definition of a toxin (given below) of a poisonous substance that causes systemic symptoms. Candidalysin produces localized symptoms and localized immune reactions during hyphal invasion of mucous membranes in superficial candidiasis. Furthermore, non-*albicans Candida* species do not produce true hyphae and, therefore, Candidalysin is not involved in their infections.

Definition of toxin: Another issue contributing to the myth about Candida toxins is the misuse of scientific terminology. *The strict definition of a toxin is a poisonous substance produced by a* *living organism that causes disease or death in humans and other animals.* To qualify as a toxin, a substance must be isolated, purified, and chemically identified in different isolates of the same biological source (Bennett and Klich, 2003).

Fungal toxins are usually large molecular weight substances called *secondary metabolites* that are produced during secondary metabolism when molds stop growing but are still carrying out biochemical reactions. Toxins produced by fungi are called *mycotoxins*; examples include aflatoxin produced by *Aspergillus flavus*, and ergot alkaloids produced by *Claviceps purpurea*.

In contrast, Candida and other yeasts produce low molecular weight metabolites, such as alcohol (*ethanol*) and acetaldehyde, which are harmful but are not considered toxins because they are *primary metabolites* that are produced during growth on glucose (see Figure 2. Sugar Metabolism). Yeast fermentation products such as alcohol and acetaldehyde can cause "brain fog" or "food coma" symptoms, which are experienced after eating carbohydrates.

So, don't believe everything you read about Candida in popular books, magazines, and on the internet. Occasionally, even scientific papers are wrong!

What can you accept as fact? The number one principle in scientific research is reproducibility. You can rely upon papers in scientific journals that corroborate and expand the published findings of other independent investigators.

Figure 2.

SUGAR METABOLISM

and symptoms caused by yeast products

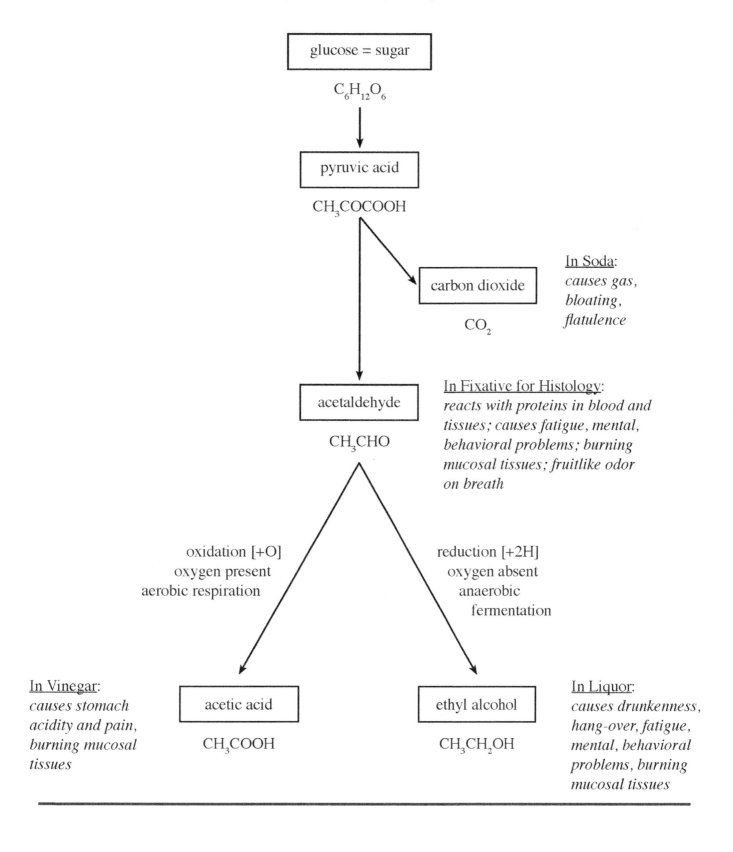

glucose = sugar

$C_6H_{12}O_6$

pyruvic acid

$CH_3COCOOH$

carbon dioxide

CO_2

In Soda:
*causes gas,
bloating,
flatulence*

acetaldehyde

CH_3CHO

In Fixative for Histology:
*reacts with proteins in blood and
tissues; causes fatigue, mental,
behavioral problems; burning
mucosal tissues; fruitlike odor
on breath*

oxidation [+O]
oxygen present
aerobic respiration

reduction [+2H]
oxygen absent
anaerobic
fermentation

In Vinegar:
*causes stomach
acidity and pain,
burning mucosal
tissues*

acetic acid

CH_3COOH

ethyl alcohol

CH_3CH_2OH

In Liquor:
*causes drunkenness,
hang-over, fatigue,
mental, behavioral
problems, burning
mucosal tissues*

How the Immune System Causes Symptoms

We have just reviewed the many ways that Candida causes disease symptoms. But that's not all. *Paradoxically, our immune system also causes symptoms while fighting yeast infections.* Immune reactions against Candida that harm our tissues include the inflammatory response, WBC activities, anti-Candida antibody reactions, Candida allergy, and Candida autoimmunity.

The Inflammatory Response

The term *inflammation* means "set on fire." Candida sufferers know this feeling very well! Yeast infections and yeast allergies produce highly inflammatory symptoms in superficial tissues. A variety of agents can cause inflammation including physical, chemical, and microbiological injuries. Tissues react to such injuries with the *inflammatory response*. It increases blood flow to the injured tissue, delivering more sugar and nutrients, and producing these clinical signs and symptoms:

- redness (*erythema*) due to an accumulation of RBCs
- swelling (*edema*) due to an accumulation of *serum*, the liquid portion of blood
- itching (*pruritus*) due to the release of histamine
- burning due to the release of proteinases by tissue cells
- sloughing off of dead tissue (*excoriation*) killed by the yeast infection
- white cheesy or creamy discharge (*exudate*) consisting of dead epithelial cells
- pain and loss of function in the infected tissue

Notice that symptoms of the inflammatory response are the same as symptoms caused by superficial candidiasis and allergic reactions. It is these symptoms that drive Candida sufferers into doctors' offices seeking relief.

"Although inflammation is an essential component of the protective response to fungi, its dysregulation may significantly worsen fungal diseases and limit protective, antifungal immune responses" (Romani and Puccetti, 2007). Inflammation promotes fungal colonization, and then fungal colonization promotes further inflammation, creating a vicious cycle (Kumamoto, 2011). Healing of tissues damaged by Candida infections is promoted by treatment with anti-inflammatory corticosteroid drugs together with antifungal drugs.

White Blood Cell Reactions

The two most important WBCs that defend us against Candida are neutrophils and T cells (Clemons et al., 2000).

Neutrophils are our first line of defense against infections. Neutrophils are called an *innate* defense mechanism because they are always ready to search out and destroy microbes. Neutrophils attack germs in the bloodstream and in tissues. The neutrophil surrounds (*engulfs*) a pathogen, ingests (*phagocytizes*) it, and kills intracellular microbes with degradative enzymes and caustic chemicals. Then the neutrophil dies and lyses, liberating its intracellular contents, which injures the infected tissues. Dead neutrophils accumulate, forming *pus* during bacterial infections, but not in yeast infections. This distinction—*no pus formed in yeast infections*—is an important diagnostic criterion.

T cells are our second line of defense against infections. T cells are called an *acquired* defense mechanism because they cannot function until after they have been exposed to Candida. Time must elapse after initial contact during which T cells divide and form a clone of T cells with newly synthesized receptors on their surfaces that recognize Candida. This process, called *sensitization, induction, activation,* or *priming,* takes several days to weeks. Once formed, sensitized T cells are *cytotoxic,* and can kill Candida.

T cells produce messenger molecules called *cytokines* and *interleukins.* Both are protein molecules that communicate with other WBCs. Some are *proinflammatory,* whereas others are *anti-inflammatory.* Interleukin IL-23 and IL-17A defend against Candida, but cause fatigue and other symptoms typical of infection.

B cells are WBCs that synthesize antibodies. Reactions between antibodies and bacteria are protective. However, reactions between antibodies and Candida produce disease symptoms.

Anti-Candida Antibody Reactions

Antibodies are blood proteins called *immunoglobulins* (Igs) that are synthesized by B cells against foreign substances. The major classes of immunoglobulins are IgA, IgG, IgM, and IgE antibodies. IgG refers to gamma globulin, which is the main antibody in the blood. The presence of anti-Candida IgG antibodies in blood indicates either a current yeast infection or a past exposure to Candida. An abnormally high level of Candida IgG in the blood indicates a current intestinal yeast infection because if the exposure was in the past, the person would not now be in the doctor's office requesting diagnostic testing.

Antigens are foreign substances that induce the synthesis of antibodies. *Foreign* means *nonself,* and refers to external antigens. Most antigens are proteins, but some are polysaccharides. Antigens and antibodies are complementary macromolecules that fit together like a lock and key.

Candida immune complexes are formed when anti-Candida antibodies combine with Candida antigens. The presence of Candida immune complexes and/or Candida antigens in blood is definitive evidence for a current, active yeast infection in the intestine.

Complement is a group of host degradative enzymes found in blood. Complement is activated by attachment to immune complexes. Activated complement is capable of digesting the cell membranes of pathogenic microbes. However, activated complement inadvertently also digests the membranes of tissue cells resulting in inflammation and tissue injury. Complement is also activated by *mannan,* a polysaccharide antigen containing mannose found on yeast cell walls. During a yeast infection, mannan reacts with complement causing additional inflammation and tissue injury.

Candida Allergy

Another example of how antibody reactions are harmful to the host is Candida allergy. If you have allergic tendencies and experience recurrent episodes of candidiasis, you will likely have anti-Candida IgE antibodies that react with Candida and contribute to your symptoms. Hence, you should be tested for Candida allergy by scratch and intradermal testing (Step 5).

Candida Autoimmunity

Another example of the immune system gone haywire and attacking the host is *autoimmunity*. In this disorder, host tissues are attacked by *autoantibodies* or *autoreactive T cells* originally induced against foreign antigens located on the surfaces of infectious agents. When these autoantibodies or autoreactive T cells cross-react with self-antigens, the result is loss of tissue function.

Autoimmune diseases are caused by protein antigens on microbial cells that have similar amino acid sequences to self-proteins on host cells. Called *molecular mimicry* (Wucherpfennig, 2001), it allows pathogens to evade immune surveillance and survive in the body (Rappleye and Goldman, 2008; Chai et al., 2009). Autoimmune diseases associated with intestinal candidiasis include endocrine disorders, immunosuppression, celiac disease, interstitial cystitis, and anti-*Saccharomyces cerevisiae* antibodies in Crohn's disease.

Conclusions of Chapter 1
Diseases Caused by Candida

This chapter explains the expanding spectrum of yeast-connected illnesses. Understanding this diversity of Candida disorders will lead to a wider application of existing tests and treatments, and the development of new diagnostic and therapeutic avenues.

This chapter also explains how symptoms of yeast infections are produced by Candida and the immune system. All of these sources of tissue injury must be treated. Candida infections are treated with antifungals, inflammation is treated with anti-inflammatory drugs, and Candida allergy is treated with immunotherapy. The next few chapters discuss yeast infections in women, men, children, and the intestine.

CHAPTER 2

Yeast Infections in Women

Terminology

Genital yeast infections in women are known by various medical terms including *vaginal yeast infections, yeast vaginitis, vaginal thrush, vulvovaginal candidiasis, Candida vaginitis, Monilia, moniliasis, fungal colpitis*, and *colpomycosis*. All these terms refer to an *active* yeast infection called *acute pseudomembranous candidiasis* that produces a white, clumpy or creamy vaginal discharge, and highly symptomatic episodes. I call it the white form of yeast infection.

In contrast, Candida vulvitis is an *inactive* yeast infection known as *chronic atrophic erythematous candidiasis*. It produces vulvar pain (*vulvodynia*) and redness. I call it the red form of yeast infection. Chapter 1 explains both forms of yeast infection in detail.

Incidence of Yeast Vaginitis

According to a review article by an international research team based at the University of Manchester (Rautemaa-Richardson et al., 2018), about 138 million women worldwide, and 9 million in the United States, are affected by a treatable fungal infection commonly called yeast, Candida vaginitis, or vulvovaginal candidiasis each year. They anticipate that annual cases of recurrent vulvovaginal candidiasis will increase to an estimated 158 million cases by 2030.

Vaginal complaints are responsible for more than 10 million office visits per year (Wilson, 2005). Vulvovaginal candidiasis is the second most common cause of vaginitis and is diagnosed in up to 40% of women with vaginal complaints in the primary care setting (Ilkit and Guzel, 2011). About 75% of women will be diagnosed with yeast vaginitis at least once during their lifetime according to the Centers for Disease Control (CDC, 2008), and about 75 million women have multiple episodes annually (Sobel, 2007).

Yeast vaginitis occurs more frequently in women of childbearing age because they have higher levels of estrogen, which promotes the growth of yeasts in vaginal tissues. Estimates suggest that about 6% of women during their fertile years and about 14% of pregnant women have vulvovaginal candidiasis at any given time.

Relapses of yeast vaginitis occur at a frequency of about 22% in women between puberty and menopause, and 50% in pregnant women. After their first episode of yeast vaginitis, one in five women will experience recurrent episodes. These data show that once you have had a vaginal yeast infection, *your tissues are in an altered state, and you are more likely to have a yeast infection than if you have never had one.* These data are explained by yeasts remaining in your vaginal tissues after standard short-term antifungal therapy (one or three days).

Symptoms of Yeast Vaginitis

The distressing symptoms of genital yeast infections in women demand rapid and effective diagnosis and treatment. Typical symptoms of *active* vulvovaginal yeast infections are vulvar itching, burning and redness, white discharge, yeasty odor, burning during urination, and pain during intercourse. Yeast vaginitis often alternates with bacterial cystitis. During a vaginal yeast infection, typically the vaginal pH is 4.5, which is also the normal vaginal pH during a woman's fertile years. Vaginitis is cyclic, being affected by the menstrual cycle. But not all these clinical manifestations occur in every woman.

Itching

The most common symptom of an active vaginal yeast infection is itching (*pruritus*) of the vulva and vaginal opening (Anderson et al., 2004). Mild symptoms can explode overnight into incapacitating itching by the next morning. Without immediate antifungal and anti-inflammatory treatments, this condition may produce such severe symptoms that they interfere with everyday activities. Itching is also the hallmark symptom of allergic reactions. In fact, allergic reactions to Candida can contribute to the symptoms of yeast infections in women who test positive for Candida IgE antibodies.

All that itches is not yeast! Vaginal itching can be caused by other infections, as well as allergic reactions to latex condoms, substances in semen, feminine hygiene products, dust mites, and/or pets in your bed. Witkin et al. (1988) detected allergic IgE antibodies in vaginal fluid to Candida, seminal fluid, and spermicides.

Burning and Redness

Vaginal yeast infections cause inflammation of the vaginal wall and inner vulvar lips (*labia minora*) that surround the vaginal opening. Inflammation produces vulvar pain, burning, redness, and swelling. Tiny blisters (*vesicles*) can develop due to liquid (*serum*) collecting under the skin. Inflammation can encompass the entire urogenital area (*vulvar vestibule*) that starts below the clitoris and covers the opening to the bladder (*urethra*), and the opening to the vagina. Inflammation can extend to the *perineal* area between the vaginal opening and the anus and around the anus (*perianal area*). Pain caused by inflammation can be much greater than what clinicians might think based just on what is seen.

White Clumpy or Creamy Discharge

Vaginal epithelial cells that are killed by vaginal yeast infections turn white and form a false membrane, called a *pseudomembrane*. It is comprised of dead tissue that sloughs off the vaginal wall forming the vaginal discharge. This white secretion can resemble clumpy cottage cheese or smooth heavy cream. When examined under the microscope, only a few yeast cells or mycelia are seen relative to the large mass of dead vaginal epithelial cells. Sometimes the vaginal discharge drips down and spreads the yeast infection to the inner thighs (*intertrigo area*), where an itchy red rash can develop.

Yeasty Odor

If the vagina is heavily overgrown with yeasts, vaginal discharge may smell like baking bread. This odor is due to products of yeast fermentation, primarily organic esters, which have a fruity smell. If vaginal discharge smells fishy, this indicates either a bacterial or Trichomonas vaginitis. See your doctor to receive an accurate diagnosis.

Burning during Urination

Yeasts in vaginal discharge can contaminate the urethra causing *Candida urethritis*. Inflamed urethral tissues are further irritated by waste products in urine. Urethral swelling may slow the stream of urine, or even block urination in extreme cases. Residual urine left in the urinary bladder allows bacteria to overgrow causing a bladder infection (*cystitis*).

Pain during Intercourse

Women normally do not suffer pain during vaginal intercourse if they are well lubricated and prepared for sex by foreplay. But women with yeast vaginitis typically experience pain during vaginal intercourse (*dyspareunia*). That's no mystery! If your vulvar and vaginal tissues are already irritated, then pain will be exacerbated by physical friction during sex. Condoms and sex toys can cause trauma to delicate vulvar and vaginal tissues. Spermicides on lubricated condoms or in contraceptive creams, jellies, and foams can cause irritation, and worsen vaginal soreness.

Vaginitis Alternating with Cystitis

Bacterial cystitis often occurs after a woman's first sexual experience because bacteria are forced up the urethra during intercourse. Hence, the term "honeymoon cystitis." Birth control methods such as spermicides and the diaphragm also predispose women to develop bladder infections. Bacterial cystitis is treated with antibiotics, which cause vaginal yeast infections, which irritates the urethra, making you susceptible to another bacterial bladder infection, and so on in a self-perpetuating cycle of cure and relapse. Subsequent episodes can lead to chronic inflammation of the entire urogenital and anal area.

Vaginal pH

The pH of a liquid is a measure of its acidity, and it is calculated by a mathematical formula. The higher the acidity, the lower the pH. For example, a decrease from pH 6.5 to 4.5 is a 100-fold increase in acidity.

Measuring vaginal acidity with pH indicator paper is an easy and rapid way to distinguish between types of vaginitis. Gynecologists and family doctors should keep wide range (pH 1-14) and narrow range (pH 3-5.5) indicator paper in their examination rooms. Rolls of pH indicator paper can be purchased online from laboratory or medical supply companies and from www.nutrablast.com/collections/feminine-health. Use these test strips to measure your vaginal pH at home. OTC test kits for vaginitis contain indicator paper that measures vaginal pH values between 4 and 7. Here's what different pH values mean in clinical terms:

> pH 2.5 = Lactobacillus vaginosis
>
> pH 4.5 = normal estrogenized woman, or Candida vaginitis
>
> pH 6.5 = postmenopausal woman, prepubescent girl, Trichomonas vaginitis, or bacterial vaginosis
>
> pH 7.2 = menstrual blood

Vaginal acidity is controlled by a woman's estrogen levels. *Estrogen* is a female steroid hormone produced by the ovaries. Estrogen stimulates glycogen synthesis inside vaginal epithelial cells (Tyler and Woodall, 1982, page 31; Dennerstein and Ellis, 2001). *Glycogen* is a complex carbohydrate polymer of glucose produced by animals, similar to starch produced by plants. Glycogen is broken down into glucose by enzymes inside vaginal epithelial cells, by *Candida albicans*, and by *Doderlein's bacillus*, the normal strain of *Lactobacillus acidophilus* found in the vagina. Then lactobacilli ferment glucose into lactic acid, which determines the pH of the vagina. You cannot control vaginal pH with douches or gels contrary to claims made by manufacturers of these vaginal products.

> *Vaginal acidity protects against yeast vaginitis.*

FACT: Women in their fertile years, between 12 and 55 years old, who are menstruating regularly, have high estrogen levels and, therefore, high vaginal acidity because of the large amount of lactic acid produced by the lactobacilli. The normal vaginal pH in estrogenized women of childbearing age is 4.5. During a vaginal yeast infection, the pH of vaginal fluid is also 4.5. These observations dispel the myth that vaginal acidity protects against yeast vaginitis!

Susceptibility to yeast vaginitis is determined by your estrogen level, which in turn controls the amount of glucose available to feed vaginal yeasts. Both before puberty and after menopause estrogen levels are low, little lactic acid is produced, and the vaginal pH is 6.5, which is close to neutral pH. Nonestrogenized women have a low frequency of yeast vaginitis because little glucose is available in the vaginal epithelium. However, if postmenopausal women are prescribed estro-gen replacement therapy, they again become susceptible to vaginal candidiasis (Dennerstein and Ellis, 2001).

If your vaginal pH is below 4.5, you have probably caused this abnormally high acidity by insert-ing probiotics into your vagina to increase *Lactobacillus acidophilus* numbers in an attempt to protect against yeast vaginitis. I advise against this home remedy. Billions of lactobacilli inserted into the vagina produce so much excess lactic acid that the vaginal pH can drop as low as 2.5. This high acidity causes a condition known as *cytolytic vaginitis*, which produces symptoms similar to yeast vaginitis. The acidity causes the vaginal epithelial cells to burst (*lyse*) producing a white, clumpy vaginal discharge comprised of dead vaginal cells. The high acidity also causes vulvar burning. Thus, symptoms of Lactobacillus vaginitis resemble the symptoms of Candida vaginitis.

Cyclicity

Women who have regular menstrual cycles often experience recurrences of yeast vaginitis follow-ing ovulation during the two weeks before menstruation. This is the *luteal phase* when estrogen levels are elevated (Eckert et al., 1998; Ilkit and Guzel, 2011). Symptoms of yeast vaginitis may improve during menstruation, which is the start of the *follicular phase*, when estrogen levels are lower, and the vaginal acidity is raised by menstrual blood to around pH 7. If you experience cyclic monthly recurrences of yeast vaginitis, you should be treated with prophylactic antifun-gals for three days each month at ovulation (days 12, 13, and 14) for about six months to prevent another relapse (Step 10).

Self-Tests for Yeast Vaginitis

In an interview with Sepah (1998), Nyirjesy suggested that self-diagnosis kits should accompany the sale of OTC vaginal antifungals. That would enable women to make sure they had yeast vag-initis, and not some other gynecological disorder before self-treating.

Self-Tests for Vaginal pH

In 2006, the Vagisil Screening Kit® and Fem-V™ self-tests became available for sale off the shelf. Both measure the acidity of vaginal discharge with test strips that detect pH values from 4.5 to 7.5. Another self-test kit called VS-Sense OTC™ (Sobel et al., 2009; Donders et al., 2010) uses vaginal swabs coated with a pH indicator.

If the pH of your vaginal fluid is 4.0 to 4.5, and your symptoms are consistent with yeast infec-tion, you need oral and/or vaginal antifungal treatment.

If your vaginal pH is 6.0 to 6.5, and your discharge has an unpleasant odor, you may have bac-terial or Trichomonas vaginitis, or a mixed infection (Ilkit and Guzel, 2011). See your doctor to obtain a medical diagnosis by microscopy and culture in order to receive appropriate antibiotic prescription medication.

Unfortunately, these self-test kits use narrow-range pH indicators that do not measure pH values below 4.5. Hence, they do not detect Lactobacillus overgrowth (*cytolytic vaginitis*), which produces so much lactic acid that it can lower vaginal pH to 2.5.

Self-Tests for Candida DNA

In 2010, a self-test called Viaguard Diagnostix Trichomonas/Candida Yeast Infections became available from www.accu-metrics.com. It detects Candida and Trichomonas DNA in swabs of the vagina in women, or the urethra or foreskin of men. A positive test can indicate the presence of either Candida, or Trichomonas, or both together.

In 2018, myLAB Box introduced two new at-home tests: one includes self-tests for bacterial vaginosis and Candida yeast; another is the V-Box, which detects vaginal yeast infections, bacterial vaginosis, trichomoniasis, chlamydia, and gonorrhea.

Pros and Cons of Self-Testing

Self-test kits are useful and cost effective (Gaur et al., 2009), but have problems. The self-test for pH does not distinguish between Trichomonas and bacterial vaginosis, and the self-test for DNA does not distinguish between Candida and Trichomonas. If you perform both self-tests, and the results are pH 4.5 and positive for DNA, then you have yeast vaginitis. But if you have a vaginal pH of 6.0 to 6.5, you need to obtain a medical diagnosis to distinguish between Trichomonas and bacterial vaginosis.

Another problem with self-testing arises when symptoms do not improve after self-treatment. Antifungal medication in your vagina will prevent the doctor from collecting a useful specimen for laboratory testing. If this is your first episode of vaginitis, or if you are not in a monogamous sexual relationship, you should see a physician to rule out a sexually transmitted disease, or an infection that mimics yeast vaginitis. *Test <u>before</u> treating!*

Medical Diagnosis of Yeast Vaginitis

Before your doctor's visit, don't douche because it washes out vaginal discharge that contains pathogenic microbes and host cells. These cells, when viewed under the microscope, are used to make a diagnosis. Also, don't use any prescription or OTC vaginal medications or herbal remedies before seeing your doctor because self-treatments may interfere with your diagnosis, or may even be the cause of your vaginal symptoms. Your gynecologist or family doctor will perform a pelvic examination, and collect vaginal swabs or vulvar scrapings for microscopy, culture, yeast identification, and antifungal susceptibility testing.

Vulvovaginal candidiasis that has become chronic is defined by the presence of at least five of the following criteria: soreness, dyspareunia, positive vaginal swab at presentation or in the past, previous response to antifungal medication, exacerbation with antibiotics, cyclicity, swelling, and discharge (Hong et al., 2014).

Genital yeast infections in women are diagnosed based on clinical signs and symptoms, risk factors for candidiasis, microscopy, and culture with species identification and antifungal susceptibility testing (Step 2).

In addition to errors made by patients in self-diagnosis, sometimes even medical doctors misdiagnose Candida vulvovaginitis (Schwiertz et al., 2006). Over diagnosis and under diagnosis result from the absence of rapid, simple, and inexpensive diagnostic tests for vulvovaginal candidiasis (Sobel, 2007).

In 2015, Lab Corp developed "nuswab" that tests for various types of vaginitis based on DNA identification (https://www.labcorp.com/tests/related-documents/L9603). Test #180068, called Vaginitis Plus (VG+) detects six species of Candida, measures their antifungal susceptibilities, and also detects bacterial vaginosis, Chlamydia, gonorrhea, and Trichomonas.

Hologic.com has developed the Aptima Vaginal Health Panel, which detects bacterial vaginitis, Candida vaginitis, and Trichomonas vaginitis by collecting vaginal swabs and analyzing them on the automated Panther system.

While microscopy, culture, and DNA testing are considered the gold standards for diagnosing Candida vaginitis, the ultimate gold standard is the patient's favorable response to antifungal therapy.

Medical Treatment of Yeast Vaginitis

The distressing symptoms of genital yeast infections in women require rapid and effective treatment. If tests are positive for a vaginal yeast infection, you should be treated with an antifungal agent administered as an oral pill, or a vaginal cream or suppository. Oral and intravaginal antifungal agents are equally effective for treatment of uncomplicated vulvovaginal candidiasis. In contrast, difficult-to-cure yeast vaginitis should be treated with both topical and systemic antiyeast medications at the same time. Most women prefer oral systemic antifungals for treating yeast vaginitis because:

- Inserting antiyeast medication into the vagina several nights in a row is inconvenient, and the next day the leaks are messy.
- Using vaginal antifungals at the same time as sanitary protection for menstruation is complicated.
- Vaginal antifungal preparations contain chemicals such as alcohols and detergents that can irritate sensitive vaginal tissues.
- Inserting antifungal medication into the vagina is difficult for women who are virgins.

In addition to antifungal therapy, an anti-inflammatory steroid cream should also be prescribed to treat vulvar itching, burning, swelling, and inflammation caused by yeast infections.

If you have recurrent episodes of yeast vaginitis, you may be allergic to Candida and/or have poor immunity against Candida. Therefore, ask your doctor for a written referral to an allergist to obtain intradermal testing for diagnosing Candida allergy and Candida immunity (Step 5).

Women with a high rate of recurrent vulvovaginal candidiasis often have concurrent intestinal Candida infection (Lin et al., 2011). Therefore, ask your doctor to order a stool culture for Candida, with identification of the yeast species, and determination of its antifungal susceptibility. Usually the male partner of a woman with yeast vaginitis is not tested for Candida or treated with antifungals unless he is experiencing urinary or genital symptoms. The protocol I recommend for treating vulvovaginal candidiasis is outlined in Step 2.

Self-Treatment of Yeast Vaginitis

Before 1991, if women developed a vaginal yeast infection, they usually had to wait several days to see their doctor and obtain an antifungal prescription. During this delay, the vaginal yeast infection might suddenly worsen. Mild symptoms might fulminate overnight into incapacitating vulvovaginal itching, burning, and pain. I experienced this scenario many times.

In January of 1991, Gyne-Lotrimin and Monistat vaginal antifungals were approved by the Food and Drug Administration for OTC sale. This has been a major advance in women's health because yeast vaginitis can now be treated early on while symptoms are still mild. Women who have been medically diagnosed with yeast vaginitis several times can usually recognize a recurrence. If their symptoms go away after treatment, their self-diagnosis is confirmed.

Of 258 female college students surveyed, most believed that OTC availability of vaginal antifungals was a good idea because it gives women access to prompt treatment and saves money by not having to pay for a doctor's visit; 92% said OTC vaginal antifungals cured their yeast infections (Lipsky and Taylor, 1996). However, some women expressed concern over the possibility of an inaccurate self-diagnosis. Their concern was well founded. Here's the evidence.

Misdiagnosis of Yeast Vaginitis

As foreseen, OTC vaginal antiyeast preparations are overused because women self-treat gynecological symptoms that are not yeast-related. Incorrect self-diagnosis delays obtaining an accurate diagnosis and effective treatment.

A survey of 601 women found that only 35% could accurately identify a vaginal yeast infection even though they had previously been diagnosed with yeast vaginitis by a physician (Ferris et al., 1996). Furthermore, of women who had never received a medical diagnosis of yeast vaginitis, only 11% correctly identified their symptoms. These discouraging findings suggest that most women are misusing OTC antifungals, and sales figures bear out this conclusion.

After vaginal antifungals became available OTC, annual sales almost doubled from 13.7 million prescriptions to 25.3 million prescription units plus OTC units (Ferris et al., 1996). Had an epidemic of vulvovaginal candidiasis suddenly developed? Or were millions of women self-treating vaginal symptoms inappropriately? The latter is most certainly the answer.

A study of 105 women attending Temple University Vaginitis Referral Center reported that most women thought they had yeast vaginitis, yet only 28% actually had this infection (Nyirjesy et al., 1997). The most common medical diagnoses in the remaining women were vulvar vestibulitis

(17%), irritant dermatitis (15%), bacterial vaginosis (11%), and normal physiological vaginal discharge (7%). The consensus from all these studies is that OTC antimycotic agents are overused.

The reason women have difficulty with self-diagnosis is because symptoms of different types of vaginitis overlap (Sepah, 1998). While itching is generally considered the hallmark of yeast vaginitis, it is present in only about a third of cases. Moreover, itching can occur in other gynecological disorders such as herpes simplex virus, contact dermatitis, human papillomavirus, pinworms, lice, and vulvar lichen sclerosis (Ferris et al., 1996). Because vaginal symptoms are nonspecific, they are not reliable for self-diagnosis. This is why yeast cultures are the gold standard for diagnosing vulvovaginal candidiasis (Hoffstetter et al. (2008).

If a delay occurs before obtaining an accurate diagnosis and appropriate treatment, adverse consequences might result. Untreated bacterial vaginosis in pregnant women can cause preterm labor, premature rupture of membranes, postpartum endometritis, and postsurgical infection. Because women commonly confuse the symptoms of bacterial vaginosis with yeast vaginitis, Ferris et al. (1996) suggested that pregnant women should always seek a medical diagnosis of vaginal symptoms to avoid complications.

Treatment Failures

If your symptoms do not improve after a week of antifungal treatment, possible explanations include yeast die-off, which makes symptoms worse, non-*albicans* Candida, which is antifungal resistant, misdiagnosis, allergy, contact irritation, or lack of concurrent treatment with anti-inflammatory cream. Go back to your gynecologist. Discuss the guidelines in this book and identify the risk factors that make you susceptible to candidiasis. Request additional testing, and more intensive treatments.

If yeast vaginitis is not treated with a large enough dosage of an antifungal for a long enough time, it can get progressively worse, evolving into recurrent vulvovaginal yeast infections, and then into chronic vulvar pain. The longer treatment is delayed, the longer it will take for damaged tissues to heal and symptoms to resolve once you obtain effective therapies.

Recurrent Yeast Vaginitis

"Oh, no! Not another yeast infection!"

Is this what you say every time you feel that old familiar vaginal itch again? I did—for more times than I want to remember. Eventually, I got fed up, and decided to find out how to beat my yeast problem. By means of my personal history of recurrences and my professional academic research, I identified dozens of risk factors and lifestyle activities that predispose women to develop yeast vaginitis. Of these, the number one risk factor for candidiasis is treatment with antibiotics. Pirotta et al. (2003) reported that 23% of women who experienced vulvovaginal candidiasis had taken antibiotics in the previous month.

Incomplete cures account for most recurrences. Once you have had a yeast infection, your tissues are in a different state. After short-term antifungal treatment, some yeasts remain in your tissues in a latent, nongrowing state. Next time you are exposed to a risk factor for candidiasis, these dormant yeasts start to grow again.

Repeated episodes of yeast vaginitis take their toll on a woman's emotional state. She complains about burnout, stress, and imbalance between work and leisure time (Ehrström et al., 2007). After several bouts of antibiotic-induced yeast vaginitis, women become anxious and obsessed with preventing relapses. They may even refuse to take antibiotics prescribed by their physicians (Pirotta et al., 2003). To avoid noncompliance with medically necessary antibiotics, physicians should ask patients if they have a history of yeast infections. If so, antiyeast medication should also be prescribed for concurrent use with antibiotics as a preventative (Step 10).

Vulvodynia

Vulvodynia is a symptom, not a diagnosis! The term vulvodynia means vulvar pain, and says nothing about the underlying cause. Vulvodynia was first used as a term to describe the symptom of vulvar pain by Friedrich (1983) and independently by Woodruff and Parmley (1983). Women with vulvodynia experience pain, burning, and redness of the inner lips of the vulva (*labia minora*) and the skin surrounding the vagina (*vestibule* or *introitus*).

In 1987, Friedrich coined the term *vulvar vestibulitis syndrome*. It refers to vulvar pain, burning, and redness at the entrance to the vagina due to inflammation of the skin and mucous secreting glands (*lesser vestibular glands*). Sometimes the term *focal vulvitis* is used to describe pain that is localized in one place, most commonly in the lower (*posterior*) half of the vaginal vestibule called the *fourchette*.

An Epidemic of "Burning Bottoms"

The incidence of vulvodynia is highest in sexually active women between puberty and menopause when estrogen levels are highest. Estimates of the prevalence of vulvodynia range from 4% to 20% (Goetsch, 1991; Harlow and Stewart, 2003; Reed et al., 2004; Bachmann et al., 2006a; Petersen et al., 2008; Sutton et al., 2008; Nyirjesy, 2008; Reed et al., 2012).

Judging by these reports, and by the large number of women who have contacted my business, Yeast Consulting Services, for information about vulvodynia, there appears to be an epidemic of "burning bottoms." As a result, a lot of couples are going without sex. So, vulvodynia affects men too—albeit indirectly!

Categorizing Vulvodynia

Types of vulvodynia were originally classified based on whether vulvar pain was localized or generalized, provoked or unprovoked (Haefner et al., 2005). But Bachmann et al. (2006b) pointed out that these categories are neither standardized, nor evidence-based. In this book, vulvar pain is classified into two types depending on whether vulvar redness is absent or present.

Vulvar Pain without Redness

The term *dysesthetic vulvodynia* refers to a painful sensation induced by a gentle touch of the vulvar skin, but the area is a normal pink color. Women with vulvar pain without redness must seek medical care from clinics specializing in neurological pain. This type of vulvodynia is not discussed further in this book.

Vulvar Pain with Redness

When women describe their discomfort of vulvodynia as painful, burning, stinging, stabbing, irritated, or raw, typically, their pain is limited to a specific site (*focal point*) where the vulvar tissue is red. Others say their pain is just inside the vaginal opening, or their pain is felt throughout the entire crotch area (*vulvar vestibulitis*), and may radiate to the thighs, buttocks, abdomen, or bladder. Their referred pain makes diagnosis difficult.

A survey of women with vulvodynia by Kahn et al. (2009) found that 80% also have urinary pain, urgency, and frequency (*interstitial cystitis*). Vulvodynia is also associated with irritable bowel syndrome. All these conditions typically develop after antibiotic treatment led to vulvovaginal candidiasis. Hence, they can be considered *yeast-related medical sequelae.*

Clinical signs of vulvar vestibulitis seen by physicians include redness, swelling, small sores, ulcers, tears, cracks, or fissures, and sometimes small bumps or water blisters beneath the skin. Inflammation can extend and include the urethra and/or anus. Equally important is what is not seen: there is no white vaginal discharge. This indicates that the vulvar pain and redness is not due to an active, pseudomembranous yeast infection.

The hallmark symptom of vulvar vestibulitis syndrome is burning pain, especially during and after vaginal intercourse (Spadt et al., 2007). Pain varies from mild to disabling, and may be constant, or occurs only when pressure is applied to the vulva. Other painful activities include urination, walking, biking, horseback riding, wearing tight pants, and inserting tampons. Even sitting may be uncomfortable. Some women sit on only one buttock, or on a donut-shaped pillow.

Bachmann et al. (2006a) pointed out that chronic vulvar pain detrimentally affects women's work, family, and social life. It may develop into depression, which drags a woman down into a whirlpool of negative feelings while she unsuccessfully seeks symptomatic relief. Typically, women with vulvodynia have seen many physicians, and tried multiple medical treatments and self-remedies without success. Usually, testing and treatment for yeast infection is not offered. As a result, women with vulvodynia may suffer physically and emotionally for months or years.

Before developing sexual pain, most vulvodynia sufferers did not differ from healthy controls in terms of their incidence of depression, sexual abuse history, sexual promiscuity, or sexual dysfunction (Spadt et al., 2007). Thus, vulvodynia is not *"All in your head!"* as some unenlightened and unsympathetic physicians exclaim when they fail to identify its etiology.

Pathogenesis of Vulvodynia

Most women with chronic vulvar pain were previously treated for vulvovaginal candidiasis (Friedrich, 1987; Mann et al., 1992; Bazin et al., 1994; Nyirjesy and Halpern, 1996; Ridley, 1998; Sarma et al., 1999; Nyirjesy, 2000; Tchoudomirova et al., 2001; Smith et al., 2002; Witkin et al., 2002; Scheinfeld, 2003; Ramirez De Knott et al., 2005; Bachmann et al., 2006a; Pagano, 2007; Nguyen et al., 2009; Farage et al., 2010; Farmer et al., 2011; and many other references too numerous to cite).

Since so many physicians have made this same observation, we can conclude that a prior episode of yeast vaginitis followed by standard, short-term, antifungal treatment is the main cause of vulvodynia.

Q: The burning question is (pun intended): *Why are women left with residual vulvar inflammation and pain after standard antifungal treatment for yeast vaginitis?*

A: In my opinion, vulvodynia is caused by the failure of short-term antifungal therapy. Standard-of-care treatment for vulvovaginal candidiasis is one or three 150 mg tablets of Diflucan. While this may reduce vaginal itching and discharge, it does not eradicate the intracellular yeast infection inside vaginal tissues. Goswami et al. (2006) reported that living yeasts persist in about half of the women treated. Further proof of the inadequacy of only one or three days of Diflucan treatment is that the recurrence rate is high.

In my review article (Crandall, 1991a), I presented evidence for intracellular yeast infection, and proposed that yeasts remain inside vaginal and vulvar epithelial tissues after short-term antifungal therapy. Even though intracellular yeasts are not actively growing, they continuously shed antigens, which react with anti-Candida antibodies, complement, and sensitized T-cells to provoke inflammation and vulvar pain.

Romani et al. (2008) pointed out that fungal persistence in tissues is associated with chronic inflammation. Nyirjesy (2008) indicated that most women with vulvodynia show hyperimmune responses consistent with infectious or postinfectious processes. Hence, hyperreactivity in the vulva and vestibule is a core issue that needs to be addressed.

The obvious conclusions from these findings is that yeast vaginitis should be treated daily with Diflucan until symptoms resolve, and corticosteroid cream should be applied to the vulva to eliminate pain and inflammation. Both the yeast infection and the inflammation (hyperreactivity) must be treated long enough to allow tissues to heal. This conclusion is also based on the fact that *all other systemic antifungals are administered daily until the infection resolves. After resolution, switch from daily antifungal treatment to weekly suppression.*

Q: Why did the FDA approve only one day of Diflucan treatment for yeast vaginitis in 1994?

A: My guess is that the medical professionals on the FDA panel who made this decision wanted to avoid the necessity of performing liver tests during daily, long-term, Diflucan therapy. In addition, there was an ongoing discussion in the literature around that time about noncompliance.

Articles blamed recurrences of yeast vaginitis on women not completing their prescribed one to two weeks of intravaginal antifungal medication that used to be standard.

In addition to incorrect reasoning leading to short-term treatment, it was not standard of care to include a prescription of corticosteroid cream for vulvar inflammation with antifungal treatment of yeast vaginitis. This inadequate medical care for yeast vaginitis has continued until the present.

Nyirjesy (2008) proposed that an initial physical, chemical, or infectious injury triggers vulvar inflammation. It does not resolve because of genetic defects in the woman's immune response. Over time, unresolved chronic inflammation damages peripheral nerve fibers, further provoking chronic pain.

Farage et al. (2010) proposed that vulvodynia is a neuropathic disorder of abnormal pain perception triggered by chronic inflammation. They suggest that possible triggers are irritating topical products or medications, prior laser or cryogenic treatments for HPV infections, allergy to seminal fluid, and infectious agents such as vulvovaginal *C. albicans*.

"Doctors' Plague"

The current epidemic of vulvodynia due to Candida vulvitis can be attributed to failure of modern medicine for the following four reasons.

1. Most vaginal yeast infections are *iatrogenic*, which means caused by physicians' treatments. Predisposing prescriptions include antibiotics, corticosteroids unopposed by antifungals, and estrogen.

2. Most cases of vulvodynia are due to failure of standard, short-term, one or three days of antifungal treatment for yeast vaginitis. *Short-term antifungal therapy leads to long-term misery!* Vaginal yeast infections should be treated with daily antifungal therapy and corticosteroid cream until symptoms resolve. Recalcitrant cases should be treated with both vaginal plus oral systemic antifungals at the same time. After resolution of symptoms, daily antifungal therapy should be switched to weekly antifungal prophylaxis for several months to prevent recurrences.

3. Most physicians do not acknowledge the fact that most cases of vulvodynia are due to latent, intracellular yeast infection (*chronic atrophic erythematous candidiasis*) remaining after inadequate treatment of vaginal yeast infections.

4. Most physicians refer women with vulvodynia to specialty clinics where Candida vulvitis is also ignored, and unproven treatments are offered—*some of which may make symptoms worse!* (See my critique of vulvar pain clinic protocols later in this chapter.)

Since the etiology of vulvodynia is mainly due to physicians' treatments and their uninformed denial of the underlying cause—Candida vulvitis, the current epidemic of vulvodynia can be called a "*doctors' plague*."

Diagnosis of Vulvodynia

While doctors are performing pelvic examinations of women's genitals and puzzling over the causes of chronic vulvar pain, the answer is usually staring them right in the face! Most cases of vulvodynia with redness are due to Candida vulvitis. Hence, the first thing that physicians should consider is a woman's past history of vaginal yeast infections, and her current risk factors for candidiasis. *Think yeast first!*

You can help your doctor *get to the bottom of your problem* by writing up a summary of your medical history, and listing your prescription medications, supplements, and OTC vaginal products. Tell your doctor what factors you think triggered your vulvar pain. A differential diagnosis must rule out various etiologies and identify the specific disease process. Vulvar pain can be caused by many conditions (Paavonen, 1995; Nyirjesy, 2008) such as the following:

- **Dermatitis** or **allergic vulvitis** caused by chemicals in personal care products such as douches, deodorant pads, colored dyes in panties and toilet paper, spermicides in vaginal jellies and lubricated condoms—even medicated creams can cause irritation!
- **Trauma** caused by friction during sexual intercourse without adequate lubrication.
- **Infections** such as:
  ○ viruses (herpes, warts, human papilloma virus, Epstein-Barr)
  ○ yeasts (Candida)
  ○ bacteria (Gardnerella, *Neisseria gonorrhea, Treponema pallidum,* Chlamydia, Streptococcus)
  ○ parasites (Trichomonas)

- **Cytolytic vaginosis** also called **desquamative inflammatory vaginitis** caused by an overgrowth of Lactobacillus due to intravaginal insertion of probiotics.
- **Neurologic** pain caused by proliferation of nerve cells, damage to intraepithelial nerve endings, Herpes neuralgia, or spinal nerve compression.
- **Systemic or autoimmune diseases** such as psoriasis, erosive lichen planus, lichen sclerosus, Crohn's Disease, Herpes zoster, postherpetic neuralgia, histiocytosis, aphthous ulcers, Behcet's syndrome, cicatricial pemphigoid, Sjogren's syndrome, systemic sclerosis, or postcandidal autoimmune cross-reactions with tissue cells.
- **Elevated estrogen levels** due to ovulation, pregnancy, fertility treatment, oral contraception, or estrogen replacement therapy for menopause.
- **Vulvovaginal ulcers** caused by drugs such as Ikorel (nicorandil).

The diversity of conditions that can lead to vulvar pain is further demonstrated by this prospective study in which 74 women were followed forward in time: 14 with a positive fungal culture improved on antifungals; 11 with a positive bacterial culture improved on antibacterials; 8 improved with dietary modification; 10 benefitted from tricyclic antidepressant medications; 13 improved after gabapentin therapy; and 13 showed no improvement (Ventolini et al., 2009).

Sometimes the cause of vulvodynia can be quite obscure and requires extensive testing. Here's a case report of a woman who worked in a hospital and developed recurrent vulvar and vaginal pain. After ruling out a multitude of possible etiologies, investigations into her home and work environments determined that her vulvar pain was due to a specific IgE-mediated allergy to **inhaled** particles of latex from rubber gloves (Chiu et al., 1999). Notice the word "inhaled." Surprisingly, her vulvodynia was not due to direct vulvar contact with latex gloves.

Take home message: You and your doctor must do careful detective work to identify the specific cause of your vulvar symptoms. Only then can you decide what medical care and self-help steps described in Part II are needed to treat your condition and prevent recurrences.

Diagnostic Tests for Vulvodynia

Because the clinical signs and symptoms of vulvodynia are *nonspecific* and could be caused by many different factors, specific diagnostic tests are needed to identify the etiology. But, since Candida vulvitis is due to intracellular yeast infection, its diagnosis presents a conundrum. Because *Candida is in the tissues, not on the surface*, cultures from swabs of tissue surfaces can be falsely negative. For this reason, Pagano (2007) utilizes the following two sensitive methods for diagnosing Candida vulvitis.

1. **Vulvar scraping for yeast culture:** A scalpel is used to scrape vulvar skin and collect tissue cells (as described by Dennerstein, 1968). Scrapings are more likely to yield positive yeast cultures than swabs because yeasts reside inside epithelial cells. The diagnostic code numbers for a "vulvar scraping thin prep" is 88142 and 88143. The Current Procedural Terminology (CPT) code 88142, as maintained by the American Medical Association, is a medical procedural code under Cytopathology Procedures. Unfortunately, it seems that very few gynecologists have learned this procedure!

2. **Colposcopy for acetowhite lesions:** After collecting a vulvar scraping, Pagano (2007) examines the inner vulvae with a *colposcope* (a microscope with a light on the end). Dilute acetic acid solution is applied to vulvar tissue. If it turns white, the tissue is abnormal, infected, or dead. *Acetowhite lesions* indicate the presence of vulvar candidiasis or another disease condition. Acetowhite lesions in women with vulvar vestibulitis were also reported by Chaim et al. (1996).

Pagano (2007) successfully treated women who had vulvodynia and acetowhite lesions with long-term, weekly Diflucan. Women who also had positive Candida cultures from vulvar scrapings had a 93% improvement rate, whereas women with negative cultures had a 60% improvement rate. While I applaud Pagano's approach to diagnosis, I take issue with treating only once a week with Diflucan. *All other systemic antifungals are given daily until symptoms resolve, and then treatment is switched to weekly maintenance.*

Positive results from yeast cultures of vulvar scrapings or from acetic acid testing, taken together with symptoms and history of yeast infections, allow an accurate diagnosis of Candida vulvitis to be made. This diagnostic approach should become standard-of-care for vulvodynia with redness.

Unfortunately, most vulvodynia clinics appear to be ignorant of the above findings, and instead perform the following two tests after ruling out other clinical diagnoses:

1. **Q-tip test:** In this low-tech test, a saline-moistened, cotton-tipped swab is firmly pressed on vulvar and vestibular areas to find the location of the pain.

2. **Vulvar biopsy and histology:** Useful information about the pathogenesis of vulvodynia has been obtained from research studies of vulvar tissue biopsies collected during controlled clinical trials. Biopsies of vulvar tissue were sliced into thin sections, stained, and examined under the microscope in a procedure called *histology*. Researchers observed that vulvar tissues from women with vulvar vestibulitis had increased numbers of these three cell types:

   - **WBCs** called lymphocytes (Pyka et al., 1988; Prayson et al., 1995; Chaim et al., 1996).
   - **Mast cells** (Chaim et al., 1996; Nyirjesy et al., 2001; Bornstein et al., 2004). However, Pyka et al. (1988) observed mast cells in only 21% of vulvodynia patients.
   - **Nerve cells** (Westrom and Willen, 1998; Bohm-Starke et al., 1998; Tympanidis, 2003; Bornstein et al., 2004).

Proliferation of intraepithelial nerve endings (*vestibular innervation*) occurred in the painful area around the entrance of the vagina. Inflammation and growth of nerve tissue in response to noxious environmental stimuli results in hyperactivity of nerve receptors (Ekgren, 2000). The end stage of this multistep process is hyperreactivity to pain.

Most physicians specializing in vulvodynia take a punch biopsy of the painful area on the vulva or vestibule for histological examination. I oppose this standard approach for several reasons. First of all, results from biopsies just indicate inflammation, which is observable with the naked eye. Secondly, research on biopsies has already been done, and we know what the results will be. Thirdly, vulvar cancer is rare, whereas Candida vulvitis is common. Fourthly, biopsies just add to the misery.

It is unwarranted to perform a vulvar biopsy to look for intracellular yeasts because it would be like looking for a needle in a haystack. Even during active vaginal yeast infections (*acute pseudomembranous candidiasis*), very few yeasts are present in histological sections of biopsies. Even fewer yeasts would be present in inactive yeast infections (*chronic atrophic erythematous candidiasis*).

The cause of vulvar inflammation can usually be identified by reviewing the woman's history of vaginal yeast infections, antifungal treatments, and use of topical products. A biopsy can always be performed later if there is a strong index of suspicion of a viral infection or cancer.

Genetic Predisposition and Immune Dysregulation in Vulvodynia

Most women with vulvodynia show a hyperimmune response consistent with an infectious or postinfectious process (Nyirjesy, 2008). The most likely etiological agent involved in this process is Candida. If vulvovaginal candidiasis is not treated long enough with an adequate dosage of antifungals, it may evolve into chronic vulvar inflammation. Immune reactions responsible for inflammation continue long after the active yeast infection has been treated. Progression to vulvodynia is also governed by a woman's genetic background and immune responses.

Genetic Predisposition

Early researchers reported that vulvodynia occurs predominantly in white women (Peckham et al., 1986; Chaim et al., 1996; Sarma et al., 1999). Later researchers focused on production of inflammatory cytokines (Petersen et al., 2008). *Cytokines* are small protein molecules secreted by epithelial cells and WBCs, and are involved in intercellular communication between WBCs. Many researchers have reported that women with vulvodynia have gene alterations that result in the production of more proinflammatory cytokines, and less anti-inflammatory cytokines. Proinflammatory cytokines were produced by vestibular fibroblasts isolated from women with vulvodynia when provoked with *C. albicans* antigen (Foster et al., 2007). Prolonged inflammatory responses are postulated to induce localized peripheral nerve damage, and increased pain sensitivity.

Immune Dysregulation

Alterations in genes affecting mucosal immune responses against fungi can lead to an increased susceptibility to recurrent vaginal yeast infections (Ferwerda et al., 2009; Jaeger et al., 2013). Women prone to recurrent vulvovaginitis candidiasis and chronic vulvodynia often develop allergy and autoimmunity to Candida.

Candida allergy: Allergic reactions to Candida exacerbate symptoms of yeast vaginitis, and make women more susceptible to recurrences (Crandall, 1991a; 2008). Repeated episodes of vulvovaginal candidiasis can lead to vulvodynia. Chronic vulvar pain might also result from *idiopathic (Id) reactions*, which can be explained by the vulva being the target organ for allergic reactions to Candida infection at another body site such as the intestines. Women who have altered immuno-inflammatory responses to environmentally induced allergic reactions may be predisposed to developing vulvodynia (Harlow et al., 2009).

Candida autoimmunity: Women who have repeated vaginal yeast infections can become hyperreactive to their own tissues. Ashman and Ott (1989) observed that antigens in vulvovaginal tissue resemble antigens in *C. albicans*. Called *molecular mimicry*, similarities between antigens in host cells and pathogens play a role in the development of autoimmunity. Immune disorders create feedback loops or self-perpetuating cycles of inflammation and pain. In turn, inflammation interferes with the body's ability to fight Candida infection (Crandall, 1991a).

Treatment of Vulvodynia

You cannot alter your genetic susceptibility to Candida infection, allergy, autoimmunity, and inflammation. But you can treat Candida vulvitis appropriately. If vulvodynia with redness is due to the failure of short-term antifungal treatment for yeast vaginitis, then long-term antifungal therapy should be used to treat Candida vulvitis (Fischer, 2014). The protocol I recommend for treating vulvodynia caused by Candida vulvitis is the same protocol I recommend for treating vulvovaginal candidiasis (Step 2).

Unfortunately, most vulvar pain specialists do not acknowledge the possibility that Candida vulvitis is the root cause of vulvodynia when redness is present. Furthermore, *some of their treatments may make yeast infections worse!* Treatments used by vulvar pain clinics are discussed next, and my critique of their protocols follows afterwards.

Vulvar Pain Clinics

Nyirjesy (2008) treats vulvar pain with various combinations of the following therapies: counseling about self-care and lifestyle, long-term antifungal therapy for yeast infections, a low oxalate diet, calcium citrate supplements, acupuncture, surgery, electromyographic biofeedback therapy, and one or more of the following medications: topical lidocaine ointment, topical corticosteroids or other anti-inflammatory therapy, cromolyn cream, low-dose tricyclic antidepressants such as Elavil (amitriptyline), selective serotonin reuptake inhibitors such as Zoloft (sertraline), serotonin-norepinephrine reuptake inhibitors such as Effexor (venlafaxine), antiseizure drugs such as Neurotonin (gabapentin), and/or interferon-α intralesional injections. *Irrespective of treatment, some women improved, and some did not!*

Nyirjesy (2008) pointed out that *"when the cause is unknown and has been attributed to such a wide variety of diseases, many treatment options have been proposed for [vulvar vestibulitis syndrome]."* Since *"no treatment has been shown to be clearly superior to others, it makes sense to try to tailor the therapy to the individual patient."*

Peckham et al. (1986) reported that half of women with focal vulvitis experience a spontaneous remission. Nyirjesy et al. (2001) reported that some women experienced a reduction in vulvar symptoms while taking a placebo during a clinical study. Similarly, Lotery et al. (2004) reported that many cases of vulvodynia improve with time regardless of what therapies, if any, were employed. Likewise, Phillips and Bachmann (2010) reported that *"Vulvodynia symptoms resolve slowly with any therapeutic option."*

The National Vulvodynia Association stated that *"Although medical professionals report utilizing as many as 30 different therapies to manage vulvodynia symptoms, currently, women can only determine treatment effectiveness through a trial-and-error process that can take many months."*

The International Society for the Study of Vulvovaginal Disease guidelines for the treatment of vulvodynia acknowledged that *"very few controlled trials have been performed to verify efficacy of these treatments"* (Haefner et al., 2005).

Positive responses to diverse treatments can be explained this way. After women remove their risk factor(s) causing vulvar inflammation, the inflammatory processes dampen down, and tissue healing occurs gradually over time. Thus, in addition to medical treatments for Candida infection and Candida allergy, along with self-help remedies and lifestyle changes, *time seems to be the most important healer in vulvodynia!*

My Critique of Vulvar Pain Clinic Protocols

While reading the above summary of reports, did it seem strange to you that so many different treatments were tried, and they helped some vulvodynia sufferers, but not others?

The answer to this conundrum became apparent when I read this statement by Nyirjesy (2008): *"...most of the data with regard to treatment of [vulvar vestibulitis syndrome] is based on retrospective case series."* Retrospective analyses look back in time at data collected from uncontrolled studies. Outcomes are based on women's memories, not on medical records. Data are collected without identifying the etiologies, and without reporting the number of women who used each treatment but failed to recover. Therefore, their conclusions have no statistical significance.

Only prospective, randomized, controlled clinical trials yield scientifically valid results. They look forward in time at data comparing a new treatment to either a placebo or a treatment known to be effective. Controlled studies reduce the number of variables by defining the subject population with inclusion and exclusion criteria.

Most published studies of vulvodynia disregarded the possibility of chronic atrophic erythematous candidiasis and/or Candida allergy even when an increased number of mast cells in biopsies pointed to allergy.

The following treatments are used by vulvar pain clinics even though they have not been validated by controlled studies, or have been shown to be ineffective.

- **Low oxalate diet:** Vulvodynia patients are told not to eat fruits and vegetables containing high amounts of oxalic acid because urinary oxalates cause vulvodynia. Some clinics continue to recommend this diet even though a controlled clinical study by Baggish et al. (1997) proved that a low oxalate diet does not cure vulvodynia, and that dietary oxalic acid is not a cause of vulvodynia.
- **Estrogen cream:** Treatment with estrogen cream is recommended by vulvar pain clinics even though estrogen is known to contribute to the development of vulvovaginal candidiasis. In a retrospective study of 20 women with vulvodynia, seven were taking estrogen replacement therapy, and four of these had positive vaginal Candida cultures (McKay, 1993). In addition, oral contraceptives were reported to be associated with vulvar pain (Bouchard et al., 2002; Berglund et al., 2002).
- **Physical therapy:** Pelvic floor physiotherapy and biofeedback exercises recommended by Glazer (2000) decrease vulvar pain in some women, but do not address the underlying causes.
- **Antidepressants:** Elavil (amitriptyline) is a tricyclic antidepressant that shows efficacy for the treatment of neuropathic pain. It is prescribed for vulvar pain based on only one retrospective study of 20 women by McKay (1993). The antidepressant Zoloft (sertraline), a selective serotonin reuptake inhibitor, is also sometimes prescribed for vulvar pain without any controlled clinical studies. Interestingly, Zoloft (sertraline) was reported to have antifungal activity (Lass-Florl et al., 2001), and to inhibit yeast phospholipase, a virulence factor in candidiasis (Rainey et al., 2010). These discoveries may explain how

antidepressants work against vulvar pain and support my hypothesis that vulvodynia with redness is due to Candida vulvitis.

- **Surgery:** Despite reports that surgical removal of vulvar tissue (*vestibulectomy*) is successful in some women, other women are worse off due to complications. Women have told me their nightmare stories about unnecessary surgeries to remove parts of their genital and urinary tracts in ill-advised attempts to lessen chronic pain remaining after vaginal yeast infections. Secor and Fertitta (1992) opined that surgery is a last resort for management of vulvar vestibulitis syndrome.

Resources for vulvodynia

Physicians who specialize in the treatment of vulvar pain are listed on the websites of the National Vulvodynia Association (**www.nva.org**), the International Pelvic Pain Society (**www.pelvicpain. org**), and the International Society for the Study of Vulvovaginal Disease (**www.issvd.org**).

Unfortunately, most of these doctors are unaware that vulvodynia with redness is due to chronic atrophic erythematous candidiasis and, therefore, they do not follow my protocol for Candida vulvitis. Therefore, I urge you to bring the scientific documentation in this book to the attention of your personal physicians who know your medical history. Ask for tests and treatments described in this chapter and in Steps 1, 2 and 5.

I also encourage you to sign up for e-mail updates from the above organizations and enroll in their controlled studies and treatment registries. In this way, you can contribute to the advancement of knowledge about vulvodynia.

Conclusions of Chapter 2
Yeast Infections in Women

You don't have to *"Learn to live with it!"* If you develop a vaginal yeast infection, obtain an early diagnosis, effective treatments, and preventive methods. In this way, you can reduce the chances of developing vulvodynia. *Nip it in the bud!*

Learn about the countless pitfalls in a woman's path that can trigger yeast vaginitis by reading Step 6. Identify your individual susceptibility factors in order to prevent recurrences. Follow all of the medical care and self-help guidelines for yeast infections and yeast allergies in my ten-step program in Part II. *You can conquer Candida!*

CHAPTER 3

Yeast Infections in Men

Symptoms

The distressing symptoms of genital yeast infections demand rapid and effective diagnosis and treatment. Genital yeast infections in men can occur on the skin of the penis, scrotum, and groin area, and inside the urethra and prostate.

Penis

Candida infection of the glans penis is called *penile candidiasis* or *Candida balanitis*. It is characterized by a painful rash, which produces redness (*erythema*), itching (*pruritus*), swelling (*edema*), and burning on the head (*glans*) and shaft of the penis. A painful rash under the foreskin (*prepuce*) of the penis due to a yeast infection is called *Candida balanoposthitis*.

A rash on the skin of the penis can have red patches that are either flat (*macular*) or raised (*papular*), with companion (*satellite*) lesions or red bumps around the edges, as well as tiny water blisters, flaky or scaly white skin, white, moist, curd-like accumulations, and white plaques seen upon retraction of the prepuce, painful urination (*dysuria*), bleeding, and ulceration of the glans penis.

Symptoms and clinical signs on the skin of the penis can be caused by:

- infections, inflammatory dermatoses, or skin cancer
- irritation from soaps, spermicides, medicated creams, or other chemicals
- physical friction from rubbing against a diaphragm or sex toys during vaginal intercourse
- allergic reactions to yeasts in the vagina, mouth, or anus of sexual partner

Urethra

A yeast infection on the skin of the penis can extend inside the urethral opening at the tip (*meatus*) of the penis. Urethral burning after ejaculation indicates a yeast infection in the prostate.

Scrotum

"Jock itch" in men is a yeast infection of the skin in the groin (*inguinal*) area. It can affect the penis, the pouch that contains the testes (*scrotum*), the area between the scrotum and anus (*perineum*), the skin around the anus (*perianal* area), and the inner thighs (*crural* or *intertrigo* area). Its colloquial name comes from the fact that athletes ("jocks") sweat a lot while exercising, and heat and moisture in the genital area promotes the growth of yeasts.

Prostate

Prostatitis is the most common urological diagnosis in men older than 50 years, and is the third most common urological diagnosis in men younger than 50 years. Pain in the prostate results in at least two million office visits per year. The vast majority have *chronic nonbacterial prostatitis,* also called *nonspecific prostatitis* because no specific urinary pathogens is detected in culture.

Yeast infection of the prostate (*Candida prostatitis*) rarely occurs in healthy men (Indudhara et al., 1992), but can occur in men with diabetes (Bilo, 2006), or other immune compromising conditions. Candida prostatitis causes urethral burning after ejaculation, pain at the base of the penis, and pain in the prostate gland. Prostate pain (*prostatodynia*) is also called *chronic pelvic pain syndrome.*

Candida Balanitis

The following information about superficial mycotic colonization and infections of the penis and scrotum is summarized from the review article by Aridogan et al. (2011) unless otherwise noted.

The normal microflora of the human male genitalia includes bacteria, yeasts (Candida and Malassezia), and fungi (*dermatophytes*). Infections are caused mainly by Candida. A higher prevalence of yeasts was found in samples from the prepuce and glans penis of uncircumcised boys.

Diagnosis

Genital yeast infections in men are diagnosed based on clinical signs and symptoms, risk factors for candidiasis, microscopy, and culture with species identification and antifungal susceptibility testing (Step 1). *Test before treating!*

Methods of collecting specimens depend on the site of infection.

Candida balanitis is diagnosed by collecting samples for microscopy and culture from the groove around the head (*glans*) of the penis (*coronal sulcus*), and under the foreskin (*subpreputial sac*). Skin scrapings yield positive yeast cultures more often than swab specimens because yeasts grow inside the cutaneous epithelial cells. Microscopy results are more accurate if samples are collected by adhesive tape pressed on the skin than by swabbing. Direct impression of the glans on an agar surface resulted in a higher Candida recovery rate than from the swab method (Lisboa et al., 2010). When balanitis persists and the cause remains unclear, a biopsy is warranted to rule out malignancy (Edwards, 1996).

Candida urethritis is diagnosed by a swab culture from the opening (*meatus*) of the urethra.

Candida prostatitis is diagnosed by culture and microscopy of prostatic fluid collected by prostate massage. In this procedure, the physician inserts a finger into the rectum, and exerts pressure on the infected or inflamed prostate from inside. It may be painful and carries the risk of forcing an infection into the bloodstream. Magri et al. (2005) recommended testing urine collected after prostate massage. Positive Candida cultures are obtained more often when prostatic fluid is collected in a condom during intercourse (Gilpin, 1967). Advance arrangements must be made with the urologist before bringing in this type of specimen for testing. Semen can also be collected during masturbation by ejaculating into a sterile cup during an office visit.

Yeasts can be seen directly in semen under the microscope. The diagnosis of Candida prostatitis can be improved by incorporating these sensitive and specific methods:

- Immunofluorescent stains consisting of fluorescent dyes attached to antibodies against specific microbes detect nongrowing or latent germs (Mårdh and Colleen, 1975).
- DNA gene sequencing and polymerase chain reaction technology detect nonculturable or occult microbes (Watson and Irwin, 2009).

Yeasts might enter the prostate via the following routes:

- *Ascending migration* of Candida cells up the urethra after antibacterial treatment or unprotected intercourse with an infected partner.
- *Reflux* of infected urine into the prostatic ducts.
- Backwards (*retrograde*) ejaculation of semen contaminated with yeasts.
- *Hematogenous* inoculation of the prostate with yeasts from a blood infection (*candidemia*).
- Yeasts carried inside WBCs (*lymphocyte transport*) from an infection at a distant site, most likely the intestines.
- Contamination during urological procedures such as prostate biopsies or surgery.
- Invasion of Candida from an intestinal yeast infection, through the wall of the rectum, into the prostate, via a connecting tunnel (*fistula*) between juxtaposed organs.

Cases of Candida prostatitis might be missed if yeasts found in prostatic fluid are dismissed as contamination by normal flora. I suggest this by analogy with the following statement by Watson and Irwin (2009): Gram-positive staining bacteria have traditionally been dismissed as normal flora in prostatic fluid cultures, but they could be disease agents. Normal defense mechanisms in healthy men render Gram-positive bacteria harmless, but men with chronic prostatitis may have defective immune responses. This theory helps explain why prolonged courses of antibiotics sometimes provide symptomatic relief.

Watson and Irwin (2009) further stated that *"Tailoring the diagnostic workup to meet the needs of a specific patient is a skill that defies textbook codification. The art of medicine comes into play in deciding, together with the patient, which possibilities to pursue and how vigorously to pursue each of them."*

Difficulties inherent in diagnosing prostatitis caused by fungal infections were explained by Wise and Shteynshlyuger (2006): *"Each fungus can cause changes in the prostate that mimic bacterial infection, benign prostatic hypertrophy, or neoplasm. Diagnosis can be established by urine cultures or needle biopsy of the prostate. Prostate surgery for carcinoma or benign enlargement may detect latent fungal infection. Different fungal species can have divergent clinical manifestations and require different treatment. In some cases, asymptomatic localized fungal prostatitis can be cured by removal of the infected gland. Symptomatic and disseminated infection may require prostatectomy and systemic antifungal therapy."*

Treatment

First-time yeast infections of the penis, scrotum, and groin area are treated with topical antifungals for one to two weeks. While several investigators have reported that single-dose Diflucan is adequate for uncomplicated yeast infections, be forewarned: based on findings with women, short-term treatment of yeast infections in men for only one day may lead to incomplete cures, frequent relapses, and long-term misery.

Recurrent yeast infections on skin are effectively treated with both topical and systemic antifungals concurrently until symptoms resolve (Step 2). When antibacterial antibiotics did not help symptoms of prostatitis or urethritis, prolonged courses of high-dose systemic antifungals might provide relief. Of course, diagnostic tests should be done first before starting treatment.

Skin infections caused by Malassezia yeasts are treated with topical antifungal agents such as selenium sulphide lotion or shampoo, sodium thiosulphate with salicylic acid, propylene glycol, zinc pyrithione shampoo, and/or ciclopirox solution.

To avoid liver problems and other side effects of systemic antifungals, follow the precautions in Step 3. Inflammation is treated with a cream that contains both an antifungal agent and a corticosteroid (Step 4). Don't use steroid cream alone because corticosteroids unopposed by antifungals cause yeast infections.

Circumcision

Approximately one-third of the world's male population is circumcised. The neonatal period is the most appropriate time for surgical removal of the foreskin. The area under the foreskin in uncircumcised men is a warm, moist environment that enables pathogens to grow, especially when penile hygiene is poor. Daily bathing of the penis with retraction of the prepuce using a mild soap is required to maintain a healthy condition.

Circumcision significantly lowers colonization by yeasts and fungi, as well as bacteria from the glans penis and prepuce. Penile rashes, infections, and carcinoma are more common in uncircumcised men, and balanitis/balanoposthitis caused by *C. albicans*, is the most frequent infection. Circumcision is sometimes performed to cure recurrent balanitis, but it can lead to other problems in adult men. Therefore, surgery should be performed only if intensive medical treatments have failed.

Predisposing Factors

Risk factors for Candida balanitis are diabetes, lack of circumcision, age above 40 years, penile-vaginal transmission, immunosuppression, atopic dermatitis, and eczema. Lifestyle conditions that predispose to genital yeast infections in men include heat and moisture in the groin area, tight-fitting garments, nylon undergarments, chemical irritants, obesity, and poor hygiene.

Sexual Transmission

About 15% of men carry Candida on the penis without symptoms (Edwards, 1996). Sexual partners carry the same yeast strains. Genotypic identity between *C. albicans* strains isolated from both sexual partners has been reported by several studies. This finding is evidence for sexual transmission of Candida.

Penile carriage (*colonization*) as well as symptomatic balanitis were primarily associated with female sexual partners who had vulvovaginal candidiasis. About 10% of men who have intercourse with women who have vaginal yeast infections later develop balanoposthitis (Oriel et al., 1972). However, male genitalia are not a reservoir of infection for recurrent yeast vaginitis. Prophylactic treatment of men did not reduce relapses of vaginal candidiasis in their female sexual partners (Fong, 1992).

If either partner has a genital infection, you should not have sex. After treatment and resolution of symptoms, you should use condoms during intercourse as a precaution to prevent sexual transmission of infections. If you have unprotected intercourse, and a rash appears on your penis or groin area shortly afterwards, it might be an allergic reaction to Candida yeasts in your partner. If so, then local treatment with steroid or antihistamine cream may be sufficient. If the rash persists, see your doctor to obtain testing for a yeast infection. If your rash is recurrent, you may be allergic to Candida or have poor immunity against Candida. In this case, ask your doctor for a written referral to an allergist to obtain intradermal testing to determine Candida allergy and Candida immunity (Step 5).

Pathogenesis of Prostatodynia

After men are treated with antibiotics for bacterial prostatitis, and then retested, results from microscopy and culture of urine are usually negative for bacteria. However, prostate pain often persists. Since antibiotics are known to cause yeast infections, it is likely that a connection exists between prostatodynia and Candida.

Supporting this suggestion, Mårdh and Colleen (1975) found that antibiotic treatment often leads to positive yeast cultures from urethral specimens. De Rose et al. (2004) found that mepartricin, an antifungal agent (Bacigalupo et al., 1983), effectively treated nonbacterial prostatitis at 40 mg (150,000 IU) daily. Mepartricin is a macrolide polyene that is useful for treating urethra, prostate, and bladder disorders, as well as chronic pelvic pain syndrome and benign prostatic hyperplasia. Mepatricin is available as a urological preparation to be used as an instillation into the bladder, and is also available as oral enteric-coated pills. Mepartricin resulted in clinically and statistically significant reduction in symptoms of chronic prostatitis/chronic pelvic pain syndrome (Cohen et al., 2012).

Diflucan at high dosages (2 x 400 mg daily) resulted in improvement in 70% of men with chronic prostatitis/chronic pelvic pain syndrome (Dybowski, 2013). Kotb et al. (2013) reported similar results.

Culture-negative prostatodynia may be analogous to a similar condition in women called vulvodynia, which is due to a hyperimmune response after a yeast infection. Some men with chronic nonbacterial prostatitis have an autoimmune component to their disease. Alexander et al. (1997) found evidence of T cell reactivity with normal prostatic proteins. Hence, molecular mimicry between host and pathogen may play a role in prostatodynia or nonbacterial prostatitis. Alternatively, prostatodynia can be due to referred pain from another site in the pelvic region (Watson and Irwin, 2009).

Progression to chronic pain after antimicrobial therapy is governed by your genetic predisposition. Recent studies of chronic pain conditions report that gene alterations produce more proinflammatory cytokines, and less anti-inflammatory cytokines. Researchers have postulated that chronic inflammation induces localized peripheral nerve damage, promotes the growth of more nerve cells, and increases pain sensitivity.

Conclusions of Chapter 3
Yeast Infections in Men

You don't have to "*Learn to live with it!*" If you develop a penile yeast infection, obtain an early diagnosis, and effective treatments with antifungal and anti-inflammatory drugs. *Nip it in the bud!*

Learn about the countless pitfalls in a man's path that can trigger Candida balanitis by reading Step 6. Identify your individual susceptibility factors. Follow *all* of the medical care and self-help guidelines for yeast infections and yeast allergies in my ten-step program in Part II. *You can conquer Candida!*

CHAPTER 4

Yeast Infections in Children

Colonization

It was previously thought that the developing fetus was in a sterile environment in the womb. But that idea is being challenged by new findings. Healthy babies were found to be born with bacteria and fungi already present in their intestines (Willis, 2019). This suggests that bacteria and fungi may cross the placenta from mother to fetus as a normal part of pregnancy. It was also found that the gut communities of several preterm infants were dominated by *Candida*.

Babies become colonized by microorganisms during birth. Yeasts and bacteria from the mother's vagina enter the newborn's eyes, ears, nose, and mouth as it travels down the birth canal. Immediately after birth, antibacterial drops are put into newborns' eyes to prevent blindness. When a newborn baby swallows, yeasts and bacteria from its mouth travel down its alimentary canal and start to grow. When girl babies defecate in their diapers, yeasts and bacteria in the feces populate her vagina.

Symptoms

Newborns are more susceptible to yeast infections than adults because their immune systems are immature. Yeast infections in children include oral thrush, colic, constipation, diarrhea, and diaper rash. These yeast infections commonly develop in babies and children when they are treated with antibiotics for ear infections or upper respiratory infections.

Oral Thrush

An active yeast infection (*acute pseudomembranous candidiasis*) of the mouth in newborns is easily recognized by a white-coated tongue. Oral thrush is characterized by white patches on the tongue that are dead tongue cells killed by Candida. When the dead tissue is scraped off, the infected tissue underneath may bleed. Oral thrush may cause the baby pain and interfere with nursing or bottle feeding. Furthermore, during breast-feeding, the yeast infection can spread from the baby's mouth to the mother's nipples, causing discomfort to both mother and child. If these dual yeast infections are not treated effectively, the baby may not get adequate nutrition and fail to thrive.

Colic, Constipation, and Diarrhea

Colic means intestinal pain. It is caused by gas produced by intestinal bacteria and yeasts during fermentation of milk sugar (*lactose*). Babies with colic cry a lot, kick their feet, and draw up their knees to their belly. This is a reflex motion that helps relieves pressure in the colon by passing gas rectally. Intestinal yeast infections can also cause constipation or diarrhea.

Colic can be caused by yeast infection of the intestinal wall or by bacterial dysbiosis, both of which are common in newborns who have not developed their normal friendly intestinal bacterial flora and whose immune systems are still immature. Babies and children can also develop these symptoms after antibiotic treatment. Some cases of sudden infant death syndrome were found to have intestinal flora dominated by *C. albicans* (Geertinger et al., 1982).

Diaper Rash

The skin in the diaper region can be infected by germs from the feces. *C. albicans* is more likely to cause diaper rash if it colonizes the alimentary tract (Dixon et al., 1969). Diaper rash (*diaper dermatitis*) is usually a mixed infection with both bacteria and yeasts. The rash affects the skin around the anus, and on the buttocks (*gluteal* region), and can spread to the genital area, and inner thighs. Chemicals in urine further irritate the rash.

Diagnosis

Yeast infections cause babies and their parents a lot of grief. Hence, it is important to obtain an accurate diagnosis. Pediatricians must consider the child's clinical signs and symptoms, history of risk factors predisposing to yeast infections, and results from microscopy, culture, yeast identification, and antifungal susceptibility testing. To save money, often testing is not offered, and the physician goes right to prescribing treatment.

Treatment

There are several liquid preparations available for treating Candida infections in infants and small children who cannot swallow pills. A spoon is supplied to measure out the prescribed dose, which is based on body weight.

Nystatin Oral Suspension

The standard treatment for oral thrush is **nystatin oral suspension**. It is also the safest treatment because it is not absorbed from the stomach and is excreted in the feces. Therefore, nystatin does not affect the liver or interact with other medications. But since nystatin is not soluble in water, it does not penetrate into tissues, and therefore it is not as effective as a systemic antifungal. For this reason, thrush often recurs after nystatin treatment is discontinued.

Nystatin suspension is flavored and sweetened with sucrose to make it palatable. Even though sugar should not be consumed by Candida patients because it feeds the yeasts and promotes symptoms through sugar fermentation, please be assured that the amount of sugar in nystatin suspension is insignificant, and this treatment is proven effective.

Diflucan and Sporanox Liquid Preparations

These antifungal preparations are used to treat oral thrush. They are absorbed from the stomach and spread throughout the body. Therefore, they are more effective than nystatin suspension because they penetrate into tissues where the yeasts grow inside epithelial cells. It may be necessary to treat children with a systemic antifungal agent such as Diflucan or Sporanox if they develop recurrent episodes of oral thrush or diaper dermatitis after being treated with nystatin. If a baby has oral thrush and the mother has a yeast infection of her nipples, they should both be treated with a systemic antifungal.

Diflucan (fluconazole) oral suspension is flavored and sweetened for infants to make it palatable. Even though sugar should not be consumed by Candida patients because it feeds the yeasts and promotes symptoms through sugar fermentation, please be assured that the amount of sugar in liquid preparations is insignificant, and these treatments are proven effective.

Active fungal infections of the mouth and/or diaper area should start to decrease after several days of oral antifungal treatment, but antifungal therapy should be continued until symptoms subside completely. Then daily treatment should be switched to weekly maintenance for several months to prevent a recurrence.

If there is no symptomatic improvement, a resistant yeast strain may be responsible. The yeast should be cultured, identified, and tested for antifungal susceptibility to determine the best antifungal agent to use. Identify the child's underlying risk factors responsible for thrush or diaper rash with the pediatrician's help and together develop a plan for prevention based on the ten-step program in Part II.

Antifungal Creams

The safest treatment for diaper rash is a cream because very little of the drug is absorbed through the skin. Some creams are available OTC, others by prescription. Since diaper rash is usually a mixed infection with both bacteria and yeasts, a cream containing both an antibacterial and an antifungal agent should be prescribed. In severe cases, a steroid cream is added to the treatment protocol.

Risk Factors

The number one risk factor for yeast infections in children and adults is treatment with antibiotics for bacterial infections. The mother may have been given antibiotics prior to, or during delivery, or while breast-feeding. Infants often receive antibiotics for bacterial infections of their ears or upper respiratory tract. Older children can develop oral thrush from using an inhaler for asthma. Work with the pediatrician to identify and eliminate your child's predisposing conditions for candidiasis. Congenital immune defects are rare, and require further testing by an immunologist.

Prevention

Pregnant women should be screened for Candida vaginal colonization prior to delivery to prevent transmission of yeast infections to babies at birth (Leli et al., 2013).

> **WARNING**
>
> Pregnant women should not be treated with systemic antifungals during the first three months of pregnancy (first trimester) unless they have a life-threatening yeast infection. During the first three months, the fetus is undergoing major developmental changes, and systemic antifungals may cause birth defects (teratogenic effects) at that time. From four months onward, the fetus is less susceptible to developing serious complications from drugs.

Safety Tip: The rate of preterm births was reduced by using vaginal antifungal treatment during the first trimester of pregnancy instead of systemic antifungal treatment (Mendling and Brasch, 2012). Vaginal antifungals should also be used between the 34th and 36th week of pregnancy to reduce the rate of oral thrush and diaper dermatitis in newborns (Schnell, 1982; Mendling and Brasch, 2012).

To prevent the development of oral thrush, children who use steroid inhalers for asthma should rinse out their mouth after each puff by gargling with water or mouthwash and spitting out the liquid.

If babies or children are being treated with antibiotics, and they have a history of thrush, colic, and/or diaper rash, they should be given nystatin suspension concurrently to prevent recurrences of yeast infections. Once antibiotic treatment is discontinued, preventive treatment with nystatin can be switched from daily treatment to weekly prophylaxis for several months to prevent the yeast infection from coming back (Step 10).

Probiotics

Another way to help prevent intestinal yeast infections in children is to administer probiotic supplements (Step 9). Parents of newborns will be especially interested in these studies.

- Hatakka et al. (2001) found that long-term consumption of probiotic milk prevented infections in children attending day care centers.
- Olivares et al. (2006) reported that intestinal symptoms such as colic in newborns can be reduced by adding probiotic supplements to baby's formula or by breastfeeding. Surprisingly, breast milk is not sterile. Rather, it normally contains friendly bacteria!

- Savino et al. (2010) reported that *Lactobacillus reuteri* DSM 17938 significantly relieved the symptoms of colic in infants. After probiotic treatment, there was an increase in healthy lactobacilli in the stools, and a decrease in the harmful strain of *Escherichia coli* associated with colic.
- Romeo et al. (2011) found that treatment of preterm newborns with probiotics prevented enteric Candida colonization, sepsis, and abnormal neurological outcomes.
- Jost et al. (2013) found the same strain of *Bifidobacterium breve* in the mother's breast milk as in the baby's feces. Presumably, this friendly bacterium passed from the mother's intestine, into her bloodstream, then into her breast milk, and from there into the baby's intestine. And this is a natural process!
- Fernandez et al. (2013) and Jost et al. (2013) explained that breast milk not only contains the mother's friendly bacterial flora, it also contains her protective antibodies. Another reason to breastfeed!
- Kumar et al. (2013) found that probiotics prevented Candida colonization of the intestine and the urine in critically ill children receiving broad spectrum antibiotics.

Is Candida Linked to Autism?

Some health care practitioners have claimed that intestinal yeast overgrowth causes autism, but there is no credible evidence for such a connection. *Autism* is a neurological disorder that affects the brain, and that develops while the baby is in utero. It is probably influenced by genetic and environmental factors during gestation and after birth.

If autistic children have intestinal Candida overgrowths, the symptoms would certainly make them uncomfortable, and they may "act out" or exhibit behavioral problems because they cannot explain their discomfort. Yeast metabolites, such as alcohol and acetaldehyde, could affect brain function. But, before putting children on a restricted diet and supplements, first obtain diagnostic tests for intestinal candidiasis. *Test before treating!*

Conclusions of Chapter 4
Yeast Infections in Children

This chapter explains the yeast-connected illnesses that develop in newborns and older children. To overcome these yeast infections, obtain medical care for your child and ask the pediatrician to follow the guidelines for yeast infections and yeast allergies in my ten-step program in Part II. Children need their yeast illnesses to be diagnosed, treated, and prevented appropriately just as much as adults. *You can conquer Candida!*

CHAPTER 5

Intestinal Yeast Infections and the Hall of Fame

Definition of the Yeast Syndrome

Intestinal yeast overgrowth produces a variety of symptoms in the gut as well as elsewhere in the body. This collection of symptoms is known by many names listed in Chapter 1. In this book, I call this disease *the yeast syndrome.*

Most of the symptoms caused by the yeast syndrome can be explained by well-understood mechanisms involving Candida activities and immune reactions to Candida. *The defining characteristic of the yeast syndrome is a worsening of symptoms after meals, especially after eating carbohydrates or yeasty foods.*

Because symptoms are nonspecific and could be due to other causes, specific diagnostic tests for Candida should be performed. Blood levels of Candida IgG, IgA, and IgM indicate a current or past yeast infection of the gut. Diagnostic tests that are definitive for a current, active intestinal yeast infection measure Candida antigens, Candida immune complexes, or Candida DNA in blood. The diagnosis is confirmed when symptoms improve with antifungal therapy.

The typical yeast syndrome sufferer is a woman in her childbearing years who has been treated with antibiotics. But anyone—male or female, young or old—can develop an intestinal yeast infection. The incidence is probably high in the general population because there are many risk factors, and a lot of people have intestinal complaints. However, no good incidence data are available because most physicians ignore this diagnosis. After reading this chapter, you will have a good understanding of how symptoms are caused in intestinal candidiasis.

"Doctors' Plague"

Most cases of intestinal yeast overgrowth are caused by antibiotic treatments (Kennedy and Volz, 1985a; Samonis et al., 1994; Ruiz-Sánchez et al., 2002; Wagner, 2005; Pappas et al., 2009; Wlodarska and Finlay, 2010; and other references too numerous to cite).

Since the etiology of intestinal candidiasis is mainly due to physicians' treatments, it is by definition an *iatrogenic disease*. Colloquially speaking, it can be called a *"doctors' plague."* Perhaps this is why doctors deny the existence of the yeast connection to disease because their treatments are responsible for causing most yeast infections!

Some antibacterial agents are worse than others in terms of causing yeast infections. For example, amoxicillin-clavulanate caused a higher increase in gastrointestinal colonization by yeasts than ciprofloxacin, sulfamethoxazole-trimethoprim, or ampicillin (Samonis et al., 1994). By far, the worst offenders in terms of causing intestinal candidiasis are penicillin, clindamycin, vancomycin (Kennedy and Volz, 1985a), and metronidazole. These antibiotics kill anaerobic bacteria, which are the "really friendly bacteria." Strict anaerobes in the gut ecosystem prevent yeast colonization by inhibiting adhesion of *C. albicans* to the gut wall.

Antibiotics also disrupt the normal population of intestinal microbes producing a condition called *dysbiosis*. Taking probiotic supplements containing "friendly bacteria" can help restore the normal flora. Other medications such as antacids and corticosteroids also promote yeast overgrowth in the intestinal tract via different mechanisms. Physicians must acknowledge these examples of inadvertent iatrogenesis before they can devise protocols to prevent yeast infections in people who are susceptible to candidiasis.

Intestinal Candidiasis

"Candidiasis of the gastrointestinal tract was first recognized in the 18th century, when it was noted that thrush could extend from the nasopharynx to the stomach and bowel" (Bolivar and Bodey, 1985). These authors reviewed the medical literature and reached the following conclusions.

- Intestinal candidiasis is diagnosed by microscopic examination of stool specimens.
- Yeast infections on esophageal mucosal surfaces appear as white patches during endoscopy, but sometimes only areas of redness or ulcerations are seen.
- Intestinal candidiasis can cause diarrhea, flatulence, abdominal pain, rectal bleeding, and anal itching.
- Allergic reactions to Candida contribute to diarrheal disease, irritable bowel syndrome, and mucous colitis.
- A yeast-free diet results in clinical improvement.
- The diagnosis of intestinal yeast infection is confirmed by the person's favorable response to the oral antifungal drug nystatin.

This article by Bolivar and Bodey is an expert academic review of the clinical characteristics of intestinal candidiasis based on medical publications up to the year 1985. Since then, many controlled clinical studies have extended our knowledge about intestinal yeast overgrowth. These studies are listed in the following Hall of Fame. It tells the inside story of the pioneering physicians who recognized that intestinal yeast overgrowth produces symptoms in the gut as well as throughout the body. The early reports based on clinical observations led researchers to perform controlled clinical studies that validated diagnostic tests and a screening questionnaire for intestinal yeast infections.

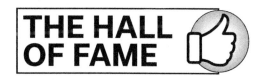

The practice of medicine progresses from initial anecdotal observations of clinical signs and symptoms, to controlled scientific investigations, to clinical applications. The timeline presented here in the Hall of Fame illustrates the discovery of a new paradigm in medicine: *a disease with multiple manifestations caused by a single etiological agent.* The clinical and scientific evidence for the yeast syndrome is presented by citing the publications. These findings have changed the way yeast infections are viewed today by "physicians-in-the-know."

Antibiotics discovered in the 1940s were in widespread use by the 1950s. Then reports started appearing about antibiotic-induced Candida infections. Brabander et al. (1957) were among the first to recognize that intestinal yeast overgrowth was associated with multiple local as well as systemic symptoms such as bloating, itching, and skin rashes. By the 1960s, it was well established that antibiotics increased the incidence and severity of candidiasis, as well as altering immunological defenses (Seelig, 1966).

Pioneering Discoveries

An astute community-based physician, C. Orian Truss, described a syndrome of physical and mental symptoms caused by Candida overgrowth of the intestine in a series of papers published in 1978, 1980, 1981, and 1984, and in a 1983 book aptly named, *The Missing Diagnosis.* His description of the yeast syndrome was based on early reports of antibiotic-induced yeast infections in the medical literature and on his clinical observations of patients. Truss called his book, *The Missing Diagnosis*, because other medical professionals had not recognized this yeast-related syndrome as a real disease.

Also, in 1983, another astute community-based physician, William G. Crook, reported his independent clinical observations of intestinal candidiasis in a book aptly named, *The Yeast Connection.* Crook's book gave credit to Truss for his original discoveries, but *The Yeast Connection* book was more popular because Crook offered a questionnaire and treatment plan in easy-to-understand language.

Many other books followed on the coattails of Truss and Crook. Noteworthy is *The Yeast Syndrome* by Trowbridge and Walker (1986). While all these trade books offered much useful information, they also ignited a controversy among establishment physicians that continues until today (Chapter 6).

Development of Diagnostic Tests

Up until 1983, when these two pioneering books were published, intestinal yeast infections were diagnosed based on clinical signs and symptoms, history of risk factors for candidiasis, and microscopy and culture of stool specimens. But in response to the barrage of Candida patients seeking help for their yeast symptoms, medical professionals saw the need for more rigorous diagnostic standards. So, researchers sought an immunological footprint left by intestinal yeast overgrowth. The early diagnostic tests detected anti-Candida antibodies in blood. Later tests measured Candida immune complexes and Candida DNA in blood.

Anti-Candida antibodies: Many controlled clinical studies found that people with intestinal candidiasis had elevated levels of anti-Candida antibodies in their blood compared to healthy controls (Munoz et al, 1980; Hopwood et al., 1985; Wojdani et al., 1986; Bunting et al., 1988; Crayton et al., 1989; Bauman and Hagglund, 1991; Lewith et al., 2007).

Skeptics who denied the existence of the yeast syndrome criticized this test saying, *"Everyone has antibodies to Candida in their blood."* While this is true, their statement overlooks results from all these controlled clinical studies showing that levels of anti-Candida antibodies above normal correlate with intestinal yeast infection. Furthermore, the higher the levels, the worse the symptoms. If skeptics had read these published studies, they would have learned that *results were statistically significant in all studies.* Obviously, the skeptics were ignorant of all these reports.

Another incorrect argument made by skeptics was that abnormally high levels of anti-Candida antibodies in blood just indicate a past intestinal yeast overgrowth. While it is true that antibodies persist for many years after the infection has been cured, common sense tells you that if a person has fully recovered, she or he would not now be in the doctor's office complaining about yeast-related symptoms. And if common sense does not work for skeptics, then the massive amount of scientific evidence discussed in this book should persuade them.

Candida immune complexes: *Definitive diagnostic tests for a current, active intestinal yeast infection detect Candida antigens or Candida immune complexes in blood.* Immune complexes are formed when antigens bind to antibodies. Several controlled clinical studies have shown that people with intestinal candidiasis have elevated levels of Candida immune complexes in their blood compared to healthy controls (Lehmann and Reiss, 1980; Lanson, 1997; Broughton and Lanson, 1997).

Broughton and Lanson validated the identification of Candida immune complexes in blood as a way to diagnose a current, active, intestinal yeast infection. The blood test for Candida immune complexes was developed through the Antibody Assay Laboratory Reference Laboratory originally based in Santa Ana, California. AALRL later moved to Austin, Texas, and eventually turned over their blood test to be distributed through Genova Diagnostics. More recently, Genova Diagnostics discontinued offering this test. AALRL was listed in Quackwatch.com, founded by Stephen Barrett, M.D., who specializes in denouncing practices considered nonstandard by establishment medicine. Some laboratories offering tests for Candida were closed down by state medical boards. Today, blood tests for Candida immune complexes, Candida antigens, anti-Candida antibodies, and Candida DNA are available from labs listed in Table 7.

Crook's Candida Questionnaire

Symptoms drive patients into doctors' offices seeking relief. To screen people for intestinal candidiasis, Crook (1983) developed a *"Candida Questionnaire and Score Sheet"* to screen patients with symptoms of intestinal yeast overgrowth and published it in various editions of his book, *The Yeast Connection*. Crook's 1995 questionnaire contained 70 questions about symptoms and risk factors for yeast infections. It became popular with the public because it provided a numerical score that *allegedly* indicated the likelihood of having intestinal yeast overgrowth. But Crook's questionnaire was not based on a controlled clinical study. Furthermore, since most of the symptoms are nonspecific, they could be due to other illnesses.

Several groups of physicians and researchers independently undertook controlled clinical studies to evaluate Crook's questionnaire using blood tests and patients' responses to antifungal therapy as objective criteria (Sehnert et al., 1990; Bauman and Hagglund, 1991; Lanson, 1997; Broughton and Lanson, 1997; Santelmann et al., 2001; Lewith et al., 2007). Here is a summary of their findings.

- All studies reported that high scores for intestinal and systemic symptoms correlated with abnormally high levels of anti-Candida antibodies and/or Candida immune complexes in the blood.
- Physical and mental symptoms of the yeast syndrome improved *in concert* with oral nystatin therapy.
- People with high symptom scores, but normal levels of anti-Candida antibodies had intestinal diseases unrelated to yeast such as Giardia, Ascaris, Epstein Barr virus, food intolerances, hyper-IgE, or inflammatory bowel disease (Bauman and Hagglund, 1991).

Yeast Questionnaire (Santelmann et al., 2001)

In a landmark, randomized, double-blind, prospective, placebo-controlled study, Santelmann et al. (2001) found that only seven out of the 70 questions in Crook's 1995 questionnaire were valid indicators of yeast-related disease. For this study, people were selected if their symptoms decreased on a sugar-free, yeast-free diet. After they filled out Crook's questionnaire, they were treated with either oral nystatin or a placebo. Answers from people whose symptoms improved on nystatin therapy were compared to answers from people who did not improve on nystatin and to answers from people on placebo, and then the results were statistically analyzed. Only seven questions from Crooks' questionnaire predicted a positive response to nystatin in 95% of the subjects. These seven validated questions are listed below in Table 3.

In a follow-up study (Lewith et al., 2007), Santelmann and coworkers found that people with high scores on this seven-item questionnaire had abnormally high concentrations of serum anti-Candida IgG antibodies. Thus, the Candida Questionnaire in Table 3 is a scientifically validated tool for screening people who may have intestinal yeast overgrowth. To arrive at a diagnosis, further evaluation with blood and stool tests is required (Step 1). Fill in your answers on Table 3, show it to your doctor, and ask her or him to order tests for intestinal yeast overgrowth.

Table 3. Yeast Questionnaire (Santelmann et al., 2001)

Score: 0 = none
1 = occasional or mild
2 = frequent or moderately severe
3 = severe or disabling

Circle the number that applies to your yeast condition:

1. Have you, at any time in your life, taken broad-spectrum antibiotics?	0 or 3
2. Have you taken broad-spectrum antibiotics for one month or longer?	0 or 3
3. Are your symptoms worse on damp, muggy days or in moldy places?	0 or 3
4. Do you crave sugar?	0 or 3
5. Do you have a feeling of being "drained"?	0, 1, 2 or 3
6. **Women:** Are you bothered with vaginal burning, itching, or discharge?	0, 1, 2 or 3
Men: Do you have burning, itching, or discharge from the penis?	0, 1, 2 or 3
7. Are you bothered by burning, itching, or tearing of eyes?	0, 1, 2 or 3

Total Score: 0-3 = unlikely
4-9 = probable
10-21 = almost certain

Is the patient positive for the yeast syndrome?   Circle one: No   Yes

Heroes of the Yeast Revolution

The physicians who discovered the yeast syndrome, and the researchers who later validated questionnaires and laboratory tests for intestinal candidiasis are credited here in the Hall of Fame for starting a yeast revolution. These groundbreaking papers have shaped our current understanding of the manifestations of the yeast syndrome, and set a new paradigm in the diagnosis and treatment of chronic intestinal candidiasis. Their clinical and laboratory findings have shown that *the yeast syndrome is a real disease, and it makes patients really sick.*

Many of the manuscripts describing these controlled clinical studies were initially rejected by skeptical academic reviewers at establishment journals (read about the controversy in Chapter 6). These rejections forced researchers to send their manuscripts to alternative medical journals for publication. Peer reviewers at these alternative medical societies were professionals knowledgeable about the yeast syndrome. But, unfortunately, some of these journals were not indexed or abstracted online. Consequently, these papers are difficult to find. I found out about these papers because I networked extensively with scientists and physicians studying the yeast syndrome. You might be able to obtain reprints by ordering copies through the lending library at your local public library. You might try to contact the journals directly and ask them to post these papers on their website for download. Or you can search for the abstract or full text of these papers on Google Scholar (https://scholar.google.com).

Symptoms of the Yeast Syndrome

Yeast overgrowths in the intestine produce symptoms locally in the gut as well as systemically throughout the body. But just because some symptoms are systemic does not mean that yeast cells are spread throughout your body. The yeast infection is localized in the intestine. Therefore, you should never use the colloquial term "systemic yeast," or you will lose credibility with your physician. Systemic symptoms arising from bowel diseases are called *extraintestinal symptoms*, and are observed in other inflammatory bowel disorders such as Crohn's disease and ulcerative colitis (Larsen et al., 2010). Typical symptoms and test results for the yeast syndrome are summarized in Table 4.

Table 4. Checklist of Yeast Syndrome Symptoms

People with intestinal yeast overgrowths typically experience many of the clinical signs and symptoms and associated diseases listed here. But not everyone with the yeast syndrome experiences all of these manifestations, and some of these signs and symptoms can be caused by other diseases unrelated to Candida. That is why you need diagnostic tests that measure specific Candida-related components to determine if you have intestinal candidiasis.

Circle the features of your illness listed below and show this checklist to your physician. It will help her or him to decide what diagnostic tests to order from Step 1. Signs and symptoms that improved with antifungal therapy in controlled studies were attributed to Candida infection. **Note**: Clinical signs are what the doctor sees; symptoms are what the patient feels.

Intestinal Signs and Symptoms

Mouth, throat, and esophagus: Clinical signs include white thrush patches and/or red areas seen on tongue, gums, inside cheeks, throat, and esophagus during endoscopy. Symptoms include burning tongue, bitter metallic taste, bad breath, sore throat, hoarseness, laryngitis, difficulty swallowing, and gastroesophageal reflux.

Intestines: Clinical signs include mucus and/or white clumps of dead tissue in stools; perianal redness; white thrush patches and/or red areas seen on walls of small intestine and colon during colonoscopy or sigmoidoscopy. Symptoms include constipation alternating with diarrhea; intestinal gas (*flatulence*), bloating, and abdominal pain (*colic*); and perianal itching and burning, especially after a bowel movement.

Genital and Urinary Symptoms

Women: Clinical signs include redness of vaginal opening, vulva, vestibule, perineum, and urethra; white vaginal discharge that is cheesy or creamy; white thrush patches or red tissue observed on vaginal wall during colposcopy. Symptoms include itching and/or burning of vaginal opening, vulva, vestibule, perineum, and urethra; vulvar pain (vulvodynia) during intercourse and everyday activities.

Men: Clinical signs include redness on skin of penis and scrotum; discharge from urethra. Symptoms include itching and/or burning on skin of penis and scrotum; urethral burning after ejaculation.

Bladder: Clinical signs of interstitial cystitis include pinpoint hemorrhages (petechiae) seen in bladder wall during cystoscopy. Symptoms of interstitial cystitis include frequent and burning urination in the absence of a culturable bacterial infection.

Symptoms at Other Body Sites

Skin: Itching, burning, red rashes, "jock itch," body odor.

Eyes: Itching, burning, redness, tearing, and scratchy feeling on surface of eyeball (conjunctiva) like you have sand in your eyes.

Lungs: Wheezing (asthma) and difficulty in getting a breath deep in the lungs, especially after eating.

Systemic (Extraintestinal) Symptoms

Fatigue: Tiredness, lethargy, feeling drained of energy, and muscle weakness, especially after eating.

Mental: "Brain fog," inability to concentrate, confusion, forgetfulness, depression, mood swings, headaches, dizziness, and feeling drunk or hungover.

Allergies and Id (*idiopathic*) reactions: Allergic and Id reactions to Candida include asthma, conjunctivitis, and rashes. They are triggered by allergic reactions to foods and airborne, contact, and internal (endogenous) allergens, especially yeasts and molds.

Adverse food reactions: Occur minutes or hours after eating a food.

Chemical sensitivities: Reactions are triggered by irritating chemicals and food additives.

Nutritional deficiencies: Low blood levels of minerals (iron, magnesium, selenium, and zinc); vitamins (A, B6, and C, biotin, and folate); and fatty acids (omega-6 and omega-3). These low levels are observed in people with "leaky gut" caused by intestinal yeast infections, which causes poor absorption of nutrients.

Autoimmune Diseases found in Candidiasis Patients

Endocrine disorders: Glands such as the thyroid, adrenals, ovaries, or testes secrete less hormones.

Associated auto-antibody disorders: Celiac disease and gluten sensitivity; interstitial cystitis; and anti-*Saccharomyces cerevisiae* antibodies in Crohn's disease.

Candida immunosuppression: Candida infection suppresses T cell-mediated immunity to Candida resulting in more proinflammatory and fewer anti-inflammatory cytokines produced.

APICH: Yeast syndrome sufferers with associated diseases have **A**utoimmune **P**olyendocrinopathy **I**mmune dysregulation **C**andidiasis **H**ypersensitivity.

Explanations of Symptoms

In order to learn how symptoms of the yeast syndrome are caused, first read about the molecular basis for the development of this disease summarized in Table 5.

Table 5. Development of the Yeast Syndrome

The main cause of intestinal yeast infections is medical treatment with drugs such as antibiotics, antacids, and/or corticosteroids.

↓

Intestinal yeasts metabolize sugar and carbohydrates producing alcohol and acetaldehyde, both of which have adverse effects on the gut and brain.

↓

Candida enzymes digest intestinal mucosa allowing yeasts to invade intestinal tissue and grow inside epithelial cells.

↓

Disruption of the intestinal wall structure destroys its selective permeability function, producing "leaky gut syndrome," which allows passage of candidal, bacterial, and food antigens into the bloodstream.

↓

Leaked antigens induce the synthesis of specific antibodies and T cell receptors, which then react with leaked antigens causing intestinal and systemic symptoms.

↓

Anti-Candida antibodies and T cells sensitized to Candida cross-react with common antigens on tissue cells causing autoimmune diseases such as endocrine disorders and Candida-specific T-cell immunosuppression.

Worsening of Symptoms After Meals

The defining characteristic of the yeast syndrome is worsening of symptoms after eating carbohydrates or yeasty foods. Physical and mental symptoms of the yeast syndrome worsen after eating sugar, complex carbohydrates, and yeasty and moldy foods, and improve during fasting. The medical term for this phenomenon is *postprandial exacerbation* of symptoms. Since after-eating worsening is the hallmark of intestinal candidiasis, it can be called *pathognomonic*, which means a clinical sign or symptom that is indicative of a particular disease or condition.

But symptoms that are typical of intestinal candidiasis are *nonspecific* and could be caused by other diseases. That is why you need to obtain testing with diagnostic tests that have been validated for intestinal candidiasis in controlled studies (Step 1).

> **WARNING**
>
> If you follow a diet that is low in carbohydrates, yeasts, and molds, and self-treat with antifungal supplements, and later obtain testing for Candida, your results may be falsely negative. So, remember: *Test <u>before</u> treating!*

Constipation Alternating with Diarrhea

Some people with the yeast syndrome have constipation so severe that they feel as if their colon is paralyzed. Lack of bowel contraction (*peristalsis*) that normally stimulates defecation can be due to invasion of the intestinal wall by Candida. Another possible cause of constipation is an overly restrictive Candida diet that forbids fruits, starchy vegetables, and whole grains in order to avoid carbohydrates. It is unwise to omit these fiber-rich foods because they are necessary for proper bowel function. You can self-treat for constipation by taking a prebiotic fiber supplement (Step 9).

Other people with intestinal yeast infections develop severe diarrhea. Most people with the yeast syndrome alternate between constipation and diarrhea. Physicians label this condition *irritable bowel syndrome*. But IBS is just a descriptive term; I called it a garbage-pail diagnosis because it does not indicate the underlying cause. Several authors have suggested that the yeast syndrome and IBS may be related (Caselli et al., 1988; Santelmann and Howard, 2005; Schulze and Sonnenborn, 2009). IBS may also be caused by illnesses such as food allergies and intolerances, other intestinal infections, and celiac disease.

As you would expect, inflammatory bowel diseases (IBDs) are worsened by Candida. For example, ulcerative colitis heals more quickly with antifungal and probiotic treatments (Zwolinska-Wcislo et al., 2009), and Crohn's disease is diagnosed by high levels of anti-*Saccharomyces cerevisiae* antibodies (ASCA), which are formed against the immunogen *Candida albicans* (see below). So, if you have intestinal symptoms, it might be useful to obtain a blood test for ASCA in addition to testing for anti-Candida antibodies (Step 1).

Gas and Bloating

A small amount of intestinal gas is normal. Some air is swallowed when you eat and drink, and gases are produced during normal digestion. But people with the yeast syndrome can have excessive gas, which causes abdominal bloating, bowel sounds (*borborygmus*), burping, flatulence, and foul-smelling gas passed from the anus.

Intestinal gas is mainly carbon dioxide (CO_2) produced by yeasts and bacteria during the fermentation of carbohydrates. The more yeasts in your intestine, the more carbon dioxide will be produced. Other gases are produced by intestinal bacteria including hydrogen sulfide (which smells like rotten eggs), plus methane and hydrogen (which are odorless, but flammable). Many a little boy who tested this idea, wished he hadn't! (Little girls don't do things like that!)

You can decrease gas and bloating by treating your intestinal yeast infection with antifungals, probiotic supplements containing Lactobacillus and Bifidobacterium, and an enzyme supplement like Beano.

Body Odor

Some people with intestinal yeast overgrowth have an offensive body odor (Zwerling et al., 1984). No amount of showering removes it. These people need to follow all ten steps in my program in Part II.

Sugar Cravings

Craving sweets is a common feature of the yeast syndrome as shown by the study reported in Table 3. Sugar cravings were found to be present in 95% of people who improved on nystatin treatment. But people who do not have the yeast syndrome also crave sweets. Anyone would crave sugar if they followed a low carbohydrate diet, and their blood sugar levels were low. Therefore, sugar cravings are not a specific diagnostic symptom of the yeast syndrome.

Auto-brewery Syndrome

Yeasts in the intestine ferment sugar producing alcohol, acetaldehyde, and other noxious metabolites. These fermentation products can enter the bloodstream, and travel to the brain where they produce "brain fog," "food coma," fatigue, spaciness, forgetfulness, dizziness, impaired judgment, emotional problems in adults, and behavioral problems in children.

People who are heavily colonized with intestinal yeasts produce so much ethanol after eating carbohydrates that it is detectable in their blood and breath. This condition is called the *auto-brewery syndrome*. The Japanese call it *Meitei-sho* or "drunken disease" (Kaji et al., 1984; Davies, 1985). It commonly occurs in people of oriental and Native American descent with impaired genes for the liver enzymes, *alcohol dehydrogenase* and *acetaldehyde dehydrogenase*. People with intestinal candidiasis and defective dehydrogenases cannot break down alcohol and/or acetaldehyde, and may flush red, become drunk, or even pass out after drinking only one alcoholic beverage. They can develop blood ethanol levels of more than 0.20% after eating a normal rice meal (Kaji et al., 1984). In the U.S., you are considered driving drunk at 0.080%.

A simple test for auto-brewery syndrome was developed by Hunnisett et al. (1990). It measures ethanol in the blood before and 60 minutes after the fasting subject swallows 5 grams of glucose. Using this test, Eaton (1991) found that normal blood alcohol remained at 0.0005% in healthy control subjects, but Candida sufferers showed an increase in blood alcohol from 0.001 to 0.007% after one hour. Presumably, Eaton's subjects were Caucasians with normal liver dehydrogenase levels.

This would explain why the elevation in blood alcohol levels was low. Studies of auto-brewery syndrome could be done by collecting blood specimens and testing them for alcohol if a person, who has fasted overnight, undergoes a 50-gram oral glucose tolerance test for diabetes.

Edenberg (2007) suggested that people with genetic variants in dehydrogenases might be at risk for alcoholism. Sehnert and Mathews-Larson (1991) tested alcoholics at a chemical dependency facility with a Candida questionnaire and an anti-Candida antibody blood test. Half of 213 alcoholic subjects were positive for intestinal candidiasis, and most of these responded favorably to nystatin treatment, plus a diet restricting sugar and yeast. Therefore, Larson and Sehnert (1992) proposed an alcoholism recovery program that recognized Candida as a contributing factor. Since many alcoholics crave sugar, Kallmyer (2011) proposed that auto-brewery syndrome could lead to "Candida alcoholism." Thus, sugar cravings in people who are genetically predisposed to alcoholism might actually be due to alcohol cravings!

"Leaky Gut Syndrome"

Normally, the integrity of the intestinal wall is maintained by the constant movement of new intestinal epithelial cells (*enterocytes*) along the extracellular matrix to the villus tips (Wagner, 2005). However, when intestinal yeasts invade the gut wall, its structure is disrupted and it becomes more permeable (Broughton and Lanson, 1997). This increased permeability, colloquially called "leaky gut syndrome," explains many of the physical and mental symptoms of the yeast syndrome.

In healthy people, only small molecules such as nutrients are allowed to pass through the intestinal epithelium into the bloodstream. Retention of certain types of substances inside the intestinal contents is called *selective permeability*. But inflammation caused by infections or allergic reactions in the gut makes capillaries more permeable or leaky. This allows larger molecular weight substances such as partially digested food particles and microbial antigens to pass through the damaged intestinal lining into the circulatory system.

In severe cases of intestinal candidiasis, even whole bacterial and yeast cells can pass through damaged intestinal mucosa into the bloodstream via processes known as *translocation* and *persorption*. *C. albicans* can also penetrate enterocytes directly from the lumen of the intestine (Alexander et al., 1990).

Food and microbial antigens that leak through the intestinal wall into the circulatory system stimulate B cells to synthesize antibodies and induce T cells to produce receptors on their surfaces against those antigens. The next time a person with intestinal candidiasis eats the same foods, those antigens leak into the bloodstream, react with their specific antibodies and T cells, and cause systemic immune symptoms. Likewise, Candida antigens that leak into the bloodstream also react with their specific antibodies and T cells causing symptoms of the yeast syndrome. Intestinal inflammation and increased permeability are also present in Crohn's disease, ulcerative colitis, and celiac disease.

Tests for intestinal permeability involve swallowing nonmetabolized chemicals, and then measuring their levels in blood and/or urine. Leakiness of the intestinal wall is also detected by the presence of higher than normal levels of antibodies against Candida, bacteria, and food antigens in blood. If you feel worse after you eat sugary or yeasty foods, obtain testing for intestinal candidiasis (Step 1).

Adverse Food Reactions

Specific immune reactions occur when food antigens leak into the bloodstream:

- **Immediate food reactions** occur within minutes after eating and can be life threatening. They are true allergic reactions between IgE antibodies and their specific antigens. Food antigens that pass into the circulatory system, can travel to target organs such as the lungs or skin, where they exit the capillaries, combine with specific IgE antibodies attached to mast cells in tissues, and trigger the release of histamine and other mediators of allergic inflammation.
- **Delayed food reactions** occur hours after eating. They can be caused by reactions between IgG antibodies or T cells and their specific antigens. These immune reactions release cytokines that cause fatigue ("food coma").

Nutritional Deficiencies

Disruption of selective permeability of the intestinal mucosa interferes with nutrient absorption and utilization, and can leading to deficiencies in vitamins, minerals, and other essential nutrients. Galland (1985) reported that people with chronic candidiasis and Candida allergy were deficient in magnesium, essential fatty acids, and vitamin B6. Edman et al. (1986) reported that women with recurrent vulvovaginal candidiasis were often deficient in zinc. Paillaud et al. (2004) reported that elderly patients with oral candidiasis were deficient in zinc and vitamin C. Other practitioners claim that yeast overgrowth leads to deficiencies of biotin, folate, iron, selenium, vitamin A, and omega-3 and omega-6 fatty acids. But before self-treating with multiple supplements, obtain blood tests that measure your levels of vitamins and minerals.

Chemical Sensitivities

People with the yeast syndrome often complain about reactions to *inhalants* (such as tobacco smoke, fragrances, perfumes, cleaning solutions, new carpet smell, formaldehyde, organic solvents, glue vapors, automobile exhaust, smog, pesticides, insect repellent, sunscreen, etc.), as well as *food additives* (such as monosodium glutamate, hydrolyzed casein or soy protein, yeast extract, flavorings, colorings, preservatives, etc.). They have to assiduously avoid these chemicals to prevent symptoms.

Allergic Id Reactions

Many symptoms of the yeast syndrome are due to allergic Id (*idiopathic*) reactions to yeasts. *Allergy* is caused by reactions between IgE antibodies and food, airborne, contact, and microbial antigens. Id reactions are allergic reactions occurring at one location in the body to a yeast infection at a distant site (Chapter 1).

Candida asthma is the best-known example of an Id reaction in candidiasis patients. It is an allergic reaction in the lungs to a yeast infection in the intestine (Keeney, 1951; Pepys et al., 1968; Robinett, 1968; Edge and Pepys, 1980; Gumowski et al., 1987; Kroker, 1987, p. 854; Hosen, 1988; Koivikko et al., 1988; Tanizaki et al., 1992; Akiyama, 2000; Palma-Carlos et al., 2002; Simon-Nobbe et al., 2008; Khosravi et al., 2009).

Drugs such as antibiotics, antacids, and/or corticosteroids predispose people to develop intestinal yeast infections, which cause increased gut permeability. Candida antigens leak into the bloodstream and induce WBCs to synthesize antibodies in all immunoglobulin classes (IgG, IgM, IgA, and IgE). Allergic IgE anti-Candida antibodies travel the lungs, where they attach to mast cells, and then combine with Candida antigens circulating in the bloodstream. The immune complexes formed trigger mast cells to release histamine and other mediators of inflammation that produce edema in the bronchioles. Tissue swelling closes off air spaces making it difficult to draw air into the deeper portions of the lungs. Wheezing occurs when airways are partially closed.

People with bronchial asthma have impaired T cell reactivity, which leads to an increased production of allergic IgE antibodies to Candida. Noverr et al. (2004) published evidence from animal studies showing that both antibiotics and fungal colonization promote the development of allergic airway disease. Goldman and Huffnagle (2009) proved evidence that gastrointestinal fungi promote allergic inflammation and asthma. Thus, events in distal mucosal sites such as the GI tract can regulate immune responses in the lungs.

Other examples of allergic Id reactions to Candida overgrowth in the intestine are urticaria (James and Warin, 1971), psoriasis (Ereaux and Craig, 1949; Crutcher et al., 1984; Rosenberg, Noah, Skinner, 1994), atopic dermatitis (Savolainen et al., 1993), conjunctivitis (Santelmann et al., 2001), and food allergies and allergic rashes (Yamaguchi et al., 2006).

Thus, even though immune reactions help protect against microbial infections, they can also damage tissues. Antifungal treatment reduces the load of Candida antigen in the intestine, thereby reducing allergic Id reactions in target organs. Injection immunotherapy with Candida antigens reduces allergic inflammatory reactions and builds up immunity to Candida.

Candida Autoimmunity

Additional systemic symptoms associated with intestinal candidiasis are produced by autoimmune diseases, which are aberrant immune responses to Candida involving antibodies and T cells formed against Candida that cross-react with tissue cells in target organs. Auto-antibodies or auto-reactive T cells associated with intestinal candidiasis cause comorbid autoimmune diseases such as endocrine disorders, immunosuppression, anti-*Saccharomyces cerevisiae* antibodies, celiac disease, and interstitial cystitis as shown by the following research.

Endocrine Disorders

People with the yeast syndrome often have poorly functioning endocrine glands. Their thyroid, adrenals, ovaries, or testes may release lower amounts of hormone, so they have to take hormone replacement therapy. Hormonal disruptions can be caused by auto-antibodies or auto-reactive T cells that attack endocrine glands. The resulting *autoimmune endocrinopathies* are often associated with candidiasis in people with inborn immune defects (Cleary, 1985), but they also occur in immune competent individuals.

Women with recurrent vulvovaginal candidiasis were found to have high levels of anti-Candida antibodies that cross-reacted with ovarian follicle tissue and T lymphocytes (Mathur et al., 1980). Many of these women were unable to become pregnant, had lost their sex drive, and experienced early menopause in their 30s or 40s instead of in their 50s. These clinical conditions, due to low levels of female sex hormones, are caused by anti-Candida antibodies that cross-reacted with ovarian cells causing premature ovarian failure. Autoreactive anti-Candida antibodies also caused T cell-mediated immunosuppression in these women. All these autoimmune disorders are due to molecular mimicry between proteins on Candida cells and structurally similar proteins on ovarian and T cells.

High levels of anti-*Candida albicans* antibodies were found in human sera also containing antibodies against thyroid, ovary, and adrenal glands (Vojdani et al., 1996). Addition of *C. albicans* antigens to these sera removed some of the antithyroid antibodies indicating cross-reactivity. Similarly, cross-reactions between anti-Candida antibodies and food antigens were also detected. Thus, high levels of anti-Candida antibodies are related to autoimmunity, endocrinopathy, and adverse food reactions in the yeast syndrome.

Candida Immunosuppression

Candida has evolved multiple strategies for waging molecular war against immune cells. Studies have found that:

- Anti-Candida antibodies, Candida antigens, and WBCs isolated from people with candidiasis caused suppression when added to T cells isolated from healthy people.
- Anti-Candida antibodies cross-react with T helper cells.
- Candida cell wall mannanprotein allows yeast cells to persist in tissues, producing a negative delayed-type IV hypersensitivity reaction (*anergy*).
- Allergic reactions to Candida release histamine, which inhibits neutrophil chemotaxis and T cell proliferation necessary to fight infection.

These immune suppression mechanisms are specific for Candida, and do not affect immunity against other pathogens.

Anti-*Saccharomyces cerevisiae* Antibodies (ASCA)

People with Crohn's disease have high levels of ASCA in their blood (Darroch et al., 1999; Standaert-Vitse et al., 2006; Schaffer et al., 2007). Even though these antibodies react with *Saccharomyces cerevisiae*, the *immunogen* (antigen) that induces ASCA synthesis is Candida (Standaert-Vitse et al., 2006). Therefore, ASCA are actually anti-*Candida albicans* antibodies that cross-react with *Saccharomyces cerevisiae* because both Candida and Saccharomyces yeasts have similar mannanprotein antigens on their cell surfaces. When antibodies against one of these yeasts cross-react with the other yeast in the intestine, symptoms can be produced.

Corroborating these findings that ASCA are really antibodies formed against Candida, an increased prevalence of these fungi, Candida, Aspergillus, Gibberella, Alternaria, and Cryptococcus, has been found in the gut of people with Crohn's disease (Li et al., 2013), yet the prevalence of Saccharomyces was the same in healthy people as in Crohn's disease patients with inflamed intestinal mucosa.

If you have high levels of anti-Candida antibodies and/or ASCA in your blood, you may experience adverse reactions after you eat fermented foods and beverages containing baker's or brewer's yeast (*Saccharomyces cerevisiae*), as well as mushrooms, moldy cheeses, and other fungi. People with Crohn's disease identify yeasty foods, cereals, and dairy products as contributing to their symptomatic deterioration. An elimination diet that avoided these foods was found to be therapeutic in Crohn's disease (Barclay et al., 1992; Riordan et al., 1993).

Celiac Disease

Some people with the yeast syndrome also suffer from a disorder of the small intestine called *celiac disease*. It is an autoimmune disease occurring in about 1% of the population (Ciclitira, 2005). People who are genetically predisposed to celiac disease experience diarrhea and abdominal distention after eating wheat, barley, and rye, and sometimes oats. These grains contain a sticky molecule called *gluten.* Celiac disease is caused by the protein component of gluten called *gliadin.*

Autoantibodies and autoreactive T cells against gliadin cross-react with an intestinal enzyme (*tissue transglutaminase*) and with a layer of connective tissue (*endomysium*) in small bowel tissue. These autoimmune reactions lead to a shortening of tissue projections (*villi*) lining the small intestine that function to absorb nutrients. Hence, uncontrolled celiac disease interferes with nutrition.

The only cure for celiac disease is life-long avoidance of gluten-containing foods. If a person with celiac disease stays on a low gluten diet, autoantibodies against gliadin drop to low levels, and further damage to the intestine is prevented.

A surprising connection between celiac disease and Candida has recently been discovered. A protein on the *Candida albicans* hyphal wall contains amino acid sequences identical to amino acid sequences in gliadin. *C. albicans* hyphal wall protein induces auto-reactive T cell receptors and auto-antibodies as does gliadin. Cross-reactions between these anti-Candida autoimmune components damage the intestinal mucosa. Thus, Nieuwenhuizen et al. (2003) proposed that *C. albicans* triggers celiac disease via molecular mimicry. Similarly, Staab et al. (2004) postulated that *C. albicans* causes celiac disease because hyphal wall protein is a substrate for epithelial cell transglutaminase, which forms cross-links with endomysium proteins on the mammalian mucosa.

Interstitial Cystitis (IC)

Many women and some men diagnosed with IC experience pain in the urethra and bladder during and after urination, and an urge to urinate frequently. These symptoms are similar to symptoms of bladder infections (*bacterial cystitis*), but urine cultures are negative for bacteria and WBCs in IC. During cystoscopy, inflammation and ulceration within the bladder wall are seen. Lesions located within the spaces (*interstices*) of the bladder epithelium are pinpoint, round, red spots, called *petechiae*, and are due to small hemorrhages of submucosal capillaries.

Men and women with IC have usually received multiple treatments with antibiotics for urinary tract infections. In addition, women with IC frequently have vulvodynia, and a history of recurrent vulvovaginal candidiasis (Kahn et al., 2010).

Pain disorders such as vulvodynia, prostatodynia, and IC frequently arise after taking antibiotics. It is likely that the pain arises from inflammatory reactions to intestinal yeast overgrowth. Anti-Candida IgG antibodies produced in response to candidiasis react with Candida antigens forming immune complexes, which activate *complement*, a group of enzymes in blood. Mannan in the yeast cell wall also activates complement. These activated enzymes normally function by digesting cell membranes of microbial pathogens. But they might inadvertently digest holes in capillaries in the bladder wall causing minute hemorrhages. This inflammatory reaction, due to deposition of immune complexes in vascular walls, is called the *Arthus reaction* (or type III hypersensitivity).

In agreement with this idea about the role played by Candida in IC is the following report. Edwards et al. (1986) found that Candida cells have binding sites on their surface resembling complement receptors on human cells. They suggested that Candida autoimmunity, due to this molecular mimicry, might modify human inflammatory and immune responses.

To test this theory, Candida antigens, anti-Candida antibodies, and Candida immune complexes in blood should be measured in IC sufferers. Patients testing positive should be treated with Diflucan tablets plus oral nystatin powder to eradicate intestinal candidiasis (according to the protocol in Step 2). Women with IC who were treated with oral plus vaginal nystatin, diet, and allergy shots of Candida extract improved dramatically (Truss, 2009; p. 51).

APICH

People with autoimmune disorders associated with the yeast syndrome have a disease called *Autoimmune Polyendocrinopathy Immune Dysregulation Candidiasis Hypersensitivity*. The sequence of events leading to these associated diseases was summarized in Table 5.

Mention APICH to your doctor and request diagnostic tests and medical treatments for each illness. Only candidiasis responds to antifungal treatment. Other disorders associated with chronic candidiasis result from immune reactions to Candida and cross-reactions with your tissues, which are determined by your genetic background.

Genetic Predisposition

Aberrant host immune responses explain the failure to control yeast infections (MacNeill et al., 2003). Gene variations (*polymorphisms*) alter the mucosal immune response against candidiasis (Jaeger et al., 2013). Polymorphisms in the immune system are associated with recurrent vulvo-vaginal candidiasis (Smeekens et al., 2013). Genes affecting mannose-binding lectin and allergy in the white race were found to be associated with recurrent vulvovaginal candidiasis (Giraldo et al., 2007).

Genes control all bodily functions including activities of WBCs. Their ability to fight infection depends on cell surface protein receptors called *human leukocyte antigens* (HLAs). Genes coding for HLAs affect susceptibility to specific infections and autoimmune diseases (Ghodke et al., 2005; Blackwell et al., 2009). For example, immunity to Candida is controlled by HLA-D and HLA-DR (Nose et al., 1980; 1981). Variant HLA genes also make people susceptible to other disorders. Mayer et al. (1990) reported that antibodies to HLA cross-reacted with binding sites on *Candida albicans*. This example of molecular mimicry is further evidence for autoimmune diseases associated with intestinal candidiasis.

Think Yeast!

The polysymptomatic nature of chronic intestinal candidiasis presents a diagnostic dilemma to physicians. When faced with patients who have multiple symptoms and claim to be *"at the end of their rope,"* doctors are advised to *"Think yeast!"* (Zwerling et al., 1984). In other words, *rule out candidiasis first, not last!*

Even though a patient's symptomatic improvement on a sugar-free, yeast-free diet indicates the yeast syndrome, *diagnosis cannot be based on symptoms alone.* Specific tests must be performed (Steps 1 and 5). If results are positive for Candida infection and/or Candida allergy, then the treatments in Steps 2 through 5 are medically justified, and should be paid for by your health insurance. Recurrences can be prevented by following Steps 5 through 10.

Future Research on the Yeast Syndrome

The published controlled studies cited in this book have raised a number of intriguing questions about chronic candidiasis that can only be answered by further research. Unfortunately, researchers have been dissuaded from applying for grants to study the yeast syndrome by the controversy created by negative statements made by academic skeptics (Chapter 6). Because this topic is now anathema among establishment physicians, studying the yeast syndrome would be the kiss of death for any young scientist or physician wanting to advance her or his career.

Conclusions of Chapter 5
Intestinal Yeast Infections and the Hall of Fame

Once community-based physicians realize that the yeast syndrome is a real disease, the learning curve begins. Physicians who read this book will learn how to help their patients suffering from Candida infection, Candida allergy, and Candida-associated diseases.

Hopefully, clinicians who are dedicated to the welfare of their patients will ignore threats to their medical licenses and professional reputations made by academic skeptics and state medical boards, and will provide appropriate medical care to patients suffering from candidiasis based on what they have read in this book.

The wealth of controlled clinical studies presented in this book provides the evidence that physicians need to justify ordering diagnostic tests for intestinal candidiasis and associated allergies (Steps 1 and 5). Positive test results for Candida infection and/or Candida allergy justify treating patients with proven medical protocols recommended in Steps 2 and 5.

CHAPTER 6

The Candida Controversy and the Hall of Shame

Why Do Doctors Deny Patients Medical Care for Yeast Infections?

This chapter identifies academic skeptics who deny the existence of the yeast syndrome and are responsible for influencing community physicians to refuse patients medical care for this disease.

Academic experts in the field of disseminated candidiasis (such as Edwards, 1988a, and others named in the Hall of Shame below) have proclaimed that "*The candidiasis hypersensitivity syndrome is quackery!*" Most of these academic skeptics work in hospitals treating seriously ill people who have deep-seated, invasive candidiasis and low WBC counts (*neutropenia*). Hospital-based physicians don't have experience treating otherwise healthy people in the community who have intestinal yeast overgrowths with normal WBC counts.

But their inexperience did not stop these hospital-based physicians from publishing uninformed statements denying the existence of a syndrome caused by intestinal candidiasis that produces symptoms in the gut as well as throughout the body. Negative opinion papers published by academic physicians **lacked data**! Yet, they influenced doctors who practice in the community to deny patients much needed testing and treatment for the yeast syndrome.

Now that you have read the earlier chapters, you are aware of the voluminous evidence for the yeast syndrome. These studies should remove any doubt about the existence of chronic intestinal candidiasis and related allergies. But most physicians have not read the controlled clinical studies cited in this book. So, the controversy continues…

Origin of the Controversy

How did this field become so contentious? The Candida controversy was started by two revolutionary books published in 1983 and written independently by two astute physicians, Truss and

Crook (listed in the Hall of Fame in Chapter 5). When Candida sufferers read these two books about the yeast syndrome, they recognized themselves as if they were looking into a mirror. Soon millions of people were flocking into their doctors' offices, with these books in hand, demanding treatment for yeast-connected symptoms.

This onslaught triggered a backlash from establishment medicine. Instead of investigating this new paradigm, university physicians ridiculed the two community physicians who discovered the yeast syndrome. Academics spread their skeptical views far and wide, publicly in print and at conferences, and privately among their colleagues. Their negative position papers influenced community physicians to deny patients testing and treatment for intestinal candidiasis out of fear of reprisals. Being refused treatment by their personal physicians condemned Candida sufferers to needless suffering and disability.

Why did establishment medicine deny the existence of the yeast syndrome when it was reported in two 1983 books and earlier papers? Trowbridge and Walker (1986) suggested several reasons for academic skepticism. Here are my ideas about why academics were skeptical about the yeast connection to chronic disease:

- Crook's Candida questionnaire contained nonspecific symptoms, and was not supported by diagnostic test results.
- Books by Truss and Crook were based on anecdotal and clinical observations, not controlled clinical trials.
- Their books contained errors such as claiming Candida produces toxins without proof and misusing the term "systemic" to describe intestinal candidiasis.

I imagine that when university-based physicians and researchers read the unsupported claims and misuse of terminology in these two 1983 books by Truss and Crook, they were aghast. So, the academics ignored the clinically important observations about intestinal candidiasis made by Truss and Crook. Instead of being open-minded and giving credence to observations made by community physicians, the academic skeptics published opinion statements denying the existence of the yeast syndrome. Then they pulled up the drawbridges, and retreated inside their ivory towers.

What the academic skeptics did not consider is that Truss and Crook were practicing community-based physicians—not university researchers—who discovered a new disease and treatments that helped cure patients. Such anecdotal evidence always comes first before controlled scientific studies can be carried out. Instead of taking the ball and running with it, i.e., instead of designing clinical studies, academics physicians ignored this new syndrome and "threw the baby out with the bath water."

Community-based physicians, who treated yeast syndrome patients with antifungals, observed dramatic improvements in symptoms. Positive responses to antifungal therapy reported in studies (listed in the Hall of Fame in Chapter 5) have converted many physicians to the belief that the yeast syndrome is a real disease. It is time now for academic skeptics to publish retractions of their negative opinion papers (cited below in chronological order).

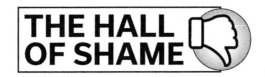

This Hall of Shame identifies the academic skeptics who quashed new ideas about a polysymptomatic illness caused by intestinal yeast overgrowth. These establishment medicine doctors are responsible for persuading community physicians to deny millions of patients tests and treatments needed for chronic intestinal candidiasis.

A few years after Truss and Crook published their ground-breaking books in 1983, an avalanche of negative position statements appeared in peer reviewed journals. Articles lacking data, but denying the existence of the candidiasis hypersensitivity syndrome were written by representatives of the following medical societies:

- American Academy of Allergy and Immunology (AAAI, 1986)
- American Medical Association (AMA, 1987)
- Infectious Diseases Society of America (IDSA; Edwards, 1988a).

Also, in 1988, Edwards presented a keynote lecture entitled "The Yeast Connection" at the annual symposium of the IDSA, and he was interviewed on a Lifetime Medical Television program called *Physicians Journal Update*. The PJU announcer introduced the program by proclaiming that "*The candidiasis hypersensitivity syndrome is quackery!*" Since Edwards was the only expert interviewed on the program, he was obviously the source of this negative statement.

Odds (1988; pp. 136, 231-2) and Renfro et al. (1989) jumped on the bandwagon and issued negative opinion statements denying the existence of the yeast syndrome. All of these negative papers were unsupported by data and ignored decades of published scientific studies about Candida infections and Candida allergy.

Even though these negative statements were uninformed opinion papers, they were very influential and set the standard of care because they were written by leaders in the field of disseminated candidiasis, which occurs only in seriously ill, immunocompromised patients. These experts on disseminated candidiasis had no experience treating chronic intestinal candidiasis in otherwise healthy patients. Yet, they sent a clear message to community-based physicians that the medical establishment was against the concept of a syndrome caused by chronic intestinal yeast overgrowth and yeast-related allergies.

After these early negative opinion papers were published, much more evidence supporting the existence of the candidiasis hypersensitivity syndrome was published. But, as yet, no negative position statement has been retracted.

The good news is that the original 1986 position statement by AAAI has been removed from their website. This group, renamed the American Academy of Allergy, Asthma, and Immunology, recently posted the following disclaimer on their website: "*AAAAI Position Statements ... are not to be considered to reflect current AAAAI standards or policy after five years from the date of publication.*" So, based on this latest statement, allergists can now resume skin testing for

Candida allergy and Candida immunity, and providing injection immunotherapy with Candida antigen as they did before the Candida controversy started.

The Infamous Dismukes Study

In 1990, Dismukes and coinvestigators published a badly designed clinical study claiming the candidiasis hypersensitivity syndrome doesn't exist even though the subjects of this study were neither tested for Candida allergy, nor treated with Candida allergy shots!

Truss diagnosed participants for this study as having candidiasis based solely on symptoms without testing. Truss also funded the study. Truss asked an academic researcher to design and perform the study with the hope that an establishment medicine physician would validate this diagnosis.

Instead, Dismukes et al. took Truss's grant money, and designed an unscientific cross-over study! Subjects were first treated with either nystatin or placebo, and then these treatments were reversed. *Nota bene:* Cross-over studies should never be used when a drug changes the subjects' condition because that approach invalidates the second round of treatment with either the drug or the placebo.

Dismukes et al. (1990) published an erroneous abstract that egregiously did not reflect their positive results. Even though nystatin was found superior to placebo, and produced statistically significant improvements in three vaginal symptoms, and four systemic symptoms, their paper ignored their positive results and concluded that the candidiasis hypersensitivity syndrome *"is not a verifiable condition."*

Despite these obvious errors and prejudicial conclusions, this poorly designed and analyzed study was accepted for publication by the prestigious *New England Journal of Medicine*. The paper by Dismukes et al. (1990) was only a pilot study, yet it was hailed as the last word on the subject and used as justification for denying people tests and treatments for Candida infection and Candida allergy. In my opinion, Dismukes and coworkers betrayed Truss.

Many criticisms of this cross-over design were published in letters-to-the-editor of the NEJM (Bennett, 1990; Crook, 1991; Truss et al., 1991; Ledger and Witkin, 1991; Crandall, 1991b; Truss et al., 1992; Santelmann et al., 2001). These physicians and scientists working in the field pointed out the errors in the Dismukes paper and deserve to be read.

My letter, Crandall (1991b), challenged the negative conclusion in Dismukes et al. (1990) because it was *"not substantiated by the results of their clinical study, which shows a strikingly positive effect of the all-nystatin regimen."*

In 1991, Dismukes and Lee replied to the letters-to-the-editor of the NEJM, saying their statistical analysis took into consideration each criticism and, furthermore, the analysis of their results was approved by their own institution and the biostatistical reviewer at the NEJM. The falsehoods in their reply and original paper were shameful.

In 1992, Truss and coworkers reanalyzed the original data from the Dismukes study using more powerful statistical methods and found additional significant improvements in systemic symptoms overlooked by Dismukes and coinvestigators. Truss's 1984 and 1992 papers are in the appendix of his 2009 book, *The Missing Diagnosis II.*

More Shameful Attacks by Academic Skeptics

In 1993, Bodey and Sobel claimed that the candidiasis hypersensitivity syndrome does not exist.

In 1996, Seebacher gave the yeast syndrome a new name: *"Mycophobia!"*

In 2002, Lacour et al. reviewed the literature published after 1990 and concluded that *"neither epidemiological nor therapeutic studies provide evidence for the existence of the so-called ... 'Candida-hypersensitivity-syndrome'."*

In 2004, I challenged the negative conclusions by Lacour and coauthors in a letter-to-the-editor. I wrote they had *"missed many papers on the candidiasis hypersensitivity syndrome (CHS) because of the narrow criteria used for their literature search. Specifically, they missed papers on CHS published before 1990 or not indexed in Medline"* (Crandall, 2004).

In 2005, Barrett, the publisher of Quackwatch.com, wrote this ignominious statement, *"I believe that practitioners who diagnose nonexistent 'yeast problems' should have their licenses revoked."*

Now do you understand why your doctor won't treat you? But wait, there's more!

In 2007, the Mycoses Study Group posted an uninformed article, *Chronic Candidiasis*, on their website, *Doctor Fungus.*

In 2009, Schulze and Sonnenborn stated that *"Controversy still surrounds the question whether yeasts found in the gut are causally related to disease."*

In 2009, Pappas et al. published the IDSA guidelines for treating candidiasis. They stated that *"... the gut as a source for disseminated candidiasis is evident from autopsy studies."* In other words, yeasts infecting the gut can escape into the bloodstream, spread to the deep organs, and cause fatal infections in seriously ill patients. Even though the Pappas et al. guidelines acknowledged that yeasts infect the gut, the bad news is they did not specifically discuss treatment of intestinal candidiasis. The good news is this state-of-the-art review of antifungal therapy for mucosal candidiasis can be followed by community physicians for treating intestinal yeast overgrowth.

In 2013, a book on fungal disease by Homei and Worboys reiterated the negative opinions of other academic skeptics, ignoring all of the scientific and clinical evidence for the yeast connection to chronic disease.

This Hall of Shame shows that, more than three decades after Truss's 1978 original journal article about localized and systemic manifestations of intestinal infection by *Candida albicans*, academics are still ignorant of the facts published in dozens of articles corroborating Truss's original findings, and the many controlled clinical studies that followed later, validating a screening questionnaire for Candida plus diagnostic blood tests for Candida antibodies and Candida immune complexes (cited in the Hall of Fame in Chapter 5).

Consequences of the Controversy

The attack on the yeast syndrome by establishment medicine has had adverse effects on doctors as well as patients.

Prosecution of Physicians and Laboratories

As a result of the controversy in this field, physicians are afraid of losing their medical licenses if they test and treat people for Candida. As evidence of this prosecution, in 1991, I presented expert witness testimony at a hearing for a physician who was being prosecuted by the New York State Medical Board because he tested patients for candidiasis. After a long legal battle, his medical license was saved.

Another physician who treated Candida patients retired rather than fight the medical board of another state.

A laboratory that offered diagnostic tests for Candida in Beverly Hills, California, was shut down.

Other labs that performed blood tests for Candida in New York and California had to move to states where this testing was permitted. Prosecution of medical professionals and laboratory owners has created havoc for patients seeking medical care for yeast-related illnesses.

The Candida Run Around

When their personal physicians won't consider intestinal candidiasis as a diagnosis, patients embark on a relentless search for relief from their distressing symptoms. They wander from doctor-to-doctor desperately seeking a cure. Along this odyssey, Candida sufferers are humiliated by establishment physicians who greet their complaints with disbelief and disrespect. At best, people receive only fragmented care because each specialist looks at only one part of their anatomy, and then refers them to another specialist. They go to the next doctor hopeful that maybe this time … you get the drill!

Doctor-shopping not only causes physical and mental stress, it also takes a financial toll on Candida sufferers. Medical costs for professionals outside the patient's health insurance network are exorbitant and usually not reimbursed. People suffering from Candida are further victimized by some alternative practitioners who offer unscientific procedures, and ineffective supplements. Furthermore, advice about Candida posted to online forums is usually unsupported by research studies. This run-around leaves Candida sufferers with no place to turn for help.

The Cover-Up

Why do physicians deny the existence of the yeast syndrome?

The simplest answer is because they cause it! Candidiasis is, in most cases, an *iatrogenic disease*, i.e., it is caused by physicians' treatments. While the following medications are miracle drugs, they cause yeast infections in susceptible people:

- antibiotics for bacterial infections

- antacids for peptic ulcers and reflux disease
- corticosteroids for inflammation, allergy, and autoimmunity
- estrogen for oral contraception, fertility stimulation, and hormone replacement therapy for menopause
- sodium-glucose cotransporter-2 (SGLT-2) inhibitors for type 2 diabetes including Invokana (canagliflozin), Farxiga (dapagliflozin), and Jardiance (empagliflozin)

Physicians must first acknowledge this inadvertent iatrogenesis before they can develop effective protocols for preventing candidiasis. Whenever they prescribe a medication that predisposes to candidiasis, physicians should ask patients if they have a history of yeast infections. If so, then doctors should also prescribe antifungal prophylaxis to protect susceptible people. In addition, physicians should provide anti-Candida immunotherapy to people who are allergic to Candida. Allergy shots of Candida extract decrease allergic reactions, increase immunity to Candida, and help prevent recurrences of candidiasis (Crandall, 1991a).

Unfortunately, most physicians do not offer preventive treatments for Candida infection and Candida allergy. Some doctors will not even test people for chronic intestinal candidiasis and/or Candida allergy—let alone treat them! Some doctors order a battery of standard tests, but no Candida-specific tests. When results come back normal, doctors say *"There's nothing wrong with you."* Thus, in addition to battling yeast infections, Candida sufferers have to battle misguided and unsympathetic physicians.

What to Do If Your Doctor Won't Listen

Many patients have told me that their doctor did not believe in the yeast syndrome and refused to test or treat them for Candida. So, they ask me for a referral to a doctor who is knowledgeable about yeast infections. I explain that I don't know physicians in every city, of every state, of every country in the world! Instead, I urge patients to stay with their primary care physician who knows their medical history, current symptoms, and risk factors for candidiasis. I explain that any doctor can follow the guidelines in my ten-step program for diagnosing, treating, and preventing yeast infections.

If your doctor refuses to consider yeast as a possible diagnosis, call customer service at your health insurance company, and ask for a referral to a physician who treats Candida infections and Candida allergy. You might also consider filing a complaint against the doctor who denied you testing and treatment.

If you cannot obtain a physician referral through your health insurance, you will have to go outside your network, and pay out-of-pocket for diagnostic testing. You can find names of providers who will order Candida tests on the websites of diagnostic laboratories listed in Table 7. Before making appointments with any doctors outside your health insurance network, ask if they offer the tests for Candida infection and Candida allergy recommended in Steps 1 and 5. Read my warning about physician referral services on my website, www.yeastconsulting.com, and follow my suggested plan of action.

If your Candida test results are positive, they provide the justification your physician needs to prescribe treatments. Take your test results back to your personal physician and ask her or him to design a treatment plan tailor-made for your specific yeast problems. Your medical care will be covered by your health insurance if prescribed by your doctor.

Keep going back to your doctor for follow-up visits to monitor your liver function and discuss your response to antifungal therapy. If you respond to antifungal therapy, but then relapse, ask your doctor for a written referral to an allergist to obtain an intradermal test that measures Candida allergy and Candida immunity. If you are positive for Candida allergy, obtain subcutaneous allergy shots of Candida extract as explained in Step 5. I sincerely hope that your physician is willing to listen to your symptoms and is open-minded about the scientific information provided in this book.

History of Science

Rejection of a new idea that contradicts the establishment paradigm is a type of cognitive bias in psychology called the "Semmelweis reflex." Dr. Ignaz Philipp Semmelweis was a Hungarian physician who, in 1847, proposed that infections are transmitted from person to person by contaminated hands. He suggested that childbed fever was caused by physicians who had performed autopsies on putrefying bodies and then did not wash their hands before performing vaginal exams on women in labor to see if their cervix was dilated. Based on supporting data collected from two birthing hospitals—one staffed by physicians where there were many deaths and one staffed only by nurses where there were less deaths—Semmelweis recommended that doctors wash their hands in disinfectant before touching patients.

Other physicians did not accept his idea. Instead, they ostracized Semmelweis whose career and health were ruined as a consequence. He died in a mental institution where he contracted the same infection from which he saved thousands of mothers. An ironic end for a brilliant physician! Fortunately, hand washing is now standard practice in medicine.

There are many other examples from the past where the entrenched scientific or medical establishment ridiculed the creators of new ideas. Years from now, what will scholars studying the history of science write about the Candida controversy? How will they answer questions such as: How could academic physicians and researchers with such extensive training and experience lack an understanding of Candida-related disorders? Why did academic physicians deny the existence of intestinal yeast overgrowth caused by antibiotic therapy and other medical treatments? How could this controversy continue for so many decades? How many millions of Candida sufferers have been harmed by the negative statements published by academic skeptics?

Conclusions of Chapter 6
The Candida Controversy and the Hall of Shame

The existence of a syndrome caused by yeast overgrowth of the mouth, intestine, and vagina should have been predicted *a priori* by the medical profession based on decades of published scientific information about the causes and cures of Candida infection and Candida allergy.

Now that the existence of the yeast syndrome has been verified by controlled clinical studies of screening questionnaires, diagnostic tests, antifungal therapy, and immunotherapy, the time has come for physicians to incorporate these findings into standard-of-care medical practice.

As time goes by, more and more doctors will recognize the yeast syndrome and its negative impact on people's lives. Doctors who are open-minded about the new Candida paradigm will learn how to prescribe long-term antifungals, anti-inflammatory drugs, and Candida immunotherapy, and improve the health of their patients.

Progress in this field would be facilitated if doctors in private practice would publish summaries of their clinical findings from Candida patients' questionnaire scores, test results, and responses to treatments. These valuable findings would stimulate more controlled clinical studies in the future by researchers based in academic institutions cooperating with physicians based in community practices where yeast syndrome patients are seen.

Advances in medicine usually proceed from initial anecdotal observations made on individual patients, to the publication of medical summaries of multiple patients, to placebo-controlled clinical studies of large numbers of patients. Even though this process has already happened, establishment medicine appears to be ignorant of the publications, or has chosen to dismiss the evidence for a yeast connection to chronic illness. I urge all Candida patients to show this book to your personal physicians and ask for the medical care you need to regain your former good health.

PART II

A Ten-Step Program of Medical Care and Self-Help for Candida Infections and Candida Allergy

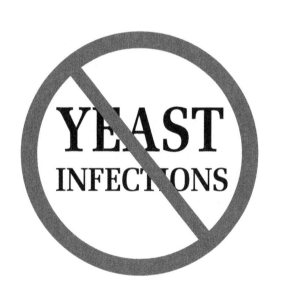

OVERVIEW

THIS TEN-STEP HEALING PROGRAM IS designed for superficial yeast infections of skin and mucous membranes in people with normal WBC counts. Guidelines are evidence-based and patient-oriented. Recommendations for diagnosing, treating, and preventing yeast infections and yeast allergies are drawn from scientifically validated tests and controlled clinical studies. Treating with both topical and systemic antifungals concurrently is recommended for hard-to-cure cases. Each protocol must be tailor-made for the individual patient. Please be assured that you can overcome yeast-related problems with proper medical care and self-help. After reading the details of this program, you will be empowered to ask your doctor for the appropriate tests and treatments. *You can conquer Candida!*

Step 1. Diagnostic Tests for Yeast Infections

Symptoms are what you feel. *Signs* are what the doctor sees. *You cannot diagnose yeast infections based on symptoms alone.* Other conditions can produce the same symptoms. Therefore, to obtain an accurate diagnosis of yeast overgrowths and yeast allergies, you need valid diagnostic testing that only a doctor can order. A preliminary clinical diagnosis can be made based on the facts of your case. These include your current signs and symptoms, history of yeast infections, recent predisposing risk factors, positive responses to antifungal therapy in the past, current medications and supplements, and for women: what birth control method you are using, and what time of the month your symptoms are the worst.

Diagnostic tests identify the cause (*etiology*) of your symptoms. Specimens collected for culture and microscopy include: swabs of oral, vaginal, and rectal mucosae; scrapings of skin, tongue, and vulva; and feces collected at stool. Yeasts isolated from cultures should be subcultured to identify the yeast species and determine its antifungal susceptibility. If your yeast is antifungal resistant, it will grow in culture even if you are being treated with an antifungal. Vulvodynia caused by Candida vulvitis is diagnosed by cultures of vulvar scrapings, and acetowhite lesions seen in colposcopy (Chapter 2).

Blood is tested for Candida antibodies, antigens, immune complexes, and DNA. Urine is tested for yeast metabolites. High levels of Candida antibodies in blood indicate a current or past yeast overgrowth of the intestine. Detection of Candida antigens and/or Candida immune complexes in blood is a *definitive* indication of a current, active Candida infection of the intestine.

Don't self-treat with natural antifungal supplements or prescription antifungal drugs before collecting specimens for yeast culture, or your test results might come back falsely negative. *Test before treating!*

Step 2. Antifungal Treatments

If your diagnostic tests are positive for Candida infection, ask your doctor for antiyeast treatments. *Antifungals are administered daily until symptoms resolve.* First-time yeast infections of the mouth, vagina, or skin should be treated for at least a week, preferably two weeks. One or three-day treatments are inadequate. A positive response to antiyeast medication confirms the diagnosis.

Recurrent or chronic yeast infections are treated more intensively with both topical and systemic antifungals concurrently. Topical antifungals treat the intracellular yeast infection from the tissue surface inward, and systemic antifungals treat the latent yeast infection from inside the tissues outward. Since every patient is different, it is impossible to predict how long your yeast condition should be treated. Enough antifungal medication should be prescribed for daily treatment until symptoms resolve, and then treatment is switched to weekly maintenance for up to six months to prevent a recurrence.

Long-term treatment for one to two months is often necessary because older, commonly prescribed antifungals are *fungistatic* and just inhibit growth, but don't kill the yeasts. If yeasts isolated from cultures are proven resistant by laboratory testing, you can be treated with higher doses of azole antifungals, or with two older systemic antiyeast medications that act synergistically and kill yeasts, or with one of the newer, more expensive, systemic antifungal agents that are *fungicidal.*

Inflammation of skin, vulva, penis, scrotum, and anus is treated with a cream containing both an antifungal and a steroid. *Always use an antifungal together with a steroid because if steroids are used alone, they predispose to candidiasis.* Intestinal candidiasis is treated simultaneously with oral nystatin powder that attacks yeasts in the intestinal contents, plus Diflucan (fluconazole) that attacks yeasts in the gut wall.

You might experience a worsening of symptoms when you take your first dose of an antifungal. This is due to immune reactions to products released by killed yeasts, and is called the Jarisch-Herxheimer reaction. Colloquially, this reaction is referred to as "yeast die-off" or a healing crisis. The good news is that "yeast die-off" means the antifungal is working. The bad news is you will have to lower the antifungal dosage, and then gradually increase the amount according to your tolerance until you reach the prescribed daily dose. Other topics discussed in Step 2 include the pros and cons of natural antifungals.

Step 3. Precautions

Systemic antifungals may cause elevations in liver enzymes or interact with other drugs or supplements. Therefore, you should obtain a liver function test before starting daily therapy, and every two weeks while on systemic antifungal therapy. Because systemic antifungals compete for degradative liver enzymes, other drugs may not be broken down and might build up to toxic levels in your blood. Therefore, you should go back for follow-up office visits so your physician can monitor your clinical improvement, liver function, and drug levels of your other medications.

To learn if Diflucan (fluconazole) interacts with the drugs you are taking, go to the websites listed under Safety Tips in Step 3 and fill in the names of your medications. If one or more of your regular medications does interact with fluconazole, one approach is to halve the dosage of drugs you take every day to prevent them from accumulating to high levels.

Don't self-treat with antifungal drugs bought on the internet, and don't take supplements together with prescription drugs unless approved by your physician. Avoid alcohol, grapefruit, and supplements that interfere with liver enzymes while taking systemic antifungals. If you plan on having an alcoholic drink in the evening, don't take your Diflucan (fluconazole) tablet that morning.

Step 4. Anti-inflammatory Drugs

Itching, burning, redness, swelling, and pain caused by yeast infections and yeast allergies are due to inflammation caused by WBCs and antibodies. These symptoms are treated with anti-inflammatory corticosteroid creams applied to skin, vulva, penis, scrotum, and anus.

If tissues are badly inflamed, first apply an anesthetic ointment such as lidocaine to numb the area before applying steroid cream. Since steroids suppress WBC-mediated immunity needed to fight infection, *always treat with an antifungal at the same time as an anti-inflammatory steroid to prevent your yeast infection from becoming worse.*

Creams such as Mycolog and Lotrisone are ideal because they contain both a steroid and an antifungal. Allergic inflammation can be treated with oral antihistamines plus allergy shots.

Step 5. Candida Allergy

Allergic reactions release histamine, which inhibits neutrophil chemotaxis and T cell proliferation. Because these two WBC activities are required for Candida immunity, *Candida allergy makes you more susceptible to Candida infections.* If Candida allergy is not treated, this sets you up for a self-perpetuating cycle of cure and relapse.

If you have repeated yeast infections or experience bad "yeast die-off" during antifungal treatment, you are most likely allergic to Candida. Hence, you should obtain skin testing for allergy to Candida and other substances. In addition to scratch (prick) tests on your back, also obtain the Candida intradermal test on your forearm.

If results from the intradermal show you are allergic to Candida (wheal and flare after 15 minutes) and/or you have poor immunity to Candida (no induration after 2 days), obtain allergy shots (subcutaneous injection immunotherapy) with Candida plus your other allergens. Immunotherapy reduces allergic reactions, boosts immunity to Candida, and helps prevent relapses of candidiasis.

Step 6. Avoid *All* Risk Factors

If you have had yeast infections in the past, you are susceptible to candidiasis—by definition. The key to preventing yeast infections in the future is avoiding *all* risk factors that predispose you to develop candidiasis. *Don't wait until you develop another yeast infection. Nip it in the bud!*

Yeast infections can be caused by medical, hospital, physiological, disease, and transmission risk factors. If you avoid all risk factors except one, then that one will eventually trigger another yeast infection. If a risk factor is unavoidable, then you must follow a maintenance protocol of antifungal prophylaxis to prevent recurrences (Step 10).

Step 7. Lifestyle Changes

Specific behavioral activities, sexual practices, and birth control methods can be risk factors for genital yeast infections. Avoid these lifestyle risk factors by following the safety tips provided.

Step 8. Candida Diet

Yeast infections cannot be cured by diet alone. To overcome yeast infections, you need diagnostic testing and medical treatments that only a physician can provide. While some yeast-related symptoms can be decreased by not eating sugary and yeasty foods, eliminating all carbohydrates is unhealthy. Such a diet is high in proteins and fat, and low in fiber, and may cause constipation, unwanted weight loss, kidney problems, and contribute to stroke and heart attacks. A balanced diet includes a variety of whole grains, fruits, vegetables, proteins, and unsaturated fats. Dietary advice for yeast infections can be summarized in one sentence: *If you eat or drink something that makes you sick, don't eat it again! If everything you eat makes you sick, you need medical attention.* Myths about Candida and diet are dispelled, and scientific facts are presented.

Step 9. Probiotics and Prebiotics

Probiotics are supplements containing "friendly" bacteria that help restore normal intestinal flora killed by antibiotics. The ideal probiotic contains species of Lactobacillus and Bifidobacterium. These bacteria produce lactic, acetic, propionic, and butyric acids needed for a healthy intestinal environment. They also produce cyclic dipeptides that are natural antifungals, which inhibit yeast growth. Meta-analysis of studies show that oral probiotics treat and prevent an amazing multitude of diseases. But inserting probiotics intravaginally is advised against because it can cause Lactobacillus vaginosis.

Prebiotic supplements contain fructooligosaccharides that promote the growth of Bifidobacterium. Instead of buying expensive prebiotics, it is better to eat fruits and vegetables that contain fructooligosaccharides, as well as vitamins, minerals, and fiber.

Step 10. Antifungal Prophylaxis

To prevent yeast infections, you must identify your susceptibility factors and assiduously avoid *all* of them. If you have a predisposing condition is unavoidable, then you must obtain preventive antiyeast treatment. For example, when you are being treated for a difficult-to-cure bacterial infection such as Lyme Disease or peptic ulcers, use a vaginal antifungal preparation plus oral nystatin powder while taking an antibacterial antibiotic. After completing antibacterial therapy, switch from taking topical oral and vaginal antifungal prophylaxis every day to taking a systemic antifungal on a weekly basis for maintenance or suppression. If you have monthly recurrences of yeast vaginitis caused by estrogen surges at ovulation, use an antifungal for three days at mid-cycle each month. Other predisposing conditions such as AIDS may require weekly antifungal suppression.

How to Benefit from this Ten-Step Program

When you are at your doctor's office, explain your current signs and symptoms, your history of yeast infections, your recent predisposing risk factors, and your positive responses to antifungal therapy in the past. Fill out Tables 1, 3 and 4, and give copies to your primary care physician.

Ask for the diagnostic tests for Candida explained in Step 1 that are relevant to your condition. Also request a written referral to an allergist-immunologist to test you for Candida allergy and Candida immunity as explained in Step 5. Positive test results justify prescribing the treatments described in Steps 2 through 5. Recurrences can be prevented by following Steps 6 through 10 with a physician's assistance.

Don't skip any steps! To achieve a cure for your yeast infection, you must follow *all* ten steps. If you follow only a few, you may experience a recurrence. I learned this the hard way. I share my personal experiences with yeast infections in the Preface so you can avoid the pitfalls that trapped me in a self-perpetuating cycle of cure and relapse.

One size does not fit all! Since every patient is different, your medical treatments and lifestyle changes must be tailor-made for your particular yeast condition. A favorable response to treatment confirms your diagnosis.

Throughout this book, myths are dispelled, and facts are substituted. You must understand why certain dogmas are incorrect before you can devise a healing program that works for you. Please be assured that you can overcome yeast infections and regain your former good health if you follow *all* of the steps in this program that are relevant to your case.

This ten-step program is tried and true. It is a new paradigm for overcoming superficial yeast infections of the skin and mucous membranes in people with normal WBC counts. As more and more doctors achieve success curing their patients by following these evidence-based guidelines for Candida infection and Candida allergy, this scientific program will eventually become standard medical practice.

STEP 1

Diagnostic Tests for Yeast Infections

You don't have to *"Learn to live with it!"* Scientifically validated tests and treatments for yeast infections are available. Therefore, you must take charge of your health, and obtain an early diagnosis from a physician. Don't self-treat with antifungal supplements or medications before specimens are collected for testing. If you do try self-treating first with OTC products, and later obtain testing, your results might come back falsely low or negative. This will ruin your chances of receiving a correct diagnosis and necessary treatment. *Test before treating!*

Yeast infections cannot be accurately diagnosed based on symptoms alone! Infections caused by bacteria, viruses, and parasites can produce the same symptoms as yeast infections. Furthermore, other diseases can predispose you to develop candidiasis. Therefore, you need laboratory testing to diagnose Candida infection and identify your predisposing disorders.

Symptoms are what you feel. *Signs* are what the doctor sees. A preliminary clinical diagnosis can be based on your current signs and symptoms, physical examination, recent predisposing risk factors, history of yeast infections, and past responses to antifungal therapy.

But a diagnosis is only as good as the tests performed. Not all tests offered by practitioners are valid. Request the tests recommended here in Step 1. Just say "No!" to tests that seem unscientific. If a practitioner offers you a test that seems phony, it probably is. After results are obtained from scientifically validated tests plus your clinical evaluation, your doctor will be able to arrive at an accurate diagnosis.

Standard Diagnostic Tests for Superficial Candida Infections

Candidiasis of skin and mucous membranes is diagnosed by microscopy and culture (Centers for Disease Control, 2008). Additional diagnostic tests are performed for specific yeast conditions.

Specimens

Swabs of mucous membranes, skin scrapings, and stool specimens are the usual specimens sent to laboratories for microscopy, culture, yeast identification, and antifungal susceptibility testing. When moistened cotton swabs are rubbed on mucosal surfaces of the throat, buccal membrane, gums, vagina, and rectum, they pick up some yeasts from infected surfaces. But scrapings of skin, tongue, and vulvar surfaces done with a scalpel are necessary to pick up tissue cells that have yeasts inside them. Scrapings yield positive Candida cultures more often than swabs. Dermatologists routinely perform skin scrapings to collect specimens for microscopy and fungal culture. Gynecologists and family doctors should learn how to perform vulvar scraping in order to obtain positive yeast cultures from vulvodynia patients. This will allow more accurate diagnoses of Candida vulvitis to be made.

Microscopy

Swabs, scrapings, and stool specimens are smeared on glass slides, mixed in a drop of saline or potassium hydroxide, and a cover slip is placed on top of the drop. This is called a wet mount or a smear. In some cases, instead of adding a drop of liquid, the smear is dried, and a Gram stain is prepared. Slides are observed under a microscope at 400X (using a 10X ocular lens and a 40X objective lens) to look for budding yeast cells, true hyphae, pseudohyphae, bacteria, parasites, abnormal epithelial cells, RBCs, WBCs and, in the case of vaginal smears—sperm may be seen.

The advantages of microscopy are that it is fast and accurate. When microscopy is performed in the physician's office, results are obtained while you are still in the examining room. A preliminary diagnosis can be made allowing the doctor to write an antifungal prescription right away for prompt treatment. Yeasts can be detected by microscopy even if they are nonviable and do not grow in culture. The diagnosis of Candida in specimens can be improved by incorporating these sensitive and specific methods:

- Immunofluorescent stains consisting of fluorescent dyes attached to antibodies against specific microbes detect nongrowing or latent germs (Mårdh and Colleen, 1975).
- DNA gene sequencing and polymerase chain reaction technology detect nonculturable or occult microbes (Watson and Irwin, 2009).

The main disadvantage of direct microscopic observation of specimens is that it is not as sensitive as culture and can produce false negative results. Microscopy needs a concentration of at least 10^5 yeast cells/ml to be seen whereas cultures can detect as low as 10^3 yeast cells/ml. False-positive diagnoses can be made from microscopy by inexperienced personnel who confuse cotton fibers from swabs with hyphae, or confuse bubbles, nuclei from epithelial cells, sperm heads, or platelets with yeast cells. Hence, it is a good idea to obtain a second opinion in complicated cases from a supervisor.

Tissue scrapings collected with a scalpel yield positive results for microscopy and yeast cultures more often than do swabs of tissue surfaces because inactive yeasts reside inside tissue cells in chronic infections even if they are not actively growing on tissue surfaces.

Results from microscope smears are interpreted in the following ways:

- High numbers of yeast cells and hyphae indicate an infection by *Candida albicans*.
- High numbers of yeasts, but no hyphae indicate an infection by a non-*albicans* Candida species.
- Low numbers of yeasts and/or hyphae indicate normal flora, or hypersensitivity caused by Candida allergy.
- The presence of eosinophils in vaginal smears from women with recurrent vaginitis is correlated with the occurrence of IgE allergic antibodies to *Candida albicans* in vaginal fluid (Witkin et al., 1989).
- The presence of WBCs indicates a bacterial infection. *Pus* (dead WBCs) is not observed in yeast infections because histamine, released by inflammatory reactions to Candida, inhibits migration of WBCs into yeast-infected tissues.

Culture

Yeast cultures are considered the "gold standard" for diagnosing yeast infections (Centers for Disease Control, 2008). Reflex (secondary) tests should be ordered along with the initial order for yeast cultures in order to identify the yeast species and determine its antifungal susceptibility (Nyirjesy et al., 1995). These secondary test results will tell you the *best drug for your bug*.

Swabs, scrapings, and stool specimens are inoculated into yeast culture medium containing antibacterial agents. Growth is normally negative or slightly positive for yeasts from healthy people, but if cultures are heavily overgrown, then yeast infection is present.

Cultures can detect very low cell concentrations (10^3 yeast cells/ml), whereas higher cell concentrations (10^5 yeast cells/ml) are need for detection by microscopy. Even though yeast cultures are more sensitive, they can yield incorrect results.

False-positive cultures can be obtained from healthy people because Candida is a normal inhabitant of the body. Hence, a positive culture *by itself* is not diagnostic even though the Centers for Disease Control (2008) calls a positive culture the gold standard for diagnosis. The amount of growth should be quantified on a scale from 0 to 4+.

False-negative cultures can be obtained from people who have yeast infections if the following conditions occurred:

- If antibacterial agents were not added to the yeast culture medium. Bacteria in specimens inhibit yeast growth in laboratory culture just as bacteria inhibit yeast growth in the body. Antibiotics such as gentamicin plus chloramphenicol, or penicillin plus streptomycin, should be added to yeast culture medium (such as Sabouraud's dextrose agar) to kill bacteria and allow yeasts to grow (Guzel et al., 2011a; Cateau et al., 2012).
- If people were treated with antifungals before specimens were collected for testing. *Test before treating!*
- If people are allergic to Candida, then even low numbers of yeasts provoke inflammation.
- If yeasts in specimens are dead, but alive inside tissues (Caselli et al., 1988; Lee, 1995). In these cases, tissue scrapings collected with a scalpel yield positive yeast cultures more often than do swabs of tissue surfaces because live yeasts reside inside tissue cells.

Cultures from swabs may be falsely negative if yeasts are inside tissue cells, but not on the surface. Scrapings will be culture-positive if yeasts are inside epithelial cells (*chronic atrophic erythematous candidiasis*; Chapter 1).

Thus, even though yeast culture is considered the gold standard, erroneous results can lead to misdiagnoses.

Yeast Identification

Yeast cultures are usually not identified by general practitioners to save money. Besides, most infections are caused by *C. albicans*, and it is sensitive to most antifungals. If hyphal filaments plus yeast cells are seen in microscope smears, they identify *C. albicans* because no other Candida species produces true hyphae (germ tubes). Furthermore, yeast identification studies report that most recurrences are *endogenous relapses* caused by the person's own yeast strain (El-Din et al., 2001). Rarely are recurrences due to Candida strains contracted from outside (*exogenous*) sources.

However, it is important to identify the causative agent in difficult-to-cure cases because some *C. albicans* strains have become resistant to Diflucan (Dorrell and Edwards, 2002), and some Candida species (such as *C. glabrata, C. tropicalis,* and *C. krusei*) are naturally less sensitive to Diflucan (Fridkin, 2005; Gygax et al., 2008; Panizo et al., 2009).

The prevalence of vaginitis caused by non-*albicans* species increased from 9.9% in 1988 to 17.2% in 1995 (Spinillo et al., 1997). In 2011, Amouri et al. reported the incidence of *Candida glabrata* was 19.3% in uncomplicated vaginitis, and 34% in recurrent vaginitis. This increased incidence occurred because Diflucan (fluconazole) eliminates sensitive *C. albicans* strains, and selects for resistant species (Chaim, 1997).

Since Diflucan (fluconazole) is the drug-of-first-choice for yeast infections (Marchaim et al., 2012), emergence of resistance highlights the importance of identifying yeasts and determining their antifungal susceptibility—*before treating!* Treatment of Diflucan-resistant *C. albicans* and non-*albicans* Candida species requires treatment with higher doses of Diflucan (fluconazole) for longer times, or with other more effective antifungals (see protocols in Step 2).

Diagnosis and treatment are further complicated by the common occurrence of multiple yeast species in one specimen. Different yeast species can be identified by their colony color on culture media containing dyes such as Hardy ChromTM Candida agar, CHROMagar Candida, and chromID Candida agar (Hospenthal et al., 2006; Guzel et al., 2011a). Most mixed yeast infections of the vagina contain *C. albicans* plus *C. glabrata*.

Antifungal Susceptibility

If your yeast infection recurs frequently or does not improve on antifungal therapy, then your yeast strain should be cultured, identified, and tested for antifungal susceptibility (Shahid and Sobel, 2009). In vitro resistance correlates well with clinical resistance (Dorrell and Edwards, 2002). Testing for antifungal susceptibility will tell you the *best drug for your bug.*

Many people think their yeast is resistant if symptoms do not improve after short-term (one or three days) antifungal therapy. But when swab specimens are cultured, the results are usually negative because yeasts are inside the tissue, not on the surface. If cultures do grow, yeasts are usually found to be sensitive (MacNeill et al., 2003). In contrast, resistant yeasts will grow in culture even if you were taking antifungals when the specimen was collected.

Thus, you must distinguish between *yeasts that are resistant to antifungals, and infections that are resistant to cure*. If symptoms persist, most likely you were not treated long enough with high enough doses, you did not use both topical plus systemic antifungals concurrently, you did not use anti-inflammatory steroid cream, and you did not follow the other recommendations in this ten-step program.

Candida DNA

If microscopy and yeast cultures are negative, and clinical signs and symptoms persist after antifungal therapy, then ordering a polymerase chain reaction (PCR) test for Candida DNA is justified. PCR is the most sensitive test for Candida (Mardh et al., 2003; Weissenbacher et al., 2009; Baykushev et al., 2014), and it is useful for detecting nongrowing (latent) yeasts. Scrapings of skin and vulva are better than swab specimens for testing.

Scope Examinations

Candidiasis is diagnosed by performing internal exams with a light and camera on a tube. Scope exams for Candida infection include *endoscopy* of the upper GI tract; *colonoscopy* or *sigmoidoscopy* of the lower GI tract; and *colposcopy* of the vulva and vagina. White thrush patches or lesions seen on mucosal surfaces are dead tissue killed by an active yeast infection (*acute pseudomembranous candidiasis*; Chapter 1). Red patches seen on mucosal surfaces are due to inflammation caused by an intracellular yeast infection (*chronic atrophic erythematous candidiasis*; Chapter 1). Infected red or white patches are biopsied for microscopy, culture, yeast identification, and antifungal susceptibility testing. Biopsies are sectioned for histology, stained for fungi, and observed under the microscope.

Vulvar and Vaginal Tests

Microscopy and Culture of Vulvar Scrapings plus Observing Acetowhite Lesions during Colposcopy are useful tests for diagnosing vulvodynia caused by Candida vulvitis (Pagano, 2007; Chapter 2). Vulvar cutaneous candidosis and ringworm (a fungal infection of the skin called dermatophytosis) cannot be reliably distinguished by routine histopathology or specific PCR. The best approach to differentiating between these two infections, which impacts on counseling, treatment, and prognosis, is a high index of suspicion combined with adequate microbiological assessment (Day et al., 2016).

Measuring the pH of Vaginal Fluid is a fast and easy way to screen for various infections (Chapter 2). Measuring the pH of vaginal discharge with indicator paper is also a way to determine whether a woman is susceptible to developing yeast vaginitis because she is estrogenized. All gynecologists and family doctors should keep wide range (pH 2-12) and narrow range (pH 4-7) indicator paper in their examining rooms. Rolls of pH indicator paper can be purchased online from laboratory or medical supply companies. OTC diagnostic kits for vaginitis contain pH indicators, which allow patients to measure their own vaginal pH.

Tests for Intestinal Candidiasis

The lament of yeast syndrome sufferers is aptly captured in this book title, *Why Do I Feel So Bad (When the Doctor says I'm O.K.)?* by Hagglund (1984). If doctors do not order specific tests for intestinal candidiasis, then people with the yeast syndrome will not receive the proper diagnosis or treatments.

When faced with polysymptomatic people who have risk factors for intestinal candidiasis, doctors should *"Think yeast!"* (Zwerling et al., 1984), and order tests from labs that specialize in Candida.

"When you hear hoofbeats in the night, look for horses—not zebras" (unless you live in Africa!). If you have symptoms characteristic of yeast infections, ask for laboratory testing for candidiasis. Be assertive. Don't let your doctor order every test under the sun—except for Candida!

Stool Analysis

Standard tests for diagnosing intestinal candidiasis are microscopy and culture of fecal specimens collected at stool. Complete stool analyses for Candida include yeast culture, identification of yeast species, antifungal susceptibility testing, culture of bacterial flora, detection of parasites by microscopy and enzyme immunoassay (EIA) testing, and evaluation of digestion, absorption, and the colonic environment (Barrie, 1986). Laboratories that perform complete stool analyses are listed in Table 6. Usually the same yeast species is found in the rectum and vagina of women who have recurrent vulvovaginal candidiasis (Guzel et al., 2011b).

Blood Tests

- **Candida Antigens, Candida Immune Complexes, and Candida DNA:** Abnormally high levels of these specific molecules from *Candida albicans* in blood **definitively diagnose a current, active intestinal yeast infection**.
- **Anti-Candida Antibodies:** Abnormally high levels of IgA, IgM, and IgG antibodies against *Candida albicans* in blood **indicate a current or past intestinal yeast infection**. Abnormally high levels of IgE antibodies against *Candida albicans* in blood **indicate Candida allergy**. An advantage of measuring antibody levels is that they are unaffected by prior antifungal treatment.

Interpretation of Tests for Intestinal Candidiasis

Even though stool and blood tests for intestinal yeast infections have been validated in controlled clinical studies (Chapter 5), the syndrome caused by yeast infection of the gut is still contested by establishment medicine (Chapter 6). Skeptical doctors contend that the blood test for anti-Candida antibodies is meaningless because everyone has anti-Candida antibodies. While it is true that healthy people have antibodies against Candida in their blood, their levels are within the normal reference range, whereas people with intestinal yeast overgrowth have higher than normal values. In fact, the higher the level, the worse the symptoms.

Skeptics also argue that high levels of anti-Candida antibodies could indicate a past yeast infection. While it is true that antibodies persist for years, common sense dictates if the yeast infection were in the past, the person would not now be in the doctor's office complaining about symptoms of yeast infections!

In addition to the lack of knowledge about testing methods for yeast infections on the part of most physicians, laboratories sometimes make errors interpreting anti-Candida antibody levels. For example, some labs incorrectly claim that past yeast infections can be distinguished from current yeast infections by comparing the levels of IgM and IgG. While it is true that IgM is synthesized early in a new infection before IgG is induced, this applies only to a new infection with viruses and bacteria. Since all of us were colonized by Candida at birth, we already have WBCs that produce anti-Candida antibodies even if we never develop a yeast infection. New yeast infections stimulate these memory WBCs to produce more anti-Candida antibodies in all immunoglobulin classes (IgA, IgG, IgM, and IgE).

Some laboratories use the wrong reference antigen for Candida tests. Bauman and Hagglund (1991) reported that cytoplasmic antigens from *C. albicans* stimulated antibody production in intestinal candidiasis. Unfortunately, some labs use cell wall antigens from *C. albicans* as the reference antigen, which produces false-negative blood test results even when symptoms and risk factors indicate intestinal candidiasis.

In addition, it seems that there was an epidemic among my clients of labs "losing" specimens collected for diagnosing intestinal candidiasis.

For all these reasons, a stool analysis should be performed in addition to blood tests. If the stool culture indicates that the patient is infected with a non-*albicans* Candida species, positive blood test results will still be obtained because antibodies to *C. albicans* cross-react with other Candida species.

While the anti-Candida antibody test is diagnostic, it is not prognostic. Therefore, repeatedly performing this blood test looking for a decrease in antibody titers is a waste of money because antibodies persist for years after the infection is cured. In fact, antibody levels may increase during treatment. On the other hand, levels of Candida antigens and Candida immune complexes in the blood are prognostic because they do decrease with effective antifungal treatment.

Blood Tests to Check for Risk Factors

WBC Counts

Normal white blood cell counts are 3.4 to 9.6 billion cells/L. I have noticed in people who consulted with me that they have borderline low WBC counts (just above or below the lower end of the normal range) when they developed intestinal yeast infections after being treated with antibiotics. The question is: Were the WBCs destroyed by the bacterial infection, the antibacterial drug, the yeast infection, or the antifungal drug? Or did low WBC numbers preexist?

Diabetes and HIV

These two medical conditions and others mentioned in Step 6 predispose people to develop candidiasis. Hence, tests for these risk factors should be performed and these conditions must be treated before you can cure yeast infections.

Liver Function

You should obtain a liver function test before starting daily systemic antifungal therapy to make sure you do not have hepatitis or elevated liver enzymes. Then, you should get your liver tested every two weeks during treatment because systemic antifungals compete for degradative liver enzymes. Therefore, other drugs may not be broken down and might build up to toxic levels in your blood. Go back for follow-up office visits so your physician can monitor your clinical improvement, liver function, and drug levels of your other medications (Step 3).

Tests for Candida Allergy

Scratch (Prick) Test with Candida Antigen

This skin test is scored positive if a red, itchy bump (*wheal* and *flare*) develops after 15 minutes indicating IgE-mediated allergy to Candida. A positive skin test result makes patient a candidate for Candida allergy shots (*subcutaneous injection immunotherapy*; Step 5).

Intradermal Test with Candida Antigen

This skin test is scored positive for candidiasis hypersensitivity syndrome if a wheal and flare reaction develops after 15 minutes indicating IgE-mediated allergy (*immediate hypersensitivity*) to Candida, and no reaction develops after two days indicates poor T cell-mediated immunity (*anergy*) against Candida. Patient is a candidate for Candida allergy shots (*subcutaneous injection immunotherapy*; Step 5).

If no allergic reaction develops after 15 minutes and a small, flesh-colored bump (*induration*) develops after two days, this intradermal test indicates good T cell-mediated immunity (*delayed hypersensitivity*) to Candida. However, if a large, red, swollen reaction develops after two days that may blister and last for days or weeks, then the intradermal test antigen is too concentrated or the test result indicates *hyperreactivity* and is a contraindication for Candida allergy shots (Step 5 and Table 8).

T Cell Proliferative Responses to Candida Antigen

If patient exhibits allergy and anergy to Candida in the intradermal test, then follow-up blood tests should be performed to measure T cell function. A negative result in the blood test for T cell proliferation to Candida antigen indicates poor immunity (*anergy*) to Candida, and normal proliferation to mitogens in this test means the immune defect is specific for Candida.

Research Tests for Intestinal Candidiasis

The following tests are not standard for measuring yeast overgrowth in the gut, but are useful for learning more about the patient's diagnosis, especially for research studies.

Anti-*Saccharomyces cerevisiae* Antibodies (ASCA)

The presence of ASCA in blood is diagnostic for Crohn's disease, an inflammatory bowel disease (Kaila et al., 2005). Even though the ASCA test detects antibodies to baker's yeast in the laboratory, the antigen (*immunogen*) that induced the synthesis of ASCA is actually *C. albicans* (Standaert-Vitse et al., 2006). *Thus, ASCA are really anti-Candida antibodies that cross-react with other yeasts.* Since ASCA cross-reacts with both yeasts (*Saccharomyces cerevisiae* and *Candida albicans*), its presence indicates intestinal Candida overgrowth just like elevated levels of anti-*Candida albicans* antibodies indicates intestinal Candida overgrowth.

> *People with Crohn's disease may actually have intestinal candidiasis that has gone undiagnosed.* Tests for antibodies against both Candida and Saccharomyces should be performed because both are a measure of chronic intestinal candidiasis.

Cytokines

Increased interleukin-17 (IL-17) production occurs during Candida infection, whereas other cytokines (IL-1B, IL-6, IL-10, IFN-y, TNF-a) are unaffected.

Ethanol and Acetaldehyde

Detecting these metabolites in blood and breath after patient consumes sugar indicates intestinal fermentation by yeasts.

D-Arabinitol, Arabinose, and Tartaric Acid in Urine

Elevated concentrations of these yeast metabolic products in urine after ingesting sugar indicates intestinal fermentation by yeasts. Advantages of this test are that:

- urine is easier to collect and analyze than blood
- results give a quantitative estimate of the amount of yeast overgrowth
- decreasing levels of metabolites are prognostic and indicate a positive response to antifungal therapy

Unfortunately, different labs disagree about which metabolites are diagnostic. Lord et al. (2004) claim that urinary D-arabinitol indicates intestinal yeast overgrowth. Shaw et al. (1995; 2000) claim that urinary arabinose and tartaric acid are specific biomarkers of intestinal candidiasis.

Other researchers reported elevated concentrations of other organic acids in urine from people with yeast overgrowth in the gut.

Intestinal Permeability

Inflammation and structural disruption of the intestinal wall caused by yeast infection increases permeability, allowing gut contents to leak into the bloodstream. *Hyperpermeability* or "leaky gut" explains many of the symptoms of the yeast syndrome. Testing intestinal permeability involves drinking solutions containing lactulose and mannitol, and collecting urine for six hours. Normally, only small amounts of lactulose pass into the bloodstream through the tight junctions between epithelial cells in the intestinal mucosa, whereas mannitol readily passes through the intestinal wall. The kidneys remove these chemicals from blood, and excrete them in urine. Increased amounts of both test chemicals in the urine indicate increased permeability of intestinal epithelium. The higher the ratio of lactulose to mannitol, the larger the pore size between epithelial cells.

Nutritional Deficiencies

Low blood levels of magnesium, zinc, iron, selenium, vitamin A, vitamin B6, vitamin C, biotin, folate, and/or omega-6 and omega-3 fatty acids have been reported in yeast syndrome patients, indicating poor intestinal absorption of nutrients.

Rule Out Other Disorders

Many other illnesses can produce the same symptoms as candidiasis. Therefore, additional diagnostic tests may be needed to exclude the following disorders.

Diseases that Mimic Oral Candidiasis

Leukoplakia and *lichen planus* produce white, thickened patches on the tongue, buccal membrane, and gums resembling oral thrush. Leukoplakia is caused by smoking and infection with human immunodeficiency virus (HIV) or hepatitis C virus (HCV). The tongue may fissure and bleed, and become malignant.

Diseases that Mimic Intestinal Candidiasis

Infections by viruses, bacteria, parasites, and other fungi produce symptoms similar to yeast overgrowth in the gut. Conditions such as irritable bowel syndrome, Crohn's disease, ulcerative colitis, celiac sprue, food allergies, and colon cancer resemble yeast syndrome symptoms.

Diseases that Mimic Genital Candidiasis

Viral, bacterial, and parasitic infections of the genitalia produce symptoms similar to yeast infections, as do leukoplakia of the vulva or penis, allergies to Candida, hypersensitivity to chemicals, and cancer.

How to Obtain Diagnostic Testing for Candidiasis

Many patients have told me that their doctor does not believe in the yeast syndrome and refused to even test them for Candida let alone treat them. So then, patients would ask me for a referral to a doctor who is knowledgeable about yeast infections. I always explain that I don't know physicians in every city, of every state, of every country in the world and, furthermore, very few doctors have extensive expertise in the area of skin and mucosal Candida infections.

It seems reasonable to think that a gastroenterologist would be the perfect physician to diagnose and treat intestinal candidiasis. But, in my consulting practice since 1988, no patient has been able to persuade a GI doctor to consider this diagnosis. One gastroenterologist dismissed what were clearly white thrush patches on a colonoscopy photo as "light reflections off the intestinal mucosa." Other patients read in their colonoscopy reports that red areas were dismissed as "non-specific inflammation." The white and/or red patches should have been biopsied and cultured for yeast; biopsies should be sectioned for histology, stained for fungi, and observed under the microscopy. Instead of following scientific methods for diagnosis, GI doctors put into practice the negative suggestions from opinion papers written by the academic skeptics listed in the Hall of Shame (Chapter 6).

I urge patients to stay with their personal physicians who know their medical history and risk factors for candidiasis. In fact, your own doctor may have even prescribed the very drugs that predisposed you to develop a yeast infection in the first place!

I suggest that patients become their own health advocate and form a partnership with their doctor. Fill in Tables 1, 3 and 4, and give copies to your doctor. Photocopy the pages in this book containing information relating to your yeast condition, highlight the applicable sentences, and give copies to your doctor. Or, buy a second copy of this book, and give it your doctor. Ask for diagnostic tests appropriate for your case.

If your physician is open-minded and interested in learning more about yeast infections and yeast allergies, she or he will appreciate reading my discussions of research findings from more than 500 controlled studies of Candida listed in the Literature Cited.

If your doctor refuses to consider yeast as a possible diagnosis, call customer service at your health insurance company, and ask for two referrals; one to a physician in your plan who treats Candida infections, and another to a board-certified allergist who will test and treat you for allergies to Candida, yeasts, and molds.

If you cannot obtain physician referrals through your health insurance, you will have to go outside your network and pay out-of-pocket for diagnostic testing. Then take your test results back to your doctor in your insurance network for treatment.

You can obtain the names of providers who will order Candida tests by visiting the websites of diagnostic laboratories listed in Tables 6 and 7. Click on their link to Patients, and then on their link to Practitioners. Request the names of doctors in your city who will order tests for candidiasis. You will have to pay for both the doctor visits and the tests.

Any doctor can follow the guidelines in my ten-step program for diagnosing, treating, and preventing yeast infections. Medical doctors (M.D.) and doctors of osteopathy (D.O.) can order the Candida tests recommended in this book. Some states authorize naturopathic doctors and/or other health care practitioners to order these tests. But doctors must first register their medical license number with the specialty lab before they can order Candida tests.

Some labs in your insurance network may perform tests recommended above, so you should not have to pay for these tests. Other tests are offered only by specialty labs listed in Tables 6 and 7. Go to the websites of laboratories, and request sample copies of their Candida test results to learn what tests they perform, if they take your health insurance, and the costs for lab tests. While some labs sell Candida tests directly to consumers, I advise you to ask your doctor to order tests and prescribe treatments.

Before making appointments with any doctors outside your health insurance network, ask if they offer the tests for Candida infection and Candida allergy recommended in Steps 1 and 5. A list of Physician Referral Services is on www.yeastconsulting.com. Go to the website of each referral service, and type in your city to find names of doctors. Read my warning preceding this list about doctors listed on physician referral services and follow my suggested plan of action.

If you are successful finding a doctor to order Candida tests for you recommended in Step 1, the lab will send your stool collection kit to the doctor. She or he will give you the stool analysis kit at the doctor's office. Follow the directions for collecting feces at home and mail the stool specimen in the container to the lab. Your doctor will draw blood and collect swabs or tissue scrapings, and send them to the lab. Test results are faxed to your doctor. When you go in to see the doctor to get your test results, request copies, and keep them in your medical file at home.

If your test results are positive, they provide the justification doctors need to prescribe treatments. Take your test results back to your personal physician and ask her or him to design a treatment plan tailor-made for your specific yeast problems. Your medical care will be covered by your health insurance if prescribed by your doctor.

Keep going back to your doctor for follow-up visits to monitor your liver function, discuss your response to antifungal therapy, and obtain refill prescriptions for medications. If you respond positively to daily antifungal treatment and weekly maintenance therapy, but then relapse, ask your doctor for a written referral to an allergist to obtain skin testing for Candida allergy and Candida immunity. If you are positive for Candida allergy, obtain subcutaneous allergy shots of Candida (Step 5). I sincerely hope that your physician is willing to listen to your symptoms and is open-minded about the scientific information provided in this book.

Table 6 lists tests for diagnosing intestinal yeast infections, and the laboratories that perform these tests. Table 7 lists the contact information for these laboratories.

Table 6. Tests and Labs for Intestinal Candidiasis

Definitive Diagnostic Tests for Intestinal Candidiasis

Candida immune complexes in blood: Alletess Medical Laboratory, Genova Diagnostics integrated with Metametrix, and Quest Diagnostics (Cambridge Biomedical, Inc.).

Candida antigens in blood: Alletess Medical Laboratory, Focus Diagnostics, Genova Diagnostics integrated with Metametrix, and Mayo Medical Laboratories.

Candida DNA in specimens: Medical Diagnostic Laboratory, and Metametrix Clinical Laboratory.

Other Tests for Intestinal Candidiasis

Anti-Candida antibodies in blood: Alletess Medical Laboratory, Cerodex Laboratories, Direct Laboratory Services, Focus Diagnostics, Genova Diagnostics integrated with Metametrix, ImmunoMycologics, Life Extension Nutrition Center, Mayo Medical Laboratories, MyMedLab and Vibrant Wellness.

Stool analyses: BioHealth Diagnostics, BIOHM Candida Report, Diagnostic Solutions Laboratory, Doctor's Data, Genova Diagnostics integrated with Metametrix Clinical Laboratory, Microbiology Reference Laboratory, MyMedLab, Quest Diagnostics, and Verisana.

Microbial products in urine: Great Plains Laboratory, Metametrix Clinical Laboratory, and Vitamin Research Products.

Intestinal permeability ("leaky gut"): Genova Diagnostics integrated with Metametrix, and Verisana.

Cytokines: Integrative Psychiatry.

Tests for Other Intestinal Disorders

Gastrointestinal Health Panel: Diagnos-Techs, and Immunosciences Lab.

Gluten and food sensitivities; celiac disease: EnteroLab, and NeuroScience.

Table 7. Addresses of Diagnostic Laboratories

Alletess Medical Laboratory
216 Pleasant Street
Rockland MA 02370
800-225-5404
www.foodallergy.com

BioHealth Diagnostics
2929 Canon Street
San Diego CA 92106
800-570-2000
www.biodia.com

BIOHM Health (BIOHM Candida Report)
Cleveland, OH 44115
216-394-0544
https://biohmhealth.com

Diagnos-Techs Inc.
6620 South 192nd Place Bldg J-106
Kent Washington 98032
800-878-3787
www.diagnostechs.com

Diagnostic Solutions Laboratory
5895 Shiloh Rd Ste 101
Alpharetta, GA 30005
877-485-5336
www.diagnosticsolutionslab.com

Direct Laboratory Services Inc.
4040 Florida St Suite 202
Mandeville LA 70448
800-908-0000
www.directlabs.com

Doctor's Data Inc.
3755 Illinois Ave.
St. Charles IL 60174
800-323-2784 / 630-377-8139
www.doctorsdata.com

EnteroLab
10875 Plano Rd Suite 123
Dallas TX 75238
972-686-6869
www.enterolab.com

Focus Diagnostics Inc.
5785 Corporate Ave
Cypress CA 90630
800-445-0185 / 714-220-1900
www.focusdx.com

Genova Diagnostics
63 Zillicoa Street
Asheville NC 28801
(Tests integrated with Metametrix)
800-522-4762 / 704-253-0621
www.gdx.net
www.metametrix.com

Great Plains Laboratory, Inc.
11813 W 77 Street
Lenexa KS 66214
913-341-8949
www.greatplainslaboratory.com

ImmunoMycologics, Inc.
Cerodex Laboratories
2700 Technology Place
Norman, OK 73071
800-654-3639 / 405-360-4669
www.immy.com

ImmunoSciences Lab., Inc.
8693 Wilshire Blvd. #200
Beverly Hills, CA 90211
800-950-4686 / 310-657-1077
www.immuno-sci-lab.com

Integrative Psychiatry
3392 Magic Oak Lane
Sarasota, FL 34232
800-385-7863
www.integrativepsychiatry.net

Life Extension Nutrition Center
5990 North Federal Highway
Fort Lauderdale, FL 33308
954-766-8144
www.lef.org/quest-com.htm

Mayo Medical Laboratories
3050 Superior Drive NW
Rochester MN 55901
800-533-1710 / 507-266-5700
www.mayomedicallaboratories.com

Medical Diagnostic Laboratory
2439 Kuser Road
Hamilton, NJ 08690
877-269-0090 / 609-570-1000
www.mdlab.com

Metametrix Clinical Laboratory
3425 Corporate Way
Duluth GA 30096
(Tests integrated with Genova)
800-221-4640 / 770-446-5483
www.gdx.net
www.metametrix.com

Microbiology Reference Laboratory
10703 Progress Way
Cypress CA 90630
800-445-0185 / 714-220-1900
www.mrlinfo.com

MyMedLab
650-434-3984 Fax
Direct to consumer www.mymedlab.com

NeuroScience Inc.
373 280th St.
Osceola, WI 54020
888-342-7272 / 715-294-2852
www.neurorelief.com

Quest Diagnostics
1290 Wall Street West
Lyndhurst NJ 07071
800-222-0446
www.questdiagnostics.com

Verisana Laboratories
818 N Quincy Street Unit 806
Arlington VA 22203
703-722-6067
www.verisana.com

Vibrant Wellness
1360 Bayport Ave. Ste. B
San Carlos, CA 94070
866-364-0963
www.vibrant-wellness.com

Vitamin Research Products
4610 Arrowhead Drive
Carson City NV 89706
800-877-2447
www.vrp.com

Walk-In-Lab
PO Box 2244
Slidell, LA 70459
800-539-6119
www.walkinlab.com

Unproven Tests and Therapies

WARNING

Some alternative practitioners offer unproven tests and therapies. Hence, you need to be proactive. Before making an appointment with any doctor, call their office and ask if the doctor offers the specific diagnostic tests and medical treatments recommended in this book. If not, call the next doctor. Also ask if they take your health insurance, and how much they charge for office visits and each test.

When you show up for your appointment, explain again what tests you want. If the doctor instead offers to perform unscientific procedures like "muscle testing" (*applied kinesiology*), just say *"No!"* If a test sounds phony, it probably is. Explain that you will not pay for the office visit because you had asked for specific tests when you made the appointment. Then they pulled a "bait and switch."

Also, don't believe everything you read on the internet. For example, the "spit test" is nonsense! In order for a lab test to be valid, it must measure a specific chemical molecule in a specimen.

Conclusions of Step 1
Diagnostic Tests for Yeast Infections

You now know what tests are available for diagnosing yeast infections. A clinical diagnosis is based on your clinical signs and symptoms, physical examination, history of yeast infections, recent predisposing risk factors, and laboratory test results. Positive test results for yeast infection and yeast allergy justify prescribing antifungal therapy and immunotherapy.

A timely diagnosis is essential for a favorable outcome. The longer you have been sick, the longer it will take you to get better. The diagnosis is confirmed when patients improve with effective antiyeast treatments, allergy shots, avoidance of risk factors, lifestyle changes, dietary control, and probiotics, and walk back into their physician's office with smiles on their faces. You don't have to *"Learn to live with it!"* If you develop a yeast infection, obtain an early diagnosis. *Nip it in the bud!*

STEP 2

Antifungal Treatments

ANTIFUNGALS ARE ADMINISTERED DAILY UNTIL *symptoms resolve.* Let me repeat this for emphasis: *Antifungals are administered daily until symptoms resolve.*

I stressed this statement because many physicians mistakenly prescribe antifungals for only one or three days, or at most, one week. These short treatment times are not long enough to eradicate yeast infections located inside tissue cells. Chapter 1 explains that yeasts do not just grow on the surfaces of skin and mucous membranes, they also grow intracellularly inside epithelial cells. This intracellular location protects yeasts from antifungals as well as from the immune system. Thus, after only short-term antifungal treatment, living yeasts remain inside your tissues in an inactive or nongrowing (*latent*) state. After a lag period, intracellular yeasts often start to grow again causing a relapse. This explains why antifungals should be administered every day for a long enough time to eradicate yeasts inside tissues, and allow time for healing and regeneration of damaged tissues. *Antifungal treatment should be continued as long as symptoms are improving.*

Another reason why antifungals should be administered daily until resolution of symptoms is because the commonly prescribed antifungals are *fungistatic*, and just inhibit yeast growth. In contrast, the newer, more expensive antifungals are *fungicidal*, and do kill yeasts.

Candida patients who were prescribed older fungistatic antifungals need to take these medications on a daily basis for a long enough time to achieve resolution of symptoms. Then, daily treatment should be switched to weekly antifungal maintenance to suppress growth of residual intracellular yeasts and prevent recurrences. *Antifungals are administered weekly for prophylaxis not for initial treatment.*

Antifungals used for treating superficial candidiasis are discussed here in Step 2. Brand names are capitalized and generic names are given in lower case inside parentheses as in this example: Diflucan (fluconazole). U.S. patents on brand name drugs expire after 20 years, at which time generic drugs can be manufactured by other pharmaceutical firms and sold for less money.

Additional information about antifungals can be found on the websites of pharmaceutical manufacturers such as www.pfizer.com/products/rx/rx_product_diflucan.jsp), and on the following general information websites: www.doctorfungus.org, and www.fungalinfectiontrust.org. To find the full text or abstracts of articles published in scientific and medical journals, search on https://scholar.google.com.

The following topics are discussed later in this Step 2: antifungal resistance, combination antifungal therapy, synergy, natural antifungal supplements (pros and cons), and protocols for treating specific yeast infections.

General Considerations for Prescribing Antifungal Drugs

When doctors prescribe antifungal medications, they must consider the following factors in choosing the best drug for a particular yeast condition: efficacy, formulation, safety, cost, convenience, dosages, and treatment time.

Efficacy: *Does it work?*

Antifungal drugs have broad-spectrum activity against most yeasts and fungi. Efficacy depends on many factors such as the patient's yeast species and its antifungal susceptibility determined by testing, as well as the patient's risk factors for candidiasis and strength of their immune system. Efficacy is judged based on improvement in symptoms. The older antifungals are commonly prescribed at low doses and just inhibit yeast growth, i.e., are fungistatic. The newer, more expensive antifungals are administered at high doses and are fungicidal. To treat resistant yeast infections, doctors must decide between treatment with high doses of one antifungal, or combination treatment with two or more antifungals.

Formulation: *How is the drug administered?*

Antifungal preparations vary depending on the route of administration:
- *Topical* formulations are applied on body surfaces.
- *Enteral* formulations are given by mouth.
- *Parenteral* formulations are administered into the body other than by mouth, such as via injection, implantation, or intravenous (IV) infusion.

Safety: *Does the drug have side effects?*

Before using medications, read the consumer information handout, and ask the pharmacist for the package insert that gives detailed instructions. Also search on the internet for the drug prescribed for you. Topical antifungals are safe because only about 5% or less of the antifungal is absorbed into the circulation through skin or mucous membranes. In contrast, systemically absorbed oral antifungals can be toxic to the liver, may interact with drugs and supplements, and cause harm to the developing fetus, especially during the first trimester of pregnancy. Tips for avoiding problems with antifungals are offered in Step 3.

Cost: *Is it affordable?*

The newer, more effective systemic antiyeast drugs are expensive. In contrast, generic equivalents of older antifungals are cheaper. If your diagnostic test results were positive for candidiasis, your health insurance should cover treatment costs for prescription drugs. Some pharmaceutical companies offer discounts on drugs to people with low incomes. Some warehouse stores sell drugs at big discounts. Check out the cost of your prescription on www.goodrx.com; it gives up to an 80% discount on medications. Discounts on drugs may also be obtained from www.mygooddays. org and www.singlecare.com.

Convenience: *How difficult is it to obtain the antifungal and use it?*

Drugs sold over-the-counter (OTC) were originally prescription drugs that were found to be safe. While it is convenient to buy vaginal antifungal creams and suppositories OTC, they contain chemicals such as alcohols and detergents that can cause vaginal irritation. Better choices for chemically sensitive women are oral systemic antifungals. Follow precautions listed in Step 3.

Dosage: *What is the correct amount of drug to take?*

Usually, doctors prescribe the standard daily dose recommended for an antifungal. However, over the years. more and more cases of candidiasis have been found that are caused by yeasts that appear to be resistant, but are actually sensitive if higher doses are prescribed. These yeast strains are called *dose dependent.* This trend toward dose dependence of yeast isolates is apparent if you look at the progression of higher standard daily doses recommended as each new antifungal comes to market, or after the drug has been in use for a while.

The correct daily dose for your yeast strain is determined by many factors. **Most important are its species and its drug susceptibility.** Other determining factors include virulence of your yeast strain, your immune status, your weight, your liver function status, your estrogen level, other concurrent drugs, allergy to Candida, predisposing risk factors, other comorbid diseases present, severity of the yeast infection, clearance rate of the drug, hypersensitivity to the medication, and your age. Because there are so many influencing factors affecting your recovery, you need to report back often to your physician for follow-up testing and adjustment of treatment based on your clinical response.

 For most yeast infections, the entire daily dose of a systemic antifungal should be taken at one time to allow it to reach its maximum concentration in the blood. For complicated cases, where high doses are needed, the systemic antifungal is sometimes taken in divided doses. Follow your doctor's orders.

Treatment time: *How long should the antifungal be taken?*

Since every patient is different, it is impossible to predict how long you should treat a yeast infection. Symptoms might resolve in a week, a month, or longer. Once you are symptom-free, you need additional antifungal medication for weekly maintenance to prevent recurrences.

The first principle of antiyeast treatment is: *Seek medical care at the first sign of a yeast infection to prevent tissue damage and immune suppression.* The longer you have been infected, the longer it will take to get better once you obtain effective antifungal treatment.

The second principle is: *Antifungals are administered daily.* Unfortunately, Diflucan (fluconazole) was approved by the FDA for only one day of treatment for uncomplicated yeast vaginitis. This short-term treatment leads to long-term misery with incomplete cures and residual inflammation that produces chronic vulvar pain (*vulvodynia*).

The third principle is: *Treat until symptoms resolve.* Continue antifungal therapy if you are still improving until a cure is achieved. But be aware that your symptoms may worsen in the beginning of antifungal therapy due to "yeast die-off." This is caused by immune reactions to dead yeast products released from yeasts killed by the antifungal agent. If you experience this reaction, decrease the initial dosage until you get over "yeast die-off," then gradually increase the dosage as you improve up to the standard amount (explained in protocol later in Step 2).

The fourth principle is: *Once symptoms resolve, switch from daily treatment to weekly maintenance for up to six months to prevent recurrences.* Just because symptoms are gone doesn't mean the yeasts are gone. Some yeast cells remain alive, but inactive, inside your tissue cells. If you discontinue antifungal therapy too early, the intracellular yeasts can start growing again.

The gold standard of antimicrobial therapy is a positive response to therapy. Since Candida is an intracellular pathogen, daily antifungal treatment is needed to eradicate active yeast infections. Watson et al. (2002) found no differences between the effectiveness of oral and intravaginal antifungal treatment of Candida vaginitis. However, they emphasized that *the most critical factor in recovery was duration of therapy.* Antiyeast medication should be taken for at least one week and preferably two weeks until symptoms have resolved completely. Then switch from daily treatment to weekly prophylaxis for several months. In order to follow this protocol, ask your doctor to prescribe one month of a systemic antifungal.

Don't expect an overnight cure! You might expect yeast infections to improve within days based on your experience with how fast most bacterial infections respond to antibiotics. Instead, you may find that your yeast infection takes weeks or months to be eradicated. The reason for this difference is that antibiotics are bactericidal and kill bacteria whereas most antifungals are fungistatic and just inhibit yeast growth but don't kill fungi.

Improvement in symptoms of yeast infections is not always steady. Occasional flare ups occur and symptoms fluctuate from day to day. But you should improve eventually with daily antifungal therapy. Once the active yeast infection is cured, it takes additional time for tissues to heal. Applying a steroid cream along with using antifungals helps healing (see Step 4).

After a while, your response to therapy may reach a plateau where symptoms stop improving. At that point, it may be necessary to add a second antifungal agent. Or you may have a relapse while on intermittent antifungal maintenance. This means you have to go back on daily treatment and maybe add a second antifungal to your treatment. This is why you should go back to your doctor for frequent follow-up visits to discuss your progress, get your liver function tested, and your prescriptions renewed.

After your symptoms are gone and you have finished weekly suppression, you need to have some antiyeast medicine on hand in case you feel that old familiar vaginal itch or other yeast symptom beginning again. *Nip it in the bud!*

Topical Antifungals

Topical medications are applied to body surfaces such as skin or mucous membranes. Yeast infections on body surfaces are called *superficial candidiasis*. Uncomplicated superficial yeast infections are usually treated with a topical antimycotic preparation.

Yeast Infections of Skin, Scalp, and Nails

Topical antifungals sold OTC include:

- body powders (tolnaftate) and skin creams (clotrimazole, terbinafine, or miconazole) for athlete's foot, jock itch, and diaper rash
- intravaginal creams (Monistat, Mycelex, or Gyne-Lotrimin) for yeast vaginitis
- boric acid suppositories for yeast vaginitis sold online
- shampoo (ketoconazole) for itchy scalp
- lotions (terbinafine or undecylenate) or ciclopirox olamine lacquer for toenail fungus

Prescription antifungal skin creams can contain nystatin, amphotericin B, econazole, terconazole, or many others. The ideal cream for itching and burning contains both an antifungal and a corticosteroid because it treats both the yeast infection and the inflammation. An example of such a cream is Lotrisone, which contains clotrimazole and betamethasone; a cheaper generic formulation is available.

Yeast Infections of the Vagina

Vaginal antifungals and oral systemic antifungals are equally effective for treating uncomplicated vulvovaginal candidiasis (Watson et al., 2002). But surveys show that women prefer oral systemic antifungal treatment, probably because taking a pill by mouth is more convenient than inserting medication intravaginally (Ringdahl, 2000; Watson et al., 2002; das Neves et al., 2008).

Standard treatments for vulvovaginal candidiasis are short-term, one- or three-day azole regimens. However, they are often not curative, and when they fail, women develop chronic or recurrent vulvovaginal symptoms that require long-term, intensive treatment with both topical and systemic antifungals (protocols are provided below).

Topical antifungal preparations for yeast vaginitis are inserted into the vagina using an applicator at bedtime. *It is better to treat vaginally for seven to 14 days with a lower dose than to treat for only one or three days with a high dose.* Wear a panty liner inside your underwear during the day because when you get up in the morning, the cream leaks out. Vaginal antifungals are safe during pregnancy because very little medication is absorbed through the vaginal wall into the bloodstream. Unmedicated homeopathic products sold OTC for vaginitis are not effective because they just temporarily cover-up the symptoms without treating the underlying infection.

Vaginal medicated creams available OTC include Gyne-Lotrimin (clotrimazole), Femcare (clotrimazole), Mycelex (clotrimazole), Gynazole (butoconazole), Monistat (miconazole), and Vagistat-1 (tioconazole). All are equally effective. Prescription creams for yeast vaginitis include Mycostatin (nystatin) and Terazole (terconazole). Terazole is more effective than the others in most cases.

A disadvantage of vaginal creams and suppositories is they contain alcohols and detergents that can cause irritation and burning in chemically sensitive women. If you have had a bad reaction to a vaginal antifungal cream, ask your gynecologist to prescribe a vaginal ointment containing clotrimazole in a hypoallergenic base to be prepared by a compounding pharmacist. A disadvantage of Monistat (miconazole topical) is that it interacts with Coumadin (warfarin).

Vaginal suppositories containing Monistat (miconazole) are available OTC. Some women find these very irritating, which may be due to the glycerin (an alcohol), or because miconazole is very effective and causes bad "yeast die-off." Monistat 1 for one-day treatment has a very high concentration of miconazole. Some women have told me that it felt like a bomb going off in their vagina. I experienced a similar reaction. Monistat 3 for three-day treatment has a lower dosage, and Monistat 7 for seven-day treatment has the lowest dosage. Use the seven-day treatment because *longer treatments with lower dosages of vaginal antifungals are more effective.*

Vaginal inserts are dry tablets that are inserted intravaginally. They are better for sensitive women because they do not contain the alcohols and detergents present in creams and suppositories that can cause vulvar irritation.

Mycostatin (nystatin) vaginal tablets used to be available by prescription, and then were taken off the market for a while. They are now available again manufactured by Duramed Pharmaceuticals, Inc., a subsidiary of Barr Pharmaceuticals, Inc., Pomona, New York 10970. Nystatin vaginal inserts, USP, are supplied as a pale-yellow, mottled, oval-shaped, flat face, beveled insert (debossed ODYSSEY on one side and 705 on the other) in packages of 15 individually foil wrapped inserts with applicator and "Instructions for the Patient." The standard dosage is one insert (100,000 units nystatin) nightly for two weeks. The inserts should be deposited high in the vagina by means of the applicator.

Vaginal inserts containing clotrimazole used to be available OTC (Vazquez and Bronze, 2011). Unfortunately, pharmaceutical companies discontinued manufacturing them perhaps because they did not sell as well as creams. I hope someday they become available again for the benefit of sensitive women because clotrimazole is more effective than nystatin.

Vaginal gel caps containing boric acid powder (600 mg) are prepared by compounding pharmacists with a prescription. Capsules containing boric acid are inserted vaginally every night for 10 days to two weeks. Continue treatment only if your symptoms are improving. Boric acid has broad-spectrum antifungal activity (Kalkanci et al., 2012), and is used to treat Diflucan (fluconazole)-resistant yeasts. Boric acid powder is sold in bottles OTC in pharmacies for use as a pesticide. Some women buy gelatin capsules and fill them with boric acid powder themselves.

However, this procedure is tedious. It is better to see a gynecologist first to get a yeast culture ordered with species identification and antifungal susceptibility testing. Then, ask for a prescription for boric acid gel caps to be prepared by a compounding pharmacist. Or you can buy Boricap or Balance Lovely vaginal suppositories containing 600 mg of boric acid online.

Beware of Yeast Arrest vaginal suppositories and Yeastaway Boiron vaginal inserts sold online. They contain homeopathic preparations of herbs plus borax (sodium borate). Disadvantages of these products are that borax is inactive against yeasts whereas boric acid is the active form against yeasts; furthermore, borax is alkaline, which promotes yeast growth in the vagina.

> **WARNING**
>
> *Boric acid is deadly poisonous if ingested by mouth.* Likewise, borax is also a poison that should not be taken orally even in small quantities as suggested inappropriately on a website. Don't believe everything you read on the internet!

Safety Tip: The probability of systemic toxicity arising from intravaginal boric acid is miniscule. Van Slyke et al. (1981) noted the absence of both local and systemic toxicity in more than 2,000 women treated vaginally with boric acid. Fail et al. (1998) stated that vaginal exposure to boric acid is unlikely to cause abnormalities of the fetus because boric acid absorption is very limited.

Vaginal douches containing boric acid can be prepared by dissolving one teaspoon of boric acid powder in a quart of warm water. Commercial douches containing acetic acid adjusted to pH 4.5 are also safe. But you should not douche often. Allow your vagina to cleanse itself naturally with secretions that carry away substances in the vaginal discharge.

Comparison of vaginal antifungals: The azoles do penetrate into vulvar and vaginal tissues, and are effective at inhibiting yeasts growing intracellularly inside epithelial cells. Nystatin and boric acid are not absorbed into vulvar and vaginal tissues, so they only kill yeasts on tissue surfaces. Nystatin vaginal cream and boric acid capsules are effective against azole-resistant yeasts.

Yeast Infections of the Eyes, Ears, and Sinuses

These superficial Candida infections are rare. Mycotic eye infections are treated with prescription antifungal eye drops containing voriconazole (Dupuis et al., 2009) taken concurrently with systemic antifungal tablets. Fungal ear infections are treated with antifungal ear drops. However, most cases of external ear infections (otitis externa) are caused by bacteria. Sinus infections are rarely caused by yeast infections because Candida does not colonize the nasal passages. Sinusitis is usually caused either by bacteria or fungal spores breathed in from moldy environments.

Oral Antifungals

All antimycotic drugs taken by mouth require a physician's prescription.

Yeast Infections of the Mouth, Esophagus, and Intestine

Oral lozenges (also called troches or pastilles) containing clotrimazole or nystatin are dissolved in the saliva, swished around the mouth, and swallowed. Antifungal lozenges are taken after each meal, and after brushing teeth at bedtime.

Oral suspensions are prescribed for babies and adults who cannot swallow pills, or who cannot follow directions for lozenges. Liquid preparations containing nystatin or an azole (Diflucan, Sporanox, Vfend, or Noxafil) are swished around the mouth and swallowed. Doses are taken four times a day to coat the mucous membranes in the mouth and esophagus. Because antifungals are bitter tasting, sugar and flavoring are added to suspensions and lozenges to make them palatable. Don't worry that the sugar in oral antifungals will make your yeast condition worse. These preparations have been proven effective in controlled clinical studies. In fact, the sugar may improve efficacy because yeasts must be growing in order to be killed by antifungals.

Oral Nonabsorbed Antifungals

Amphotericin B (AMB) and nystatin are commonly used polyene antifungals that are nearly identical in structure, function, and efficacy. Other polyenes include candicidin, pimaricin, and mepatricin. Polyenes bind to ergosterol in the yeast cell membrane and cause yeast cells to burst (*lyse*). When taken by mouth, polyenes are not absorbed from the stomach into the bloodstream. Because they do not spread systemically, polyenes do not cause liver damage, drug interactions, or affect the fetus. Polyenes just treat yeasts in the lumen of the gut and on the surface of the intestinal wall, but not yeasts inside intestinal epithelial cells.

Amphotericin B

AMB is slightly more effective than nystatin when tested in the laboratory against Candida cultures. However, this difference in antifungal activity in vitro is clinically insignificant in vivo when treating intestinal yeast overgrowth. Besides, AMB is not FDA approved for oral administration and cannot be prescribed in the U.S. An oral formulation of AMB that is absorbed was developed by Wasan et al. (2009), but it is not commercially available. AMB powder for oral administration is available overseas, but you are advised against purchasing medications on the internet because it can be dangerous. Fungizone, an intravenous formulation of amphotericin B containing deoxycholate is administered only by IV infusion in hospital to patients who have very low WBC counts (*neutropenia*) and disseminated candidiasis.

Nystatin

This oral nonabsorbed antifungal was approved by the FDA in 1954 for the treatment of mucosal and cutaneous candidiasis. It is named after its place of discovery (**New York State**). Nystatin USP is the generic name. USP stands for the United States Pharmacopeia, the organization that sets the standards for medicines. Brand names of nystatin include Mycostatin and Nilstat. Pure USP nystatin powder for oral administration is manufactured by several companies and is available in bottles containing 50 million units (MU) and 100 MU.

Compounding pharmacists usually add nystatin powder to a solution of sucrose and flavoring to make the oral suspension palatable for the treatment of oral thrush and Candida esophagitis because antifungals are bitter tasting. Don't worry about the sugar in oral antifungals making your yeast condition worse. These preparations have been proven effective in controlled clinical studies. In fact, the sugar may improve efficacy because yeasts must be growing in order to be killed by antifungals.

Dosage: The standard adult dosage of oral nystatin powder for intestinal candidiasis is two MU per day. One dose (1/8 teaspoon) equals 500,000 units. Ask your doctor to prescribe a bottle containing 50 MU of oral nystatin powder USP for suspension with 2 refills. If you don't want a suspension containing sugar and artificial flavoring, ask your doctor to write a prescription for oral nystatin USP powder in capsules. Instruct the compounding pharmacist to put 1/8 tsp of powder (500,000 units) into gelatin capsules. Take one capsule 4 times a day (before meals and at bedtime). A bottle of 50 MU will provide about one month of treatments. Store nystatin prescriptions in the refrigerator to protect it against heat and light. To decrease the worsening of symptoms at the beginning of antifungal therapy, read the protocol for avoiding "yeast die-off" below.

Efficacy: Nystatin has broad-spectrum activity against yeasts and fungi. Oral nystatin treats yeast infections of the mouth, esophagus, stomach, and intestine. Since it is not absorbed, nystatin taken orally does not reach yeast infections in the prostate, vagina, skin, or internal organs. Oral nystatin attacks yeasts in the lumen of the intestine where the food and feces are located, but it does not penetrate into the gut wall. To kill yeasts inside epithelial cells of the intestinal wall, add an oral systemic antifungal such as Diflucan (fluconazole) to oral nystatin treatment.

Formulation: Nystatin is available as oral lozenges, oral tablets, oral powder, oral suspension containing sucrose and flavoring, vaginal cream, and topical powder containing talcum powder (for skin and athlete's foot, **not** for oral administration!). Pure nystatin powder is preferable for treating intestinal candidiasis because it does not contain additives and it distributes evenly throughout the intestinal contents when taken four times a day.

Oral nystatin tablets are cheaper, but they are coated with a red dye that might make sensitive people sick, and they do not disintegrate readily in the intestine. You can rinse off the red dye, dry the tablet with a paper towel, and crush the tablet in a pill crusher purchased in a pharmacy, add powder to a small amount of water, swish suspension around in your mouth for a minute, and then swallow. Repeat four times a day to treat oral thrush and intestinal candidiasis.

Because nystatin is not soluble in water, it forms a suspension, not a solution. Therefore, it is preferable to obtain a prescription for a bottle containing 50 MU of nystatin powder for oral administration and take it to a compounding pharmacist who will put 1/8 tsp into capsules. Then take four capsules a day to treat intestinal candidiasis. To avoid the extra charge for preparing capsules, you can get the bottle of powder and take 1/8 tsp added to water four times a day.

Safety: Because nystatin is not soluble in water, it is not absorbed into the bloodstream, not toxic to the liver, and does not interact with drugs or alcohol. For this reason, nystatin is safe for babies, pregnant women (Czeizel et al., 2003), the elderly, people with liver diseases (such as cirrhosis or viral hepatitis), and people taking medications that are metabolized in the liver.

Cost: Nystatin is taken for weeks or months until symptoms clear. While oral nystatin tablets are usually covered by insurance, oral nystatin powder is not covered. This can become costly if patients have to pay for it out of pocket.

Convenience: Advantages of oral nystatin powder are that it is effective against all yeasts, and you can lessen "yeast die-off" by taking a small amount at the start of treatment. Disadvantages of nystatin powder are that it must be obtained from a compounding pharmacy, it costs extra for the pharmacist to add the powder to gelatin capsules, it must be taken four times a day, it is not soluble in water, the suspension in water is bitter, and it is unstable to heat, light, moisture and long-term storage.

Treatment Time: Some people need only a few weeks of nystatin treatment to obtain relief from intestinal yeast overgrowth, whereas others need many months of oral nystatin combined with a systemic antifungal. After resolution of symptoms, switch from daily treatment to weekly maintenance with standard dosages of both antifungals concurrently for several months to prevent relapses.

> **WARNING**
>
> Don't take an ergosterol supplement to build up vitamin D levels when taking nystatin because ergosterol interferes with nystatin activity. Nystatin works by binding to ergosterol in the yeast cell membrane and causing rupture (lysis) of yeast cells.

Mepatricin

This macrolide polyene antifungal has similar activity to AMB and nystatin. It is available as a urological preparation administered as an instillation. Mepatricin effectively treated nonbacterial prostatitis at 40 mg daily (Bacigalupo et al., 1983). Mepatricin instilled into the urinary bladder is useful for treating disorders of the urethra, prostate, and bladder, as well as chronic pelvic pain syndrome and benign prostatic hyperplasia. Mepatricin (50,000 units) is also available in enteric coated tablets for oral administration.

Oral Systemic Antifungals

Antimycotics that are taken by mouth and absorbed from the stomach into the bloodstream are called systemic because they spread throughout the body. Oral systemic antifungals attack yeasts at any site in the body by penetrating into tissue cells where yeasts grow. The following oral systemic antifungals are discussed below under their brand names: Nizoral, Diflucan, Sporanox, Lamisil, Vfend, and Noxafil. (Their generic names are given in parentheses.) All of these are azoles except Lamisil, which is an allylamine. They all work by inhibiting ergosterol synthesis in the yeast cell membrane. To learn about side effects caused by systemic antifungals, read Step 3.

Nizoral (ketoconazole)

In 1981, Nizoral was approved for treating superficial yeast infections. It is an orally administered, systemic, imidazole antifungal manufactured by Janssen. The standard daily dose is one 200 mg tablet, but difficult-to-cure yeast infections are treated with 400 mg/day. Nizoral must be taken with meals because it needs to be in the acidic form to be absorbed from the stomach. Therefore, *don't take antacids with Nizoral.*

Nizoral is more effective than nystatin, but less effective than triazoles (Diflucan and Sporanox). The advantage of Nizoral is that it is often effective against non-*albicans* Candida species that are naturally resistant to Diflucan (fluconazole; Nguyen and Yu, 1998).

Nizoral rarely has side effects (Lewis et al., 1984; Stricker et al., 1986; Cauwenbergh, 1989; Knight, 1991). Only about one out of 10,000 people taking Nizoral develop elevations in their liver enzymes. Fortunately, this side effect is reversible. When Nizoral is discontinued, liver enzyme levels return to normal.

However, at high doses, Nizoral inhibits adrenal and testicular steroid synthesis, resulting in hair loss, breast swelling, and loss of sexual function in men. Since these side effects are more problematic during puberty, teenagers should not be treated with Nizoral. Effects on testosterone levels are reversible when Nizoral is discontinued.

In August 2013, the U.S. FDA announced that medical professionals should not prescribe ketoconazole tablet as a first line therapy for any fungal infection because of the risk of severe liver injury, adverse drug reactions, and adrenal insufficiency. In July 2013, the European Union withdrew the ketoconazole tablet from the market.

Diflucan (fluconazole)

In 1990, Diflucan was approved for the treatment of esophageal candidiasis in people with AIDS. It is an orally administered, systemic, triazole antifungal manufactured by Pfizer-Roerig. Triazole antifungal drugs are second generation azoles that are more effective than imidazoles such as Nizoral. Triazoles inhibit ergosterol synthesis in the yeast cell membrane by targeting the fungal cytochrome P450 enzyme, lanosterol 14α-demethylase, which catalyzes a step in ergosterol synthesis. Diflucan is effective against most yeasts and fungi and has a good safety profile. For these reasons, *Diflucan is the drug-of-first-choice for treating superficial Candida infections.*

Drugs that interact with Diflucan (fluconazole) include oral hypoglycemics, coumarin-type anticoagulants, phenytoin, cyclosporine, rifampin, theophylline, terfenadine, cisapride, astemizole, rifabutin, tacrolimus, and short-acting benzodiazepines. Step 3 explains what precautions to take to counteract drug interactions.

Prescribing guidelines for Diflucan are recommended on www.pfizer.com/products:

- Dosage and length of treatment are based on the infecting organism, and patient's response to therapy.

- Treatment should be continued until clinical parameters or laboratory tests indicate that the active infection has subsided, and *for at least two weeks following resolution of symptoms.*
- Recurrent candidiasis requires maintenance therapy to prevent relapses.

While the standard daily dose of Diflucan is 100 mg for adults, a higher dosage of 200 mg a day is needed for many patients such as those who weigh 200 lb. or more, are infected with a non-*albicans Candida* species. or suffer from chronic or recurrent candidiasis. Patients infected with a dose-dependent Candida species that is resistant to low doses of Diflucan (100 mg or 200 mg a day), usually respond to high doses of Diflucan (400 mg daily). Diflucan does not need to be taken with meals. Visit www.PfizerRxPathways.com for assistance programs that help eligible patients access their Pfizer prescriptions.

The patent for Diflucan expired in 2005, and less expensive generic fluconazole is now available. Oral fluconazole tablets (50, 100, and 200 mg) are available in bottles of 30. Ask your doctor to prescribe 30 tablets of 200 mg (a one-month supply) with two refills to cover sufficient daily treatment to achieve resolution of symptoms followed by several months of weekly maintenance to prevent recurrences.

In 1994, the FDA approved one 150-mg tablet of Diflucan for the treatment of uncomplicated yeast vaginitis. Immediately after this approval, Pfizer-Roerig had an advertisement on TV stating that "One pill of Diflucan cures most yeast infections." My question is: *"What about the women who are not cured?"*

The answer is that approval of only one day of antifungal treatment for yeast vaginitis was an unfortunate decision. It resulted in incomplete cures for millions of women who were left with chronic vulvar pain (*vulvodynia*) and/or chronic/recurrent vulvovaginal candidiasis. Goswami et al. (2006) reported that Candida persisted vaginally in half of women treated with only one tablet of Diflucan. Prior to 1994, yeast vaginitis was routinely treated for seven to 14 days with a vaginal antifungal preparation such as nystatin or the imidazole clotrimazole. It takes a week or two of daily antifungal treatment to eradicate yeast vaginitis.

Sobel et al. (2004) recognized the failure of a single dose of Diflucan to treat vaginal yeast infections, and so they carried out a controlled study treating vulvovaginal candidiasis with Diflucan given in three 150-mg doses at 72-hour intervals. This sequential treatment induced remission of symptoms. Then 387 women were assigned to receive weekly suppression therapy with either one tablet of Diflucan (150 mg) or a placebo for six months, followed by six months of observation without therapy. They found that weekly maintenance reduced recurrences, but permanent cures were difficult to achieve with only three pills, each one given at 3-day intervals.

Experts worldwide agree that *difficult-to-cure yeast infections should be treated long-term with daily antifungals* (El-Din et al., 2001; Sobel et al., 2004; Goswami et al. (2006); Centers for Disease Control, 2008; Mendling and Brasch (2012). After symptoms resolve, daily treatment should be switched to weekly maintenance for up to six months to prevent the rebound effect that often occurs after antifungals are discontinued (Sobel et al., 2004; Donders et al., 2008; Mendling and Brasch, 2012). Despite the important results from the above-mentioned studies, Vazquez and

Bronze (2011) still recommended only one 150 mg tablet of Diflucan as standard treatment for yeast vaginitis.

In my opinion, only one day of treatment with 150 mg of Diflucan (fluconazole) is responsible for the current epidemics of vulvodynia and recurrent vulvovaginal candidiasis. Incomplete cures result in persistent vulvovaginal pain when residual latent intracellular yeasts continuously release antigens resulting in immune reactions (Crandall, 1991a; download from www.yeastconsulting.com) and/or relapses when yeasts start growing again. Another negative outcome of only one day treatment is that multiple short-term retreatments may select for fluconazole-resistant yeasts.

Take home message: *One pill of Diflucan* (fluconazole) *is not "magic" and does not cure most yeast infections. Short-term antifungal therapy leads to long-term misery! All antifungals should be administered daily until symptoms resolve and then daily treatment should be switched to weekly maintenance to prevent recurrences.*

Sporanox (itraconazole)

In 1992, Sporanox was approved for the treatment of candidiasis. It is an orally administered, systemic, triazole antifungal manufactured by Janssen. Sporanox is similar to fluconazole in structure and activity against Candida and other fungi. It is available as oral capsules containing 100 mg, and as an oral solution. Sporanox should be taken with meals because it must be in the acidic form to be absorbed. Therefore, *don't take antacids with Sporanox.*

Lamisil (terbinafine)

In 1996, Lamisil was approved for the treatment of fungal infections of fingernails and toenails. It is an orally administered, systemic, allylamine antifungal manufactured by Sandoz and Novartis Pharmaceuticals. Lamisil is active against a broad range of fungi and yeasts including *C. albicans*. It is highly active against *C. parapsilosis* (Ryder et al., 1998). Lamisil is available by prescription as 250 mg oral tablets that are taken daily for three months for nail fungus. Because fungi invade the nail bed, long-term therapy is necessary. Lamisil cream is available OTC for athlete's foot.

Vfend (voriconazole)

In 2002, Vfend was approved for the treatment of disseminated fungal infections. It is an orally administered, systemic, second-generation triazole antifungal manufactured by Pfizer. Vfend inhibits ergosterol biosynthesis in the yeast cell membrane and is more effective than Diflucan. The greater efficacy of Vfend may be due in part to its higher dosage. The standard oral dosage of Vfend for superficial candidiasis is 200 mg twice daily for two weeks. If Diflucan is administered at a dosage of 400 mg daily, it too is more effective. Vfend should be taken no longer than 28 days. Continue treatment as long as symptoms are improving.

Vfend should not be prescribed unless long-term courses of other systemic antifungals have failed, and the infection is caused by a yeast strain *proven to be fluconazole-resistant by laboratory testing.* Vfend is available as a pill and a liquid, and it is safe and well tolerated in pediatric and adult patients (Michael et al., 2010). Growth-inhibition studies demonstrated that voriconazole, like itraconazole, is fungistatic against all *Candida* species tested (Greer, 2003). Overall, voriconazole showed more potency than fluconazole or itraconazole for most *Candida* isolates studied.

Advantages of Vfend are that it has broad-spectrum activity against most fungi and Candida species including non-*albicans* species that are naturally resistant to Diflucan (fluconazole; Nguyen and Yu, 1998). However, Vfend is very expensive, and its side effects include visual disturbances and photosensitivity. To avoid an intestinal bleed, *don't take Vfend on an empty stomach*. Since fats bind to Vfend and lowers its activity, *take Vfend one hour after a low-fat meal*.

The pharmaceutical company Mylan Institutional markets generic voriconazole tablets that are cheaper than brand name Vfend (https://www.viatris.com/en-us/lm/countryhome/us-products/productcatalog/productdetails?id=0712c415-709d-4ad3-9b3f-5b5408824a5f).

Noxafil (posaconazole)

In 2006, Noxafil was approved for the treatment of disseminated fungal infections. It is an orally administered, systemic, second-generation triazole antifungal manufactured by Schering-Plough. Noxafil inhibits ergosterol biosynthesis in the yeast cell membrane and is fungicidal. It has broad-spectrum antifungal killing activity against most fungi and Candida species including strains refractory to Diflucan and Sporanox. Noxafil oral solution contains 40 mg/ml. For the treatment of oropharyngeal candidiasis refractory to itraconazole and/or fluconazole, a dose of 400 mg of Noxafil twice a day is recommended for as long as 12 weeks depending on the severity of the yeast condition and the patient's response to therapy.

Lannett Company Inc. manufactures generic posaconazole in the form of 100 mg delayed-release tablets. The loading dose is 300 mg (three 100 mg delayed-release tablets) twice a day on the first day. The daily therapeutic dose is 300 mg (three 100 mg delayed-release tablets) once a day, starting on the second day. *Posaconazole is absorbed better if taken with a high-fat meal.*

Lipopeptide Echinocandins

Newer antifungals that are fungicidal include Cancidas (caspofungin), Mycamine (micafungin), and Eraxis (anidulafungin). These lipopeptide echinocandins inhibit β-1,3-glucan synthesis in the yeast cell wall, and are very effective for treating recalcitrant yeast conditions. However, their disadvantage is that they must be administered intravenously (IV) by an attending physician who has hospital privileges.

Triterpenoids

Ibrexafungerp (formerly SCY-078) is a glucan synthase inhibitor that is undergoing clinical trials for recurrent vulvovaginal candidiasis and other fungal infections. The brand name has been conditionally approved as Brexafemme. Key attributes of Brexafemme (ibrexafungerp) are:

- Fungicidal (kills the pathogen) versus fluconazole, which just inhibits growth (fungistatic)
- Broad spectrum antifungal activity against *Candida*, including fluconazole-resistant species and echinocandin-resistant strains
- Oral therapy; 600 mg dose for one day; no concerns about liver toxicity

- Effective at pH 4.5, the acidic environment of the vagina
- No pregnancy warning

Ineffective Drugs

Ancobon or Ancotil (flucytosine) should not be taken orally for candidiasis because 50% of Candida strains are resistant. Having said that, flucytosine is used together with other antifungals to treat difficult-to-cure cases of candidiasis.

Fulvicin (griseofulvin), also called Gris-PEG, is effective against fungal infections of skin and nails. *But it does not inhibit Candida.* Sporanox and Lamisil are less toxic and more effective against fungal infections.

Nikkomycin Z is a chitin synthase inhibitor that works by interfering with the building of the fungal cell wall and results in the fungal cell bursting open. It was discovered in 1976 and has weak activity against *Aspergillus fumigatus*. Nikkomycin Z might be synergistic when used with other antifungal medications such as caspofungin, ranconazole, amphotericin B, fluconazole, or itraconazole against Candida isolates in vitro. However, its effects in vivo are not known.

Lufenuron does not possess antifungal activity (Hector et al., 2005). Ignore the nonsense you have read on the internet about taking Lufenuron for yeast infections.

Colloidal silver was banned by the FDA in 1999. It is unproven to cure anything, and if too much silver is consumed, it causes *argyria*, which is an irreversible condition that causes the skin turns bluish-grey.

Antifungal Resistance

If symptoms do not improve after antifungal treatment, people think their yeast has developed resistance. But you have to distinguish between resistant infections and resistant yeasts.

Resistant infections that are still symptomatic after short-term antifungal therapy often test culture-negative because yeasts are no longer growing on tissue surfaces and, consequently, swabs do not pick up any yeasts for culture. But yeasts remain alive inside tissue cells, and produce chronic symptoms by releasing yeast products that react with the immune system causing inflammation.

Resistant yeasts will grow in swab cultures even if you are taking an antifungal when the specimen was collected. The yeast species should be identified from cultures and tested for antifungal susceptibility to determine the best drug for your bug.

Sensitive but Dose Dependent

Some yeast infections do not improve on the standard dose of 100 mg/day of Diflucan (fluconazole) and are assumed to be resistant. But some of these seemingly resistant infections are caused by yeast species that are "sensitive but dose dependent" (S-DD) and are cured by higher doses of Diflucan that yield higher blood and tissue levels of the drug. Doctors-in-the-know have found that chronic/recurrent candidiasis patients should be treated routinely with 200 mg/day. If that is not effective, then the dose can be increased to the maximal dose of 400 mg/day in a 70-kg (154 lb.) adult with normal renal function (Pfaller et al., 2006).

Note that the newer, second-generation triazoles (Vfend and Noxafil) are prescribed at much higher dosages than the first-generation triazoles (Diflucan and Sporanox). **The higher dosages of Vfend and Noxafil undoubtedly contribute to their greater efficacy**.

The good news is that Diflucan and Sporanox can also be prescribed at higher dosages and have the advantage that their generics are cheaper than the newer drugs. Dose-dependent yeasts that appear resistant to antifungals at low (standard) doses are sensitive at high doses. Be sure to monitor liver function every two weeks while treating with systemic antifungals, especially at high dosages (Step 3).

WARNING Don't follow the bad advice published on the internet telling people to treat yeast infections with four different antifungals one at a time rotating each one every four days. This unscientific protocol selects for yeast strains that become multiply resistant to all four antifungals!

Safety Tip: To avoid the development of resistance, treat yeast infections as soon as possible after symptoms appear with a high enough dose for a long enough time to eradicate the infection. Or, treat with two antifungals simultaneously as explained next.

Combination Antifungal Therapy

Superficial yeast infections that are not cured with a single drug (monotherapy) usually respond to long-term treatment with two antifungals plus steroid cream for inflammation. After symptoms are gone, combination antifungal therapy is switched from daily treatment to weekly suppression for several months to prevent recurrences.

Another advantage of combination antifungal therapy is that it helps to prevent the development of multiply resistant yeast strains. Here's how:

Genes mutate at a rate of about one in a million (10^{-6}). The frequency of a double mutation is the product of both mutation frequencies ($10^{-6} \times 10^{-6} = 10^{-12}$ = one in a trillion). This is a very small number and, therefore, it is unlikely that two different antifungal resistance mutations will occur simultaneously in the same cell. Since combination antifungal therapy will knock down the infection quickly, it is unlikely that resistant mutations will accumulate. If one does occur, it is unlikely to persist once antifungal therapy is discontinued because mutants tend to grow more slowly than normal (wild type) yeasts. Therefore, resistant mutants cannot compete with sensitive yeasts in the absence of antifungals. Infections caused by laboratory-proven resistant yeasts should be treated with two or three antifungals concurrently.

Antifungal Synergy

Combination antifungal therapy results in *synergy*, i.e., joint action that increases each other's effectiveness. Treating difficult-to-cure yeast infections with two different antifungals together, each at standard dosages, is more effective than treating with only one antiyeast drug at a high dosage. Treatment with two antifungals that have different modes of action has great potential for enhanced fungicidal activity (Ghannoum and Elewski, 1999; Weig and Muller, 2001; Vazquez, 2003; Johnson et al., 2004; Walker et al., 2008). Here are some examples of antifungal synergy.

Topical plus Systemic Antifungals

Combining both topical plus systemic antifungals is synergistic because *topical antifungals treat yeast infections on the surfaces of skin and mucous membranes, whereas systemic antifungals treat yeast infections inside tissue cells*. In other words, the topical antifungal treats tissues from the outside in, and the systemic antifungal treats tissues from the inside out. Here are some examples of effective combination regimens:

- Yeast infections of the mouth and esophagus are treated with oral nystatin powder, oral nystatin suspension, or clotrimazole lozenges, plus an oral systemic antifungal such as fluconazole.
- Intestinal candidiasis is treated with oral nystatin powder plus an oral systemic antifungal. Since nystatin is not absorbed into the bloodstream, it only inhibits yeasts in the lumen of the intestine and on the surface of the gut wall, whereas systemic antifungals inhibit yeasts inside the intestinal epithelium. Since each of these antifungals acts at a different site or location in the gut, combination antifungal therapy is ideal.
- Yeast vaginitis is treated with both intravaginal and oral systemic antifungals, plus an anti-inflammatory steroid cream on the vulva.
- Fungal infections of skin, scalp, or nails are treated with an antifungal cream or liquid, plus an oral systemic antifungal, and an anti-inflammatory steroid cream.

Diflucan (fluconazole) plus Lamisil (terbinafine)

A case of oropharyngeal candidiasis caused by a laboratory-proven, Diflucan-resistant *C. albicans* was successfully treated daily with 200 mg of Diflucan (fluconazole) plus 250 mg of Lamisil (terbinafine) taken concurrently (Ghannoum and Elewski, 1999). This combination is synergistic and fungicidal because each antifungal inhibits a different enzyme involved in the biosynthesis of ergosterol, a steroid incorporated into the yeast cell membrane. Taking these two older drugs together is less expensive than taking one of the newer, more effective triazoles such as Vfend (voriconazole) or Noxafil (posaconazole).

Synergism was also observed in laboratory studies of voriconazole plus terbinafine in azole-resistant *C. albicans* isolates from HIV-infected patients with oropharyngeal candidiasis (Weig and Muller, 2001).

Other Synergistic Antifungal Combinations

In addition to synergy between two prescription antifungals, combinations of a prescription anti-fungal drug with another chemical can promote antifungal activity. Here are some more examples of synergistic potentiating combinations (references too numerous to list).

- Azoles combined with one of the following: lactoferrin, ibuprofen, berberine, cyclosporin, amiodarone, baicalein, Hos2 histone deacetylase inhibitor, nicotinamide, honokiol, anti-cholesterol statins, antiarrhythmic amiodarone, curcumin, allicin, statins, or doxycycline.
- Synergy between azoles and statins (Nyilasi et al., 2010) undoubtedly occurs because each drug inhibits sterol synthesis at a different site in the biosynthetic pathway.
- Polyenes combined with curcumin or flucytosine.
- Echinocandins (glucan synthesis inhibitors) with nikkomycin Z, a chitin synthase inhibitor that interferes with fungal cell wall synthesis. This combination is synergistic against Candida isolates in vitro, but their effect in vivo is unknown.
- Cinnamon oil with pogostemon oil.

Such a diversity of substances that act synergistically with antifungals is stunning, and begs for further research to uncover the multiple potentiating mechanisms. Since most reports of antifungal synergy were *in vitro* studies, we must await *in vivo* studies to learn if they have clinical relevance. Randomized, placebo-controlled, double-blind clinical trials are required to determine efficacy and either synergy or antagonism between two different drugs or chemical agents.

Natural Antifungals

Many natural substances have antifungal activity when tested against Candida in laboratory cultures. However, few have been tested on patients in clinical studies for synergy and efficacy against intestinal candidiasis. Some of these natural substances taken orally might be antagonistic and adversely interact with your prescription drugs.

- **Garlic** inhibits Candida in vitro, and probably in the intestine. But when taken by mouth, garlic does not inhibit vaginal Candida colonization (Watson et al. (2013).
- **Caprylic acid** in enteric-coated capsules is helpful against intestinal candidiasis.
- **Undecylenic acid** is effective for treating psoriasis (Ereaux et al., 1949). It is available in an oil-based gel cap or a powder in salt form for oral administration. Undecylenic acid is also used in topical preparations for nail fungus and athlete's foot.
- **Coconut oil** contains the fatty acids lauric acid, caprylic acid, and capric acid that have antifungal activity. It reduces Candida colonization of the intestine (Gunsalus et al., 2015). But don't supplement your diet with coconut oil because it contains 82-90 percent saturated fat. This explains why it is solid at room temperature. By comparison, much maligned butter is 63-64 percent saturated fat. Since saturated fats are damaging to heart health, it is better to use liquid oils for salad dressing and cooking because they contain mainly unsaturated fatty acids. Restrict your use of coconut oil to occasional Thai cooking or baking pie crusts.

- **Essential oils** that have antifungal activity are extracted from spices such as thyme, oregano, mint, cinnamon, patchouli aka pogostemon, salvia, clove, and turmeric.
- **Lactoferrin** is secreted by human cells, inhibits iron uptake in Candida, and acts synergistically with azole antifungals.
- **Aloe vera** leaf gel has antifungal and anti-inflammatory properties.

WARNING

Grapefruit seed extract (GSE) is touted to inhibit bacteria, viruses, fungi, and parasites. I advise against taking GSE because its lack of specificity with respect to the type of pathogens affected could lead to dysbiosis.

Pros and Cons of Natural Remedies

Symptoms of yeast infections drive people to try home remedies before seeking medical help. Arguments for and against self-treatment are presented here.

Pro: *Self-treating with natural antiyeast products saves time and money by avoiding doctor visits, diagnostic tests, and expensive prescription medications.*

Con: If you rely exclusively on herbal remedies to treat yeast infections, you deprive yourself of the benefits of an accurate medical diagnosis and prescription antifungal drugs that are proven effective. You might have another illness that causes the same symptoms as yeast infections. Therefore, you should *test before treating!* If you treat first, and then get tested, your results may come back falsely negative and, consequently, you would be denied appropriate medical treatment. Furthermore, costs for supplements are not covered by health insurance, and some don't even work! Here's one example: Supplements containing cellulase and other so-called yeast-eating enzymes is touted to digest Candida cell walls. However, Candida cell walls don't contain cellulose or the other substrates for these enzymes!

Pro: *Some natural substances have antifungal activity when tested on yeast cultures in the laboratory.*

Con: But where is the evidence that these remedies work against yeast infections in the body? Manufacturers of supplements do not perform clinical studies of their products, and doctors do not publish summaries of their patients' responses to supplements. In addition, it is a conflict of interest for doctors to sell antifungal supplements in their offices.

Pro: *Natural antifungal substances taken by mouth might be helpful for treating yeast overgrowths in the lumen of the intestine.*

Con: But antifungal supplements are probably not absorbed systemically. Therefore, they would not reach yeast infections at other body sites such as the genital area. Natural remedies failed when used to treat a serious type of yeast infection called systemic granulomatous candidiasis (Haas and Stiehm, 1986).

Pro: *Most nutritional supplements are categorized as "generally regarded as safe" (GRAS).*

Con: But some herbal remedies contain pharmacologically active ingredients that can adversely affect the liver or other organs and interact with other natural products or prescription drugs (University of Michigan Health System, 2008). Before taking natural remedies, get approval from your physician or a doctor trained in either Western Holistic Medicine or Eastern Oriental Medicine. *Just because it's natural, doesn't mean it's good for you!*

Protocols

Protocols are given below for yeast infections at various sites in the body. Before searching for the protocol for your specific yeast infection, reread the overview of this ten-step program at the beginning of Part II. Discuss the overview with your doctor and obtain diagnostic testing explained in Step 1. If your test results are positive for Candida infection, then obtain prescriptions for the appropriate antifungal treatment based on your results from antifungal susceptibility testing. If you cannot obtain effective treatment, your yeast condition can progress from uncomplicated, to recurrent, to chronic, to resistant.

Protocol for Uncomplicated Yeast Infections

First-time yeast infections of skin and mucous membranes usually respond to treatment with one of the commonly prescribed antifungals mentioned earlier in this Step 2.

1. Treat first-time superficial yeast infections with either a topical or a systemic antifungal every day for at least one week—ideally for two weeks. While several investigators have reported that a single Diflucan (fluconazole) tablet (150 mg) is adequate for uncomplicated yeast infections, be forewarned: only one day of treatment leads to incomplete cures and frequent relapses.

2. Topical antifungals are available OTC for various yeast infections. But it is better to obtain a medical diagnosis first (Step 1). *Test before treating!* Besides, antifungal medications prescribed by physicians are usually more effective than OTC antifungals.

3. For short-term treatment (one or two weeks) with an oral systemic antifungal, it is not necessary to test for liver function. Monitoring liver enzyme levels is recommended for long-term treatment (Step 3).

4. For symptoms of itching, burning, redness, swelling, and pain on skin, scalp, vulva, penis, scrotum, and anus, also obtain a prescription for an anti-inflammatory cream such as Lotrisone or Mycolog. Both of these creams contain a steroid plus an antifungal (Step 4). Apply cream to irritated surfaces of skin tissue twice a day for a week or so—with the stipulation that your condition is improving. *Always use an antifungal together with a steroid because steroid treatment alone predisposes to yeast infections!*

Protocol for Oral Thrush and/or Candida Esophagitis

1. Treat uncomplicated cases of oral and/or esophageal candidiasis four times daily for two weeks with Mycelex (clotrimazole) lozenges (10 mg troches), or oral nystatin suspension,

or an oral solution of either Diflucan or Sporanox. Ignore the fact that these preparations contain sugar because antifungals only kill growing yeasts, and yeasts need sugar to grow.

2. Let the clotrimazole lozenges dissolve in your saliva, swish the liquid around in your mouth for a minute or so, and then swallow. Repeat four times a day.

Protocol for Nystatin Treatment of Intestinal Yeast Overgrowth

Chronic intestinal candidiasis is initially treated with oral nystatin because it is not absorbed, but stays in the intestine, and is excreted in the feces (as explained in the section on Oral Antifungals for Intestinal Yeast Infections). When improvement reaches a plateau, add an oral systemic antifungal to oral nystatin treatment. If treatment is started with both antifungals together, the "yeast die-off" (Herxheimer reaction) might be overwhelming.

1. Obtain a prescription for a bottle containing 50 million units (MU) of oral nystatin powder USP for suspension, and instruct the compounding pharmacist not to make a suspension. Instead, add 1/8 tsp of powder (500,000 units) to gelatin capsules. Or, you can just add the powder to water and swallow the suspension. Since it tastes terrible, it is preferable to take a capsule containing nystatin powder four times a day.

2. Some health insurance companies do not cover oral nystatin powder and, consequently, some doctors will only prescribe oral nystatin tablets (500,000 units). The disadvantage with nystatin tablets is they do not dissolve because nystatin is not water soluble. That is why nystatin should be taken in powder form four times a day to distribute it evenly throughout the intestinal contents. If you cannot obtain oral nystatin powder, then fill your prescription for oral nystatin tablets and buy a pill crusher from the pharmacy. Rinse off the red dye, dry the tablet with a paper towel, crush it, suspend the powder in some water, swish the suspension around in your mouth, and swallow. Repeat four times per day.

3. If you experience a worsening of symptoms at the beginning of nystatin therapy, follow the Protocol for Preventing "Yeast Die-off" below.

4. Once you have overcome "yeast die-off" and can tolerate the full dose of nystatin powder four times daily, continue treatment for a few weeks or months—with the stipulation that you are improving.

5. Eventually, you may reach a plateau where you stop improving because nystatin only kills yeasts in the lumen of the intestine where the food and feces are located. At that point, add the systemic antifungal Diflucan to the nystatin treatment in order to kill the yeasts located inside the epithelial cells in the gut wall. A combination antifungal protocol with both oral nystatin and oral fluconazole is necessary to kill yeasts at both sites in the intestine. Follow the Protocol for Systemic Antifungal Treatment below.

Protocol for Preventing "Yeast Die-off"

A paradox of antifungal therapy is that symptoms may get worse at the beginning of treatment. Colloquially called "yeast die-off," the medical term for this phenomenon is the *Jarisch-Herxheimer reaction*. It was named after two physicians who discovered this drug side effect around 1900 while using mercury to treat syphilis. (No antibacterial drugs were available at that time.)

The Herxheimer reaction is observed during treatment of other infections as well. Exacerbation of symptoms during antimicrobial therapy is attributed to the release of toxic substances from killed microorganisms, or immune reactions to antigens released from dead pathogens. Antifungals cause yeasts to burst (*lyse*), and leak antigens into infected tissues. Then these Candida antigens react with anti-Candida antibodies and WBCs producing inflammatory symptoms.

The good news is "yeast die-off" means the antifungal is working. "Yeast die-off" is worse in people who are allergic to Candida and have high levels of allergic IgE anti-Candida antibodies, and in people who have heavy yeast overgrowths with high levels of anti-Candida IgA, IgG, and IgM antibodies. If you fall into these categories and are experiencing a worsening of symptoms since you started antifungal treatment, follow this protocol to decrease "yeast die-off."

1. Decrease the antifungal dosage. For example, open a capsule and take just a pinch of nystatin powder equal to the amount on the tip of a toothpick. Suspend it in a little bit of water, swish it around your mouth and swallow.

2. If no reaction occurs, increase the amount of nystatin powder or suspension at the next dose. If "yeast die-off" symptoms are severe, stop taking the antifungal for a day or so until you regain your equilibrium.

3. Gradually increase the amount taken each time according to your tolerance until you reach the prescribed dosage. Continue taking nystatin powder for several weeks or months—as long as your symptoms are decreasing.

4. Eventually, you will reach a plateau where improvement stops because nystatin only kills yeasts located in the lumen of the intestine. When you reach this plateau, add a systemic antifungal to your nystatin treatment to kill yeasts inside epithelial cells in the gut wall.

5. You may go through "yeast die-off" again when you add a systemic antifungal to the nystatin therapy because the two antifungals kill yeasts in different parts of the intestine. Nystatin works only in the lumen whereas systemic antifungals kill yeasts growing inside the epithelial cells of the gut wall.

6. **WARNING** *Don't start antifungal therapy with a loading dose of Diflucan* (fluconazole) *that is double the standard dose* because the "yeast die-off" symptoms might overwhelm you. Instead, crush the fluconazole tablet and take only a pinch to start with as with the nystatin powder.

7. If the "die-off" is really bad, take the systemic antifungal at bedtime so that side effects occur while you are sleeping. Or, take it every other day until symptoms diminish. Then gradually increase the dose according to your tolerance up to the prescribed daily dosage. Don't take antifungals if you have something important to do during the day. *You are in charge of your recovery!*

8. Treat with this combination of nystatin powder plus a systemic antifungal for weeks or months until symptoms resolve—with the stipulation that the treatment is working. It is

not possible to predict how long to continue daily combination antifungal therapy. The longer you've been sick, the longer it takes to achieve a cure.

Protocol for Systemic Antifungal Treatment

1. Diflucan (fluconazole) is the treatment of first choice for superficial yeast infections. Generic fluconazole is less expensive. Obtain a bottle containing 30 tablets of 200 mg. Take one tablet a day for difficult-to-cure, recalcitrant yeast infections.

2. *Don't start with a loading dose of Diflucan* (fluconazole) *that is double the standard dose* because the "yeast die-off" symptoms might overwhelm you. If your symptoms worsen at the beginning of systemic antifungal therapy, follow the Protocol for Preventing "Yeast Die-off" above.

3. Obtain a blood test for liver function before starting systemic antifungal treatment to make sure that your liver enzyme levels are okay. Repeat this test every two weeks and follow the other precautions in Step 3 while taking a systemic antifungal.

4. Treat with a systemic antifungal for weeks or months until symptoms resolve—with the stipulation that the treatment is working. It is not possible to predict how long daily antifungal treatment will take to achieve a cure.

5. Also treat itching, burning, redness, swelling, and pain on skin, scrotum, vulva, and anus with a cream such as Lotrisone or Mycolog. They contain an antifungal plus an anti-inflammatory corticosteroid as explained in Step 4.

6. After symptoms resolve, switch from daily treatment to weekly maintenance (also called suppression, prophylaxis, and prevention) with a systemic antifungal or both a topical and a systemic antifungal for about six months to prevent yeast infections from returning.

7. If you have suffered for a long time from chronic or recurrent yeast infections and you have other allergies, get skin tested for Candida allergy and, if positive, get treated with subcutaneous immunotherapy (hyposensitization) allergy shots following the procedures described in Step 5.

8. Follow the rest of the guidelines in Steps 6 through 10 to identify and avoid risk factors that predispose you to develop yeast infections, and prevent recurrences if you have an unavoidable risk factor.

Protocol for Nystatin Enemas to Treat Intestinal Candidiasis

The standard treatment for intestinal candidiasis includes concurrent administration of oral nystatin and oral fluconazole as described in protocols above. Recently, new information about treatment of Candida infection of the gut has been published in patient testimonials in an online Candida Forum at www.curezone.org. Several "long-haul" Candida patients reported finally achieving success using nystatin enemas after failing to achieve a cure using long-term treatment of their intestinal yeast infections with oral antifungals. (Thanks to Jorge Dieguez for sending me these testimonials. Jorge Dieguez currently facilitates a Candida support group for patients who speak Spanish on Facebook called "Candidiasis Cronica Grupo de Soporte.")

While such anecdotal testimonials are usually dismissed by academic skeptics as insignificant because the reports did not result from controlled clinical studies, nevertheless, patient observations are important preliminary findings that deserve to be studied further. For this reason, I mention these Candida patient testimonials here because I feel they are believable. I comment on their significance after I describe their protocol for nystatin enemas below.

1. **Cleansing enemas**. Perform several enemas each with a liter of boiled or distilled water containing sea salt until no more feces are expelled. Various ingredients added to the water were tried.

2. **Retention enema**. Then mix 500,000 units of nystatin powder with 4 ounces of aloe vera juice in a small enema bottle. Various ingredients added to the nystatin suspension were tried. Inject this suspension into the rectum with legs up in the air allowing the suspension to penetrate by gravity as deeply as possible into the intestinal tract. Retain the nystatin enema as you continue with your normal daily tasks. You won't feel any urgency to expel it after having used enemas to cleanse the colon.

Many patients have testified that they improved with this nystatin enema protocol better than with anything else they tried. They reasoned that by cleansing the intestine first and then applying the nystatin, the antifungal would make direct contact with yeasts attached to the intestinal wall and would not be diluted by mixing with food and fecal matter in the lumen as happens when nystatin is taken orally.

My Comments on Nystatin Enemas

As a researcher, I would like more information before I recommended nystatin enemas. I need to know what treatments Candida patients used before trying the nystatin enema. Did they take an oral nonabsorbed polyene antifungal along with an oral systemic antifungal and probiotics concurrently? Which ones? Dosage? How long?

Or did Candida patients first try over-the-counter remedies? The main problem patients face is that many doctors will not even test patients for intestinal yeast overgrowth let alone treat them because of the controversy over the yeast syndrome. So, Candida patients have to take charge of their own health and find a way to self-treat. If they were unable to obtain prescription oral antifungals, and instead took herbal supplements by mouth, which are not as effective, then that would explain why treatment via the oral route did not work.

Then I wonder where they got the nystatin for the enemas? Did patients continue treating with antifungals via the oral route while also performing nystatin enemas? How long did the apparent cure last? Did patients follow a weekly maintenance protocol after using the nystatin enemas to prevent recurrences?

The only way to state definitively that nystatin enemas are effective is for a large number of patients to enroll in a controlled clinical study in which subjects were distributed into two groups, with one group following the treatment protocol and the other group following a placebo-controlled protocol.

In addition to nystatin, I would like to suggest that a mepatricin preparation be studied as an enema since it is already available as a urological preparation to be used as an instillation. It effectively treated nonbacterial prostatitis at 40 mg daily (Bacigalupo et al., 1983). Mepatricin is a macrolide polyene antifungal, similar to nystatin and amphotericin B. Polyenes taken by mouth are not absorbed systemically. Therefore, they just treat yeasts in the lumen and on the intestinal wall surface, but not yeasts inside intestinal epithelial cells. Mepatricin instilled into the urinary bladder is useful for treating disorders of the urethra, prostate, and bladder, as well as chronic pelvic pain syndrome and benign prostatic hyperplasia (Chapter 3). Mepatricin is also available in enteric coated tablets for oral administration.

Until research studies of nystatin enemas are carried out, analyzed by statistical methods, and the results published in medical journals, Candida patients are on their own. Most cannot get proper medical care because of the negative opinion papers published by academic skeptics who claimed that the yeast connection and the candidiasis hypersensitivity syndrome do not exist (see the Hall of Shame in Chapter 6). Even though their negative position statements lacked scientific data, they nevertheless influenced physicians in community practices to deny patients treatment for Candida-related illnesses.

Protocol for Recurrent Vulvovaginal Candidiasis and Vulvodynia

If your first-time vaginal yeast infection responded to short-term antifungal therapy, but then came back afterwards, it is because you were not treated with antifungals long enough to eradicate the intracellular infection. After finishing your prescription for antiyeast treatment, residual nongrowing (*latent*) but living yeast cells remain inside your vulvar and vaginal epithelial tissue cells and serve as *a reservoir for reinfection.* Therefore, it is important for you to remember that: *Once you have been infected with Candida, your tissues are in a different state.*

The next time you are exposed to a risk factor that predisposes you to develop candidiasis, you will likely develop a yeast infection *at the same place* as the previous infection because yeasts are still lurking there entrenched in your tissues. The second and subsequent yeast infections may be more difficult to cure, and will require longer and more intensive treatment as described in the protocol below.

The key is long-term treatment with both topical and systemic antifungals. The topical antifungal treats from the outside of the tissue inward, and the systemic antifungal treats from inside the body outward. Latent intracellular yeast infections require longer treatment times to be eradicated presumably because the yeasts are not growing. Yeasts must be growing in order to be killed by antifungals.

To cure recurrent vulvovaginal yeast infections, you need antifungal susceptibility testing to distinguish between these two possibilities: One is that your yeast condition is recalcitrant, but your yeast strain is sensitive to antifungals. The second is that your yeast strain is dose dependent (sensitive at high doses) or resistant to antifungals (unresponsive even to high doses). You also need to determine if your vaginal yeast infections are stimulated by estrogen, or you have other predisposing risk factors.

1. After receiving a medical examination and results from diagnostic testing (Step 1 and Chapter 2), ask your gynecologist or primary care physician to prescribe:

   • A bottle of 30 fluconazole tablets each containing 200 mg. Dosage depends on your weight, your previous response to therapy, and the antifungal susceptibility of your yeast strain as determined by testing. Diflucan (fluconazole) is the treatment of first choice for superficial yeast infections. Generic fluconazole is less expensive. Take 200 mg a day for difficult-to-cure yeast infections.

   • A tube of Terazol 7 vaginal cream, or nystatin vaginal cream, or 14 capsules each containing 600 mg of boric acid powder for intravaginal administration. You can buy boric acid capsules online (Boricap or BalanceLovely).

   • A tube of Lotrisone or Mycolog cream each containing an anti-inflammatory corticosteroid and an antifungal (Step 4).

   • A tube of lidocaine ointment in a hypoallergenic preparation

2. Apply lidocaine ointment to the vulva, and wait until the area turns numb.

3. Then insert an intravaginal antifungal. Repeat every night for seven to 14 days.

4. Apply a cream containing both a corticosteroid and an antifungal to the urogenital and anal area twice a day for a week or as needed until inflammation is gone.

5. You might find coconut oil soothing when applied to the vulva. Coconut oil has weak antifungal activity.

6. Treat daily and concurrently with a vaginal antifungal and oral fluconazole (a systemic antifungal) until symptoms resolve.

7. Get a blood test for liver function before you start and every two weeks while you are taking a systemic antifungal (Step 3).

8. Daily treatment with this combination protocol should be continued long enough to eradicate the yeast infection and allow your tissues to heal—with the stipulation that you are improving. Every patient is different. So, you might improve in two days, two weeks, or two months.

   • If your symptoms have not decreased after about two weeks, a different systemic antifungal will have to be substituted based on the test results from your yeast culture, species identification, and antifungal susceptibility testing.

   • If your yeast is resistant to fluconazole, a swab culture will be positive for yeast even if collected during treatment.

   • If your yeast infection is latent inside your epithelial cells, it will not be on the tissue surface, and a swab culture will be negative. A vulvar scraping is more likely to yield a positive culture (Chapter 2).

9. Return to see your doctor every two weeks while being treated with a systemic antifungal to discuss your response to therapy, obtain a blood test for liver function, and request refills of your prescriptions.

10. After resolution of symptoms, switch from daily treatment to weekly maintenance with both an oral systemic and a vaginal antifungal together (Step 10). Rosa et al. (2012) found that maintenance with one oral fluconazole tablet (150 mg) a week for six months prevented

recurrences of vulvovaginal candidiasis if the yeast was susceptible to fluconazole. If your recurrent vaginal yeast infections are estrogen-dependent, follow monthly cyclic prophylaxis by using oral plus vaginal antifungals for three to seven days at ovulation (midcycle) each month (Step 10).

Protocols for Resistant Non-*albicans* Candida Infections

What should you do if you have a recalcitrant yeast infection that does not respond to standard antifungal therapy? Your condition may be caused by either a dose-dependent yeast or a resistant yeast. Therefore, your doctor must obtain a specimen to be cultured and at the same time also order tests to identify the yeast species and determine its antifungal susceptibility.

Treatment of "Candida long-haulers" with recalcitrant dose-dependent or resistant yeasts usually requires long-term therapy with high doses of an oral systemic antifungal plus a second or third antifungal used concurrently. Based on the results from susceptibility testing, a newer, more expensive, and more effective antifungal might be necessary.

Some Candida species are naturally less susceptible to azole antifungals (Nyirjesy et al., 1995; Sobel et al., 2003; Ray et al., 2007; Iavazzo et al., 2011; Mendling and Brasch, 2012). Other species exhibit dose-dependent susceptibility, whereas still others are completely resistant to azoles even at the highest doses. Infections caused by non-*albicans* Candida species are successfully treated with higher doses of either commonly used antifungals, or synergistic combinations of antifungals, or a newer more effective antifungal.

1. *C. albicans* causes most yeast infections, and most *C. albicans* isolates are susceptible to Diflucan (fluconazole). That is why *Diflucan is the drug of first choice for candidiasis.* However, occasional strains of *C. albicans* are resistant to Diflucan. Laboratory-proven, Diflucan-resistant *C. albicans* strains are treated daily for two to four weeks with Vfend (voriconazole) or Noxafil (posaconazole), no more than 28 days; or with nonazole antifungals; or with combinations of antifungals such as oral tablets of Lamisil (terbinafine 250 mg) plus Diflucan (fluconazole 200 mg) because these two are synergistic together (Ghannoum and Elewski, 1999).

2. *C. glabrata* is the second most common yeast species causing infections. Its incidence increased significantly after broad-spectrum antifungal usage became widespread (Fidel et al., 1999). *C. glabrata* vaginitis that is resistant to oral Diflucan (fluconazole) can be treated with intravaginal boric acid suppositories (Chaim, 1997; Sobel and Chaim, 1997; Sobel et al., 2003) or another vaginal antifungal or combination (such as nystatin, or terconazole, or flucytosine plus amphotericin B) together with oral Sporanox for seven to 14 days.

   Vaginitis caused by *C. glabrata* and other Candida species resistant to azole antifungals is successfully treated with vaginal cream containing flucytosine plus amphotericin B (Horowitz, 1986; Fidel et al., 1999; Sobel et al., 2003; San José et al., 2012). Flucytosine (1 g) is compounded from oral Ancobon or Ancotil and used together with amphotericin B (100 mg) formulated in lubricating jelly for an 8 g delivered dose daily for 14 days (White et al., 2001).

   Mendling and Brasch (2012) suggested treating *C. glabrata* vaginitis with one of these antifungals: vaginal boric acid, vaginal flucytosine, oral Diflucan (fluconazole) 800 mg/day for 2 to 3 weeks, or oral Noxafil 2 × 400 mg/day plus either vaginal ciclopirox olamine or vaginal nystatin for 15 days. Following eradication of the infection, vaginal nystatin (100,000 U) cream can be used for weekly maintenance.

3. **C. krusei, C. tropicalis, and C. parapsilosis** are often naturally resistant to Diflucan (fluconazole) as well as to flucytosine (Fidel et al., 1999). *C. krusei* is also resistant to Sporanox (Mendling and Brasch, 2012), but can be successfully treated with oral Vfend (voriconazole), intravenous amphotericin B, or an echinocandin (micafungin, caspofungin, or anidulafungin). Amphotericin B and echinocandins are administered through intravenous infusion due to their limited oral bioavailability. Vaginitis caused by these three Candida species can be treated with vaginal boric acid, or vaginal flucytosine plus another antifungal. Lamisil (terbinafine) is highly active against *C. parapsilosis* (Ryder et al., 1998). However, different isolates of this species may be resistant. That is why culture, identification, and antifungal susceptibility testing should be performed routinely with difficult-to-cure yeast infections in "Candida long-haulers."

Protocol for Genital Yeast Infections in Men

1. First-time yeast infections of the skin on the penis, scrotum, and groin area, called "jock itch," are treated with the Protocol for Uncomplicated Yeast Infections given above. If a skin scraping is cultured and observed under the microscope, often it is learned that this infection in men is caused by Malassezia yeasts, which are treated with topical antifungal agents such as selenium sulphide lotion, sodium thiosulphate with salicylic acid, propylene glycol, zinc pyrithione shampoo, or ciclopirox olamine solution.

2. Recurrent genital yeast infections of the skin are more difficult to cure and require more intensive treatment because residual nongrowing (*latent*) but living yeast cells remain inside epithelial skin tissue cells and serve as *a reservoir for reinfection*. Therefore, long-term treatment with both a topical and a systemic antifungal together are needed. Ask your urologist, dermatologist, or primary care physician to prescribe:

   - a tube of Lotrisone or Mycolog cream, which contains an antifungal plus an anti-inflammatory corticosteroid
   - a bottle of 30 fluconazole tablets containing 200 mg depending on the antifungal susceptibility of your yeast strain, and other factors discussed earlier here in Step 2 in General Considerations for Prescribing Antifungal Drugs.

3. Treat daily with the cream and the oral systemic antifungal until symptoms resolve—with the stipulation that you are improving. Daily treatment should be continued long enough to eradicate the yeast infection, eliminate the inflammation, and allow your tissues to heal.

4. If your symptoms have not decreased after about two weeks, a different antifungal will have to be substituted based on the antifungal susceptibility testing of your yeast strain.

5. Return to see your doctor every two weeks while being treated with a systemic antifungal to discuss your response to therapy, obtain a blood test for liver function, and refills of your prescriptions.

6. After resolution of symptoms, switch from daily treatment to weekly prophylaxis with one day of treatment with both topical plus systemic antifungals for six months to prevent recurrences.

7. Circumcision is sometimes performed to cure recurrent balanitis, but surgical removal of the foreskin can lead to other problems in adult men. Therefore, it should be performed only if long-term, daily, intensive medical treatments have failed.

8. If symptoms of prostatitis or urethritis were not helped by antibacterial antibiotics, prolonged courses of high-dose antifungals often provide relief. Urologists are just beginning to recognize the existence of fungal infections in the male urogenital tract, but treat only with monotherapy. It is more effective to treat with both a topical and a systemic antifungal concurrently using this protocol.

   - **Diflucan** (fluconazole), an oral systemic antifungal, when taken at high dosages (400 mg twice daily) produced a positive response in 70% of men with chronic prostatitis/chronic pelvic pain syndrome (Dybowski, 2013). Similar results were reported by Kotb et al. (2013).

   - **Mepatricin** is a urological preparation for installation that effectively treated nonbacterial prostatitis at 40 mg daily (Bacigalupo et al., 1983). Mepatricin is a macrolide polyene antifungal similar to nystatin or amphotericin B; polyenes are not absorbed systemically and only treat tissue surfaces. Mepatricin is useful for treating disorders of the urethra, prostate, and bladder, as well as chronic pelvic pain syndrome and benign prostatic hyperplasia (Chapter 3).

Checklist for Preventing Relapses

Here are key issues relating to treating and preventing recurrent yeast infections.

1. Based on clinical observations, how soon do relapses occur after discontinuing antifungal treatment? Are relapses in women estrogen-related?

2. Based on antifungal susceptibility testing, is the yeast condition recalcitrant to treatment, yet the yeast strain is sensitive to antifungals? Or is the yeast dose dependent or resistant to antifungals?

3. Collect a scraping of skin or vulva (not a swab).

4. Send specimen to the laboratory for microscopy, yeast culture, yeast species identification, and antifungal susceptibility. Culture medium should contain antibacterials (such as penicillin and streptomycin) to inhibit bacteria in the specimen that prevent yeasts from growing in culture.

5. For vulvodynia, also test with a drop of diluted trichloroacetic acid (TCA) and look for acetowhite lesions.

6. Based on results from scratch and intradermal tests, does the patient have Candida allergy and poor immunity to Candida?

7. Based on test results and clinical failure with older antifungals, choose a newer fungicidal antifungal or a combination of two antifungals that are synergistic for long-term treatment followed by weekly maintenance after resolution.

How to Obtain Medical Treatments for Candidiasis

If you were originally denied testing and treatment by your insurance network doctor, and you were forced to get tested by a doctor outside your network, and your Candida test results are positive, take copies back to your primary care physician and/or specialist, and ask for treatments explained in Steps 2 to 5 that are appropriate for your case. Your positive test results are the justification your doctor needs to prescribe necessary medical treatments for Candida infection and Candida allergy. Your health insurance should cover the treatments prescribed by your doctor. *Don't take "No!" for an answer.* It is your fundamental right to receive medical care for an illness. Fight for it!

What to Do If You Are Denied Medical Care

If your doctor still refuses to treat you for yeast infections and yeast allergies even though your tests results are positive, file a complaint with the grievance committee of your health insurance. You can file the complaint yourself without a lawyer. But you have to provide justification. Base your request for treatment on your:

- positive laboratory test results
- clinical signs and symptoms
- physical examination
- history of yeast infections (indicating your susceptibility to candidiasis)
- recent risk factors predisposing you to develop a yeast infection
- the scientific information in this book (include photocopies of relevant pages with reference citations in your complaint)

If your request for treatment is denied by the grievance committee, escalate your complaint to the appeals committee of your health insurance. If you are denied again, the next step is to hire a lawyer, and contact your state department of health and/or your state insurance commissioner. In California, you can file complaints against your physician and/or your health insurance company at this link: https://www.insurance.ca.gov/01-consumers/101-help/index.cfm.

You Need a Plan

If you are disabled by chronic candidiasis so much so that you cannot work and, therefore, do not have health insurance, *you need a plan* in order to obtain medical care. Here are some suggestions:

1. Search for free clinics where you pay according to your income.

2. Apply for state disability or federal Medicaid. You will need diagnostic test results proving you have chronic candidiasis, plus a letter from your physician. Cite information and

reference citations in this book plus your positive test results and evidence about your clinical condition to justify treatment.

3. If you have a prescription for an antifungal from your doctor, but cannot afford it, contact the pharmaceutical company. Many have programs for people with low incomes and provide free drugs.

4. There are people in your life who are financially capable of helping you. Swallow your pride. Ask them for help. Ask a friend, relative, or acquaintance to lend you money, or give you credit card privileges to be used to get testing and treatment.

5. Obtain effective antiyeast medications for Candida infection and immunotherapy for Candida allergy. Make lifestyle changes to avoid risk factors and prevent recurrences. Get your health back.

6. Get a job that provides health insurance, or purchase health insurance. Get off disability. Pay back the loan. Start living a normal, healthy, independent life again. How does that plan sound?

Conclusions of Step 2
Antifungal Treatments

You now know what antifungals are available for treating superficial yeast infections and protocols for the different types of yeast infections. You have learned that a timely diagnosis is essential for a favorable outcome. You don't have to *"Learn to live with it."* The longer you have been sick, the longer it will take you to get better. Obtain prompt treatment with high enough doses of both topical and systemic antifungals for long enough times to eradicate yeast infections. *Nip it in the bud!*

In addition to receiving antifungal treatments (Step 2), following precautions (Step 3), and using anti-inflammatory drugs (Step 4), some cases also require allergy shots of Candida antigen (subcutaneous injection immunotherapy) to decrease allergic reactions to Candida and increase immunity to Candida (Step 5).

After your symptoms have resolved, *the key to preventing recurrences is identifying your risk factors and assiduously avoiding all of them* (Step 6). Pay special attention to unrecognized risk factors such as certain medical conditions and lifestyle behaviors (Step 7), follow the Candida diet (Step 8), and take probiotics and prebiotics (Step 9). If you have recurrent or chronic yeast infections, or you have an unavoidable risk factor, follow weekly prophylaxis (Step 10).

To achieve a permanent cure, follow *all* of the medical care and self-help guidelines in this ten-step program while under a physician's supervision. Right now, take the time to reread Chapter 1, plus the chapter about your yeast condition, and the overview to my ten-step program. Promise yourself that you will follow *all* of the recommendations and steps that are relevant to your yeast condition. Only then will you be able to break free from your cycle of cure and relapse, and prevent future episodes.

STEP 3

Precautions

ORAL SYSTEMIC ANTIFUNGALS ARE ROUTINELY prescribed for superficial yeast infections of skin and mucous membranes in otherwise healthy people with normal WBC counts. Candida patients who have only minor medical problems are safely treated long-term with systemic antifungals and they experience few side effects if the precautions described here are followed.

However, systemic antifungals can pose risks for children, the elderly, women who are pregnant or breast-feeding, and people with liver disease or other serious conditions. Systemic antifungals can produce birth defects in the fetus (*teratogenesis*) if taken during the first three months of pregnancy when the baby is undergoing major developmental changes (Molgaard-Nielsen et al., 2013). Therefore, you should discuss safety issues and medical conditions that require special precautions with your physician. She or he is responsible for informing you about the potential risks and benefits of all prescription drugs and medical procedures.

Drugs can produce many different adverse reactions. But just because it has been reported that some people develop certain side effects while on systemic antifungals does not mean that you will develop these same side effects. People who have yeast infections in addition to other medical conditions can have symptoms related to their illnesses and unrelated to the antifungal drug. Therefore, don't deny yourself effective antifungal treatment out of fear of developing side effects.

Be your own advocate. Read the patient information that comes with your prescriptions as well as information about safety precautions and side effects posted on websites of pharmaceutical companies. Ask your doctor and pharmacist any questions you may have about medications.

Possible adverse reactions to systemic antifungals are discussed below under these headings: contraindications, liver toxicity, drug interactions, "yeast die-off," and other side effects. Follow the safety tips given for each topic.

Contraindications

> **WARNING**
>
> In rare cases, Candida patients being treated with an oral systemic antifungal can develop severely reddened, blistering, itching, or peeling of skin (*exfoliative skin disorders*), called Stevens-Johnson syndrome or *toxic epidermal necrolysis*. If you experience severe skin eruptions or other severe symptoms after starting a new drug, discontinue taking it, call your doctor, and go to the emergency room or, if you are having trouble breathing, call 911 for an ambulance.

Allergic reactions to drugs can be life threatening. Symptoms include an itchy rash, throat swelling, difficulty breathing, and low blood pressure. Death could follow within minutes after taking the drug. Allergic airway constriction and other serious drug reactions are referred to as *anaphylactic shock*.

Safety Tips: If you have allergic tendencies, or you have had a serious drug reaction in the past, take the first dose of a new medication in your doctor's office, or in the presence of someone who can call 911. Carry an EpiPen with you so you can inject epinephrine at the first sign of anaphylaxis, and then obtain emergency medical help.

It is not possible to predict if you will have a bad reaction to a drug. But if you do, follow the safety tips just mentioned above. At the next office visit with your doctor, ask the nurse to write a warning about this drug at the top of your medical file. This drug is now *contraindicated* for you. That means you should not take it again. Obtain a prescription for a different drug that is effective for treating your medical condition.

Liver Toxicity

In a recent study of side effects from long-term fluconazole therapy, Davis et al. (2019) did not even mention liver problems! The most common adverse effects were dry lips (*xerosis*; 16.9%), hair loss (*alopecia*; 16.1%), and fatigue (11.3%). Of the 64 patients who experienced adverse effects, 42 (65.6%) required a therapeutic intervention such as dose reduction, discontinuation, or switching to a new antifungal.

Based on this study and the clinical experience of a multitude of physicians, we could conclude that monitoring liver function during long-term treatment with fluconazole or other antifungals is not necessary. But, out of an abundance of caution, I do recommend testing for liver function every two weeks or as frequently as ordered by the attending physician.

> **WARNING**
>
> In rare cases, some Candida patients develop liver toxicity (*hepatotoxicity*) during long-term systemic antifungal therapy, especially if the antifungal interacts with other drugs being administered concurrently. Typical symptoms of liver toxicity are yellow skin (*jaundice*), yellow eyeballs, brown urine, yellow stools, nausea, and extreme fatigue. This condition is diagnosed by abnormally high blood levels of bilirubin and liver enzymes (transaminases, ALT, AST, SGOT, SGGT, SGPT, and alkaline phosphatase).

A slight increase in liver enzymes while taking a systemic antifungal is expected because more enzymes are needed to metabolize the drug. The liver responds by synthesizing higher amounts of detoxification enzymes. When the drug is discontinued, liver enzyme levels usually return to normal. Hence, the elevation of liver enzyme levels is *reversible*.

Some people with heavy intestinal yeast overgrowths have elevated liver enzymes **before** starting antifungal treatment. This elevation in liver function is attributed to the production of alcohol, acetaldehyde, and other yeast metabolites during intestinal sugar fermentation by yeasts. After starting antifungal therapy, yeast numbers and alcoholic fermentation are reduced, and liver enzymes usually return to normal.

If you have intestinal yeast overgrowth and are also infected with HIV or a hepatitis virus, or you have liver cirrhosis or liver cancer, you are more likely to develop hepatotoxicity during systemic antifungal therapy.

Safety Tips: To avoid developing hepatotoxicity during long-term systemic antifungal therapy, follow these recommendations:

- Obtain a blood test to measure your liver enzyme levels **before** starting a new drug.
- Test your liver function every two weeks while taking fluconazole or another systemic antifungal. **The upper limit of normal is 34. Liver injury is indicated by a value over 102.** If your liver enzyme levels are dangerously elevated, your doctor will tell you to discontinue taking that drug.
- Repeat this test every two weeks while under treatment. It is not necessary to monitor liver function during short-term treatment (one or two weeks).
- Go back for follow-up doctor visits every two weeks to discuss your response to antifungal therapy, obtain another blood test for liver enzyme levels, and request refills of your prescriptions for daily treatment or weekly suppression.

Drug Interactions

> **WARNING**
>
> Systemic antifungals inhibit liver enzymes and cytochrome P450 isoenzymes (CYP 2C9 and CYP 3A4), which are involved in detoxification in the liver. Therefore, if you are on systemic antifungal therapy, and are taking other drugs, herbs, or supplements, or drinking alcoholic beverages, these other substances might not be broken down by the liver and might build up to toxic levels in the blood (Bressler, 2006).

Safety Tips:

- Don't drink alcohol while taking systemic antifungals. If you want to have an alcoholic drink in the evening, don't take a systemic antifungal that morning.
- Don't consume grapefruit or grapefruit juice. They contain furanocoumarin derivatives that inhibit hepatic and intestinal cytochrome P450 isoform CYP 3A4, resulting in elevated concentrations of drugs that could reach toxic levels.
- Obtain approval from your doctor before taking other drugs, herbs, or supplements together with a systemic antifungal drug.
- Don't take a systemic antifungal with a drug known to interact with it. Metabolism of other drugs might be inhibited, and they might rise to dangerous levels. Drug interactions are listed on the websites of pharmaceutical firms. For Diflucan, go to: www.pfizer.com/products/rx/rx_product_diflucan.jsp.
- To learn if any of your regular drugs interact with fluconazole or another systemic antifungal drug, go to the websites listed below, and follow their instructions to find a drug combination that does not interact with cytochromes:
  - www.drugs.com/drug_interactions.html
  - www.webmd.com/interaction-checker/default.htm
  - http://bioinformatics.charite.de/supercyp/index.php?site=drug_interaction_checker (Preissner et al., 2010).
- Discuss your search results from these websites with your medical doctor. If you decide to take a drug that interacts at the cytochrome protein (CYP) level with a systemic antifungal, I suggest that your doctor decreases the dosage and frequency of the interacting drug, and take the systemic antifungal such as fluconazole at full dosage (200 mg/day).
- While taking a drug known to interact with your systemic antifungal, go back for frequent follow-up doctor visits to monitor your liver enzymes as well as blood levels of other drugs.
- For example, if you are taking a systemic antifungal with an antihypertensive, measure your blood pressure twice a day. If it goes down too much, lower the dose of the blood pressure medicine according to your doctor's directions. One approach is simply to halve the dosage of the drug you take every day to prevent it from accumulating to high levels.
- Likewise, if you are taking a diabetes drug, measure your blood sugar level several times a day. If it goes down too much, lower the dose of the diabetes medication according to your doctor's directions.
- After resolution of your yeast symptoms on daily antifungal therapy, start weekly antifungal maintenance and restore your other medications to their regular daily dosages.

The Food and Drug Administration encourages you to report adverse side effects of drugs and drug interactions. Call 1-800-FDA-1088 or fill out the form at www.fda.gov/Safety/MedWatch/default.htm.

"Yeast Die-off"

> **WARNING**
>
> A common complication of antifungal therapy is the development of minor skin rashes and/or other symptoms at the beginning of treatment. These symptoms are due to allergic and other immune reactions to yeast antigens released from Candida cells killed by the antifungal. The medical term for these immune reactions is the Herxheimer reaction. Colloquially, these symptoms are called "yeast die-off."

Safety Tips:

- Follow the Protocol for Preventing "Yeast Die-off" (Step 2).
- If you have a severe reaction to a drug, ask your doctor to perform a patch test on your skin to test for allergy to that drug. If there is no reaction, the initial rash was probably "yeast die-off," and you can restart oral therapy with that same drug but at a lower dose. Take your first dose in a doctor's office with an epinephrine syringe or EpiPen in hand so the doctor can administer life-saving first aid, and call 911 if necessary.
- Or, obtain a prescription for a different antifungal, and start with a low dose. If the same skin rash or other reaction occurs with a new antifungal, you are probably experiencing "yeast die-off." Don't self-treat with drugs purchased on the internet. Your response to therapy needs to be monitored by a physician.

Other Side Effects

> **WARNING**
>
> Don't take a systemic antifungal on an empty stomach. If you notice black specks in your stool, discontinue the drug, and call your doctor. These specks may be little blood clots from microbleeds in the intestinal wall.

Safety Tips: Follow the specific directions for each systemic antifungal drug about whether to take just before meals, with food, or after a meal. Candida patients who also have serious illnesses often develop dangerous adverse reactions to long-term treatment with systemic antifungals and, therefore, they must be monitored very closely by their attending physicians (Benitez and Carver, 2019).

Conclusions of Step 3
Precautions

Now you know what precautions to follow when taking oral systemic antifungals. Discuss these safety tips with your doctor, and design a management strategy for your individual case.

STEP 4

Anti-inflammatory Drugs

SYMPTOMS OF YEAST INFECTIONS ARE due primarily to the inflammatory response by the body that produces itching (*pruritus*), burning (*inflammation*), redness (*erythema*), swelling (*edema*), peeling (*excoriation*) of dead epithelial tissue, and discharge (*exudate*). These clinical signs and symptoms of yeast infections are treated with anti-inflammatory drugs in addition to antifungals.

Even though azole antifungals have some anti-inflammatory activity (Steel et al., 2008), people with severe inflammation also require anti-inflammatory therapy to promote healing. If only antifungals are used, the active yeast infections may resolve and swab cultures will become negative, but the tissues may remain inflamed.

Inflammation of skin, vulva, penis, scrotum, and anus is treated with corticosteroid cream concurrently with antifungals. In some cases, other anti-inflammatory drugs such as antihistamines, leukotriene receptor antagonists, or nonsteroidal anti-inflammatory drugs (NSAIDs) may be helpful for mucosal inflammation, which cannot be treated with corticosteroids.

Corticosteroids

Corticosteroids are large lipid molecules (*steroids*) secreted by the outer portion (*cortex*) of the adrenal gland. *Hydrocortisone* (*cortisol*) is a natural corticosteroid produced by the body. Both natural and synthetic steroids have anti-inflammatory activity, and are used to treat itching, burning, redness, swelling, and peeling of skin. Creams containing steroids are not used on mucous membranes.

Creams containing 1.0% hydrocortisone are sold OTC, but this concentration is too low to be effective. Higher concentrations of hydrocortisone (2.5%, 5%, or 10%) in creams are available by prescription. They can be prepared in a nonirritating hypoallergenic ointment by a compounding pharmacist. Synthetic steroids such as betamethasone are more active and, therefore, are formulated at a lower concentration (0.05%).

Ideally, superficial candidiasis should be treated with topical as well as systemic antifungals together with a corticosteroid cream. Unfortunately, sometimes women do not use the steroid cream when it is prescribed along with antifungals for yeast vaginitis. When I ask them why, women usually say because it stings. I reply, *"Of course it is going to sting because you are already inflamed. But one thing's for sure—if you don't use anti-inflammatory cream, it won't work!"*

The solution to this problem is to apply Lidocaine anesthetic ointment first to numb the vulva. Then insert the antifungal cream intravaginally, and then apply the anti-inflammatory steroid cream on the vulva. Brand names Lidocaine-HC Top and LidaMantle HC contain lidocaine plus hydrocortisone for treating pain and inflammation.

> **WARNING**
>
> Corticosteroids combat inflammation by suppressing WBC activities, which are needed to fight infections. Therefore, don't use a corticosteroid cream by itself, i.e., unopposed by antifungals, because corticosteroids decrease local immunity in tissues and increase your susceptibility to candidiasis

Safety Tip: Always treat yeast vaginitis with an antifungal at the same time as using a corticosteroid cream on the vulva. Opposing a corticosteroid with an antifungal prevents the steroid from making your yeast infection worse. An ideal protocol for yeast vaginitis is daily treatment with an oral systemic antifungal agent like Diflucan (fluconazole), plus an intravaginal antifungal, along with Mycolog cream or Lotrisone cream on the skin of your vulva. Each of these creams contains an antifungal plus a steroid, offering the best of both worlds.

> **WARNING**
>
> If you have a latent viral infection such as genital Herpes, don't use corticosteroid cream unopposed by an antiviral.

Safety Tip: Ask your doctor to prescribe an antiviral agent to be used at the same time as the steroid cream.

Doctors often warn that corticosteroid cream thins tissues. For this reason, they do not routinely prescribe corticosteroid cream along with Diflucan (fluconazole) for vulvovaginal candidiasis. But topical corticosteroid preparations are designed for short-term treatment of highly symptomatic allergic and inflammatory conditions. It is unlikely that tissue thinning will occur during only a week or two of steroid treatment. Besides, even if tissues do become thin, they will regenerate and plump back up when use of a steroid cream is discontinued. Therefore, women should not be deprived of relief offered by corticosteroid cream while being treated for vulvovaginal candidiasis. Ditto for men being treated for "jock itch" or balanitis caused by penile candidiasis.

Antihistamines

First-line treatment of inflammation caused by yeast infections is a steroid cream added to the antifungal regimen. If you tested positive for IgE-mediated Candida allergy, adding topical and systemic antihistamines to the steroid plus antifungal protocol might help.

Benadryl (diphenhydramine) is an oral antihistamine available OTC. It makes you sleepy, so take it only at bedtime. Benadryl cream can be applied to the vulva for allergic inflammation caused by Candida. Nonsedating oral antihistamines are available OTC such as Zyrtec (cetirizine) and Claritin (loratadine). Neves et al. (2005) reported success treating recurrent vulvovaginal candidiasis with Zyrtec every day plus Diflucan (fluconazole) weekly for six months.

Antihistamines have a good safety record when taken with other drugs. However, interactions between OTC and prescription drugs can occur. For example, men with enlarged prostates might experience urinary problems if they take systemic antihistamines. Search for potential drug interactions and side effects online and discuss your findings with your physician and pharmacist.

Antihistamines provide only temporary relief from allergic reactions to Candida, and must be taken every day. To achieve a lasting cure for Candida allergy, obtain long-term antifungal therapy plus allergy shots of Candida antigen called subcutaneous injection immunotherapy (Step 5).

Leukotriene Receptor Antagonists

Accolate (zafirlukast) and Singulair (montelukast) are leukotriene receptor antagonists taken orally for asthma. Accolate was also used successfully to treat severe recurrent vulvovaginal candidiasis (White et al., 2004). Other anti-inflammatory drugs used for asthma include corticosteroid inhalers, beta-adrenergic blocking agents, and mast cell stabilizers.

NSAIDs

Symptoms of superficial candidiasis can be reduced and recovery can be promoted by nonsteroidal anti-inflammatory drugs such as ibuprofen and benzydamine that block the production of prostaglandin or inhibit its action in the body. These two preparations are used topically.

- **Ginenorm (ibuprofen isobutanolammonium)** formulated as a vaginal douche, effectively treats vulvar and vaginal inflammation (Milani and Iacobelli, 2012). It induced a rapid reduction in redness, swelling, itching, and burning caused by vulvovaginitis in 10 clinical studies. Ibuprofen is an effective anti-COX1 and anti-COX2 inhibitor found in Advil, Motrin, and Nuprin. In addition to its anti-inflammatory activity, ibuprofen surprisingly also has antifungal activity because it acts synergistically with fluconazole (Pina-Vaz et al., 2000) and reverses fluconazole resistance (Costa-de-Oliveira et al., 2012). Skin rashes due to yeast infections could be treated with ibuprofen compounded by a pharmacist with an azole antifungal in a hypoallergenic ointment.
- **Benzydamine hydrochloride** is a locally acting analgesic drug used to treat inflammatory conditions of the mouth, throat, vulva, and vagina. Over 40 controlled clinical trials of

benzydamine were reviewed by Mahon and De Gregorio (1985) who found that benzydamine applied topically was safe and effective for relieving pain.

Other treatments prescribed for vulvar pain include:

- **Capsaicin** (Steinberg et al., 2005).
- **Anticholinergics** (Ekgren, 2000).
- **Lidocaine ointment** is used by some women who have vulvodynia to numb their vulva
  and allow vaginal penetration and intercourse without pain.

Conclusions of Step 4
Anti-inflammatory Drugs

Anti-inflammatory medications are safe and provide relief from itching and burning when used
together with antiyeast therapy. Take advantage of the best that modern medicine has to offer.
Work with your physician to find the right combination of drugs for your specific case. *Don't
suffer in silence!*

Candida Allergy

Definitions

The terms *allergy* and *hypersensitivity* both refer to overreactions of the immune system that harm the host. But the specific definitions of these two terms vary depending upon their mechanisms of action, diseases produced, diagnostic tests used, and treatments needed.

Allergy is defined as a reaction between an IgE antibody and a specific antigen that causes inflammation.

- *Antigens* are mainly proteins. Some antigens are polysaccharides. Antigens induce the synthesis of antibodies, and then react with their specific antibodies.
- *Immunogens* are substances that produce immune responses. *Immunogen* is another term for antigen.
- *Allergens* are antigens that induce the synthesis of IgE antibodies, and then react with their specific antibodies.
- *Antibodies* are globulin proteins found in blood that participate in immune reactions. An antibody is called an *immunoglobulin* (*Ig*). The different classes of immunoglobulins include IgG, IgM, IgA, and IgE.
- *Immune complexes* are formed when antibodies combine with their specific antigens.
- *Atopic* describes people who are genetically predisposed to develop allergies.
- *Allergic inflammation* is caused when allergens combine with their specific IgE antibodies attached to WBCs (*mast cells* or *basophils*). This triggers the WBCs to release chemical mediators such as histamine, leukotrienes, and prostaglandin E2 that cause inflammation.

Hypersensitivity refers to four types of exaggerated immune reactions to foreign substances causing tissue damage (types I, II, III, and IV). All four hypersensitivity reactions produce symptoms during yeast infections.

- *Type I immediate hypersensitivity* refers to reactions between IgE antibodies and allergens that occur within 15 minutes of exposure. The hallmark symptoms of allergic inflammation include itching, burning, redness, and swelling of skin and mucous membranes. These are also symptoms of yeast infections. Allergy is diagnosed by skin tests (scratch or prick tests and intradermal tests), and by a blood test called the *radioallergosorbent test* (RAST). Allergic diseases mediated by IgE antibodies include asthma, anaphylactic shock, immediate food reactions, hives, dermatitis, hay fever, tissue swelling, and allergic candidiasis. Candida allergy is treated with antifungals to reduce the load of Candida allergens in the body plus anti-inflammatory drugs and immunotherapy (allergy shots of Candida extract).

- *Type II hypersensitivity,* known as *cytotoxicity*, occurs when cells within the body are destroyed by antibodies, with or without complement.
- *Type III hypersensitivity,* called the *Arthus reaction*, involves the deposition of immune complexes in vascular walls.
- *Type IV delayed hypersensitivity* refers to reactions between T cells and allergens that occur one to two days after exposure. Delayed hypersensitivity is diagnosed by the intradermal skin test with Candida antigen, which detects these three conditions: poor immunity (*anergy*), normal immunity, and hyperreactivity to Candida. Diseases involving abnormal T cell responses to Candida include Candida allergy and asthma, poor immunity to Candida, and Candida-associated autoimmune endocrinopathy.

All four types of hypersensitivity to fungal antigens play roles in the pathogenesis of fungal infections (Fidel and Huffnagle, 2005). Fungal diseases occur in immune deficiency states as well as in hyperinflammatory conditions.

Incidence

According to the American Academy of Allergy, Asthma, and Immunology (AAAAI, 2011), about 15% of people have allergic disease. About 10% of people with asthma and rhinitis have immediate hypersensitivity to yeasts (Gumowski et al., 1987). Although the incidence of allergy to Candida is low in the general population, women who experience frequent episodes of yeast vaginitis often have high levels of allergic anti-Candida IgE antibodies (references reviewed in Crandall, 1991a; download from www.yeastconsulting.com). These women have defective suppressor T cells that cannot down-regulate IgE levels (Witkin, 1985; Witkin et al., 1988; Witkin, 1991).

Disturbances in T cell dampening result in *allergic breakthrough* in which people become sensitized to many substances (Katz, 1978). It is like the "tipping point," or the "straw that broke the camel's back." When a threshold of allergens and stressors is reached, people become "allergic to everything."

Allergens can be foods, inhalants, toxins, microbial antigens, and other substances. *Stressors* can be infectious, nutritional, emotional, and hormonal factors. Thus, allergic breakthrough explains why people with allergic tendencies and chronic yeast infections often become "universal reactors." Continue reading the rest of this ten-step program to learn how to lower your total load of allergens and stressors.

Candida Allergy

Because candidiasis is both an infection and an allergy to the infective agent, both conditions must be treated. Candida infection is treated with antifungals (Step 2 and 3). Candida allergy is treated with anti-inflammatory drugs (Step 4), and immunotherapy (described here in Step 5). Recurrences are prevented by following Steps 5 through 10.

Allergy to Candida is a predisposing risk factor for candidiasis. Therefore, if you suffer from repeated yeast infections, you should be skin tested for allergies to Candida, baker's yeast (*Saccharomyces cerevisiae*), molds, fungi, foods, and other common allergenic substances.

Candida allergy makes symptoms of yeast infections worse, slows improvement while on anti-fungal therapy, weakens immunity to Candida, and increases susceptibility to recurrences. Here's how.

Candida Allergy Worsens Your Yeast Infection Symptoms

When you have a yeast infection, your WBCs synthesize antibodies against Candida in all immu-noglobulin classes including IgM, IgG, IgA, and IgE. Their synthesis is under genetic control. More IgE antibodies against Candida are produced every time you have another yeast infection. Anti-Candida IgE antibodies produce allergic reactions by combining with Candida antigens and triggering the release of histamine and other mediators of allergic inflammation. Histamine causes blood vessels to dilate and leak serum and RBCs into tissues producing swelling, redness, burn-ing, and itching. These are the hallmark symptoms of allergic inflammation as well as of yeast infections. Hence, allergic inflammation amplifies symptoms of yeast infections.

Candida Allergy Slows Your Response to Antifungal Therapy

When you start antifungal treatment, some yeasts are killed. They burst (lyse) and release anti-gens, which react with anti-Candida allergic IgE antibodies, liberating histamine and other chem-icals that exacerbate inflammation caused by the infection. This allergic reaction to dead yeast products is called "yeast die-off." You can prevent severe "yeast die-off" by initially taking only a small amount of antiyeast medication, and then gradually increasing the dosage until you reach the standard dose according to the protocol in Step 2. Allergic reactions to yeast products are treated with oral antihistamines, steroid creams, and/or other anti-inflammatory drugs discussed in Step 4.

Candida Allergy Weakens Your Immunity to Candida

Allergic reactions to Candida release histamine and prostaglandin E2, both of which suppress WBC-mediated immunity (Witkin et al., 1988; Witkin, 1991; Crandall, 1991a; download from www.yeastconsulting.com). Two mechanisms are involved:

- Histamine inhibits the migration of neutrophils to the site of infection. Neutrophils are WBCs that are called the *first line of defense against candidiasis* because they are always ready and able to attack Candida cells. For this reason, they are referred to as *innate immunity*. Because histamine inhibits neutrophil migration, pus is not present in tissues infected by Candida. *Pus* is an accumulation of dead WBCs produced only in tissues infected by bacteria.

- Histamine and prostaglandin E2 inhibit proliferation of T cells, another type of WBC. T cells are called the *second line of defense against candidiasis* because they must first encounter Candida antigens, multiply, and produce a clone of T cells with Candida receptors on their surfaces before they can attack Candida cells. For this reason, they are referred to as *adaptive immunity*.

Candida Allergy Increases Your Susceptibility to Recurrences

Since Candida allergy inhibits both the first and second lines of defense against Candida, your Candida immunity is suppressed. As a result, each time you have another yeast infection, more anti-Candida IgE antibodies are produced. They react with Candida antigens, and release more histamine, which makes yeast infections worse, and creates a self-perpetuating cycle of cure and relapse (Crandall, 1991a; download from www.yeastconsulting.com).

Diagnostic Tests for Allergy and Immunity

Serious, life-threatening allergies and immune defects are usually identified during childhood. Adult Candida patients with chronic/recurrent candidiasis should obtain Candida-specific tests for allergy and immunity in addition to the full battery of other allergens. Ask your primary care physician to write a referral to an allergist-immunologist summarizing your case and requesting that you be tested for Candida allergy and Candida immunity.

Allergy is diagnosed by RAST blood tests, scratch (prick) tests, and intradermal tests. Immunity to Candida is measured by the Candida intradermal test and follow-up blood tests that measure T lymphocyte functions.

RAST Blood Tests

RAST stands for *radioallergosorbent test*. It measures IgE antibodies in blood. RAST is less sensitive than skin tests for allergy and, therefore, can yield false-negative results. RAST is useful for testing people who are extremely allergic and might have bad reactions to skin testing.

Scratch (Prick) Tests

Allergy is usually detected by board certified allergists/immunologists. They perform allergy testing by scratching or pricking the skin on your back multiple times with a sterile pin, and then placing a drop of Candida antigen or another allergen on different individual scratches. Many substances can be tested on your back during one office visit. If you have yeast problems, get tested with the full battery of allergens including *Candida albicans*, baker's yeast (*Saccharomyces cerevisiae*), molds, fungi, foods, pollen, animal dander, dust mites, etc.

Don't take an antihistamine or corticosteroids for two to seven days prior to skin testing because these anti-inflammatory drugs will cause false-negative results.

A positive reaction in skin tests for allergy looks like a mosquito bite. The red, itchy bump is called a *wheal* and *flare*. A wheal is a bump caused by swelling (*edema*) due to an accumulation of liquid (*serum*) in the skin. The flare is redness (*erythema*) due to an accumulation of RBCs. Itching (*pruritus*) is caused by histamine released into the tissue.

Allergic reactions are scored after 15 minutes on a scale from zero to 4+. The larger the reaction, the higher the level of IgE antibodies against a specific allergen. Reactions to allergens are compared to two controls: saline is scored as zero, and histamine is scored as 4+. A positive reaction (1+ to 4+) to Candida after 15 minutes indicates allergy (type I immediate hypersensitivity). False-positive and false-negative test results can be obtained.

The scratch (prick) test is generally considered safe, and it is unlikely that you will develop a systemic allergic reaction (anaphylactic shock) after being tested.

Safety Tips: Stay in the allergist's office for 20 minutes after your test results are recorded. If your throat starts to swell up or you have trouble breathing, epinephrine should be injected and 911 should be called.

Intradermal Tests

Results from scratch tests are confirmed by further testing with intradermal injections. The intradermal test is performed by allergists-immunologists, ear, nose, and throat (ENT) physicians, and by doctors who are members of the American Academy of Environmental Medicine. The intradermal is the most sensitive test for detecting allergy to Candida and other allergens. It also measures immunity to Candida (type IV delayed hypersensitivity) as well as monitoring responses to immunotherapy (Pepys, 1984).

The skin test antigen, CANDIN®, is the only *Candida albicans* extract-based skin testing antigen for intradermal injection licensed by the FDA to assess cell-mediated hypersensitivity to *Candida albicans*. The intradermal test is performed by injecting allergen just under the top layer of skin on your forearm.

> **WARNING**
>
> Systemic reactions can occur with skin test antigens and in certain individuals these reactions may be life-threatening or cause death. Immediate hypersensitivity local allergy reactions can include itching, swelling, pain and blistering at the test site occurring 15-20 minutes after administration. Necrosis is possible. Systemic reactions to CANDIN have not been observed, however all foreign antigens have the remote possibility of causing Type 1 anaphylaxis and even death when injected intradermally. Pharmacologic doses of corticosteroids during two weeks of therapy prior to testing may suppress the delayed skin test response.

Safety Tips: Physicians using the skin test antigen, CANDIN®, must have facilities, equipment, and medication such as epinephrine and oxygen available in the event of a serious systemic response. Patients receiving beta-blocking drugs may be refractive to the usual dose of epinephrine, in the event that epinephrine is required to control an adverse allergic reaction. Patients should be observed for at least 20 minutes following the administration of a skin test.

After receiving the Candida intradermal injection, draw a circle around the injection site with black ink, and don't wash it off during the next few days! Observe the injection site after 15 minutes and during the next two days for these reactions:

- **IgE-mediated allergy** (type I immediate hypersensitivity) is scored after 15 minutes. A positive reaction is a red, itchy bump (wheal and flare). The reaction happens immediately because allergic IgE antibodies circulate in blood and are present in skin and mucous membranes.
- **T cell immunity** (type IV delayed hypersensitivity) is scored after one to two days. A positive reaction is a hard, flesh-colored bump called an *induration* about 1/8 inch in diameter. It is due to an accumulation of T cells under the skin. The reaction is delayed because T cells migrate slowly out of the blood to the injection site.

Since the intradermal is scored after 15 minutes and then again after two days, there are four possible results: +/–, –/+, +/+, and –/–. Each is explained below and summarized in Table 8.

The normal scores are negative (–) for Candida allergy and positive (+) for Candida immunity. These results are abbreviated –/+. Most people have no immediate reaction because they are not allergy to Candida, and they have a positive delayed reaction because they have good T cell-mediated immunity against Candida.

A score of +/– is diagnostic for the candidiasis hypersensitivity syndrome in which allergy to Candida is coupled with poor T cell immunity (*anergy*) to Candida. IgE-mediated allergy to Candida prevents the development of an induration because histamine released from allergic reactions inhibits migration of T cells to the injection site.

Some people with chronic candidiasis have no immediate reaction in the intradermal, but a severely red and painful delayed reaction (–/++++). It may be one to three inches in diameter, and cause blisters that last for weeks, or cell death (*necrosis*) may occur. This *hyperimmune* reaction or hyperreactivity to Candida is due to abnormal T cells that produce inflammation instead of fighting yeast infections. Many women with vulvodynia exhibit hyperimmunity to Candida and overproduce proinflammatory cytokines.

Table 8. Test Results for Candida Allergy		
Tests with Candida Antigen	**Results**	**Interpretations**
RAST blood tests (*radioallergosorbent test*)	positive	IgE allergy to Candida
	negative	Not allergic to Candida or false-negative due to low sensitivity of test
Scratch (prick) and Intradermal tests after 15 minutes	positive (red, itchy bump = *wheal and flare*)	IgE allergy to Candida = *type I hypersensitivity*
	negative	not allergic to Candida or antigen too dilute
Intradermal test after 2 days	positive (flesh-colored bump = *induration*)	strong T cell immunity against Candida = *type IV hypersensitivity*
	negative	poor T cell immunity against Candida (*anergy*) or antigen too dilute
	strongly positive (large red bump; may blister; long lasting; rarely necrosis)	hyperreactivity of T cell to Candida or antigen too concentrated

Blood Tests for Immune Function

If your delayed reaction to Candida in the intradermal test is negative indicating poor immunity (*anergy*) to Candida, ask your allergist/immunologist to order these follow-up blood tests to measure your immune function against Candida:

- IgM, IgA, IgG, and IgE antibodies against Candida in blood
- T lymphocyte counts
- T lymphocyte proliferation in response to Candida antigen and mitogens

- T lymphocyte production of leukocyte migration inhibitory factor when induced by concanavalin A
- Blood levels of pro-inflammatory and anti-inflammatory cytokines

Invalid Tests for Food Allergy

People with the candidiasis hypersensitivity syndrome usually complain about food-related symptoms. True food allergies are mediated by IgE antibodies that are detected by skin tests and RAST.

WARNING

The following tests are not valid for evaluating IgE-mediated food allergy (Boyce et al., 2010): basophil histamine release, lymphocyte stimulation, facial thermography, gastric juice analysis, endoscopic allergen provocation, hair analysis, applied kinesiology, provocation neutralization, cytotoxicity assays, electrodermal test (Vega), mediator release assay, and the LEAP diet (Lifestyle Eating and Performance).

False-positive results from these tests may lead to unnecessary dietary restrictions, and delay in obtaining accurate diagnoses. Because these tests are not covered by health insurance, paying for them out of pocket just adds to a Candida sufferer's burden.

Safety Tips: Be an informed consumer of health care. Just say *"No!"* to unreliable tests.

Non-IgE-mediated Food Sensitivities

The following procedures were approved by Boyce et al. (2010) for diagnosing non-IgE-mediated reactions to foods: double-blind placebo-controlled food challenge, contact dermatitis patch testing, atopy patch test, intradermal testing, lymphocyte activation assay, endoscopic biopsy, and food-specific IgG testing.

However, contradictory results from IgG_4 testing for food sensitivities have been reported. Some doctors claim that IgG_4 antibodies against foods cause delayed symptoms (Mullin et al., 2010). Other doctors warn that blood tests for IgG_4 against foods lack diagnostic value (Shakib, 1987; 1988; Stapel et al., 2008; Antico et al., 2011). Since positive results may not correlate with symptoms, Stapel et al. (2008) proposed that high IgG_4 antibody levels just indicate the foods that you eat frequently.

Elevated levels of food-specific IgG_4 antibodies probably indicate "leaky gut syndrome." If more food antigens pass from the gut into the bloodstream, higher levels of antibodies against those foods will be synthesized. Only food challenges confirm the diagnoses of food sensitivities.

Treatment of Candida Allergy

If you have chronic or recurrent candidiasis, and your skin test results were positive for Candida allergy, you have the candidiasis hypersensitivity syndrome. CHS is treated with antifungals

(Steps 2 and 3), anti-inflammatory drugs (Step 4), and allergy shots of Candida extract plus your other allergens (this Step 5).

Avoidance of Candida Allergens

The key to preventing allergic reactions is to avoid contact with allergens. For example, if you are allergic to an external (*exogenous*) allergen like certain foods, don't eat them. But since Candida grows inside your tissues, it is an internal (*endogenous*) allergen and more difficult to avoid. You can lower the number of Candida cells in your body by treating yeast infections with systemic antifungals and preventing recurrences with allergy shots.

Allergy Shots Help Fight Candida Infections ·

Called *subcutaneous injection immunotherapy*, allergy shots work by:

- decreasing allergic symptoms
- boosting immunity to Candida
- preventing relapses of candidiasis

These findings were reported by early researchers in numerous controlled clinical studies that were reviewed by Odds (1979), Truss (1983), Kroker (1987), and Crandall (1991a; download from www.yeastconsulting.com). Evidence that allergy shots of Candida antigens are effective in fighting yeast infections have been corroborated by recent studies by Rigg et al. (1990), Truss et al. (1992), Moraes et al. (2000), Palma-Carlos et al. (2002), Neves et al. (2005), Weissenbacher et al. (2009), and van de Veerdonk et al. (2010). While all these studies focused on vulvovaginal candidiasis, their results apply broadly to yeast infections at other body sites in both men and women.

How Allergy Shots Work

It may seem counterintuitive to inject substances you are allergic to into your body. However, injection immunotherapy has been proven effective as shown by all of the controlled studies mentioned in the above paragraph. Furthermore, the mechanisms of action of injection immunotherapy are understood. Allergy shots are injected under the skin (subcutaneously) where Candida does not normally reside. Your immune system sees the vaccine as a foreign invader, and T cells respond to injected Candida extract by dividing and forming a clone of T cells that have receptors on their surfaces that recognize Candida. These activated T cells:

- induce the synthesis of IgG antibodies that block IgE-mediated allergic reactions
- attack Candida cells and help prevent relapses
- secrete cytokines, such as interleukin-10, that are anti-inflammatory

After receiving injection immunotherapy, fewer allergic reactions occur, less histamine is released, less inflammation is produced, and less suppression of cell-mediated immunity occurs. Often, a negative delayed hypersensitivity reaction to Candida converts to a positive reaction indicating restored T cell-based immunity to Candida (Garner et al., 1990).

> **WARNING**
>
> If you had an abnormally large delayed reaction in the Candida intradermal test, you have Candida hyperreactivity and should not receive allergy shots of Candida extract because they will make your Candida hyperimmunity worse.

Safety Tips: You can safely follow the other guidelines in this ten-step program to overcome chronic candidiasis.

Protocol for Allergy Shots

The standard Candida antigen used for allergy skin testing and subcutaneous injection immunotherapy is purified from *C. albicans* because this species causes most yeast infections. If you are infected with a different yeast, please be assured that *C. albicans* antigen will be effective for testing and treatment because it shares common antigens with other Candida species.

Candida antigens for skin testing and injected vaccines are available from ALK-Abello, Allergy Laboratories, AllerMed, Antigen Laboratories, Greer, Hollister-Stier, Nelco and other laboratories.

Candida allergy shots are injected subcutaneously (s.c.) ¼ inch under the skin in your upper arm. A s.c. allergy shot should provoke a red itchy bump like a mosquito bite after 15 minutes. The diameter of the wheal and flare reaction should be less than a dime. If it is larger, the Candida antigen is too concentrated. If you have no reaction, the Candida vaccine is too dilute, and the allergy shot will be ineffective.

> **WARNING**
>
> If the antigen is too concentrated, anaphylaxis and death might occur after an allergy shot.

Safety Tips: Before the first s.c. shot is given, dilutions of Candida vaccine should be tested intradermally starting with the lowest concentration to find a safe concentration to start immunotherapy. You should remain in the doctor's office for 20 minutes after each allergy shot.

In the beginning of immunotherapy, you may experience flu-like symptoms or itchy eyes later in the day. Don't get discouraged by minor systemic reactions to allergy shots. People who are highly allergic to Candida and develop these reactions are the very ones who need immunotherapy the most. After several injections at low antigen concentrations, these systemic reactions will disappear and the concentration of antigen in your shot can be increased based on the size of the reaction to the s.c. injection on your arm.

You should receive allergy shots two or three times a week. At each visit, your allergist will ask about your reaction to the last shot. If your reaction was larger than a dime, then the next shot should be decreased. If there was little or no reaction, the vaccine concentration can be increased.

The goal of immunotherapy is to gradually increase the antigen concentration in successive injections until you reach the maintenance dose. Then booster shots of the maintenance dose will be needed about once a month or so. The immunization process takes about six months before any symptom improvement occurs. However, the decrease in allergic reactions and increase in immunity are long lasting.

> **WARNING**
>
> *Don't give yourself allergy shots at home.* If your doctor gives you syringes and vials of antigen to self-inject at home, that means the antigen concentration is probably too low to cause an adverse reaction and, hence, probably too low to be effective!

Before you start receiving allergy shots, consider asking the allergist to prepare two vaccines: one with Candida alone, and the second with all of your other allergens. Get two allergy shots at each visit, one in each arm. This allows you to monitor your response to the Candida vaccine. Doing a separate shot for Candida is important if your strongest allergic reaction in the battery of scratch tests was, for example, 4+ to dust mites, but your reaction to Candida was only 1+. If all your allergens were in one vaccine, your reaction to dust mite antigen would overshadow your reaction to Candida. This would prevent you from increasing Candida antigen to an effective concentration. After you reach the maintenance dose for both vaccines, they can be pooled, and you would get only one booster shot thereafter.

If you also test positive for allergy to baker's yeast (*Saccharomyces cerevisiae*) and molds, your allergist will add them to your vaccine. In addition to allergy shots, you should also avoid moldy places and follow a yeast- and mold-free diet. For example, no indoor living plants, hayrides, composting, or raking autumn leaves! No pizza, beer, or blue cheese salad dressing! Ask your allergist how to avoid molds at home, work, and out-of-doors.

After six to 12 months of immunotherapy, you will reach the maintenance dose. At that point, you can try doing a food challenge by adding back yeasty and moldy foods to your diet one at a time. You may not have allergic reactions to these forbidden foods and beverages. You may also convert from negative to positive delayed hypersensitivity in the Candida intradermal indicating that your T cell-mediated anergy to has been restored to good immunity to Candida.

Sublingual Immunotherapy

Allergy treatment with oral vaccines (*sublingual immunotherapy*) is proven safe and effective for environmental allergens such as molds, pollen, animal dander, dust mites, etc. Some doctors recommend placing drops of Candida allergen under your tongue as a low-dose oral immunotherapy for people with hyperreactivity to Candida (Kroker, 2011a, b). However, no controlled clinical study of sublingual immunotherapy for Candida has been published. Since Candida is a normal inhabitant of the mouth, intestine, vagina, and skin, it is doubtful that a dilute solution of Candida antigen placed under the tongue would be effective.

NovaDigm Vaccine

A new fungal immunotherapeutic vaccine for the treatment of recurrent vulvovaginal candidiasis has been studied. One intramuscular dose of NovaDigm Vaccine (NDV-3A) increased the percentage of symptom-free patients at 12 months to 42% in vaccinated patients vs. 22% patients who received a placebo (Edwards et al., 2018). Until the efficacy of this vaccine is improved, you can help prevent recurrences of yeast infections by following the ten-step program in this book. Allergy shots of Candida antigen has been proven effective in a multitude of controlled clinical studies of recurrent vulvovaginal candidiasis (as explained above under the heading, Allergy Shots Help Fight Candida Infections).

T.O.E. Vaccine

In the early 1900s, before antifungal drugs became available, physicians used to treat fungal infections with a fungal vaccine to boost immunity. Called T.O.E., this vaccine contained antigens from the molds, Trichophyton, Oidium, and Epidermophyton. Oidium is the old name for Monilia, which is the old name for Candida. This vaccine was found to be effective based on empirical evidence.

Unproven Treatments for Allergy

The efficacy of the following procedures and products is not established: provocation and neutralization; supplements touted to boost the immune system; and homeopathic oral drops sold at health food stores. The FDA banned enzyme-potentiated desensitization in 2001. Be an informed consumer of health care. Just say "No" to untested treatments.

How to Obtain Candida Allergy Testing and Treatment

Testing and treatment of Candida allergy used to be standard medical practice until 1986 when the AAAI published an opinion paper—**lacking data**—but declaring that the candidiasis hypersensitivity syndrome (CHS) does not exist (see Hall of Shame in Chapter 6). Their paper ignored all of the scientific studies demonstrating the role of Candida allergy in chronic candidiasis. Yet, it persuaded practicing allergists to discontinue testing and treating Candida allergy out of fear of losing their medical licenses.

Likewise, researchers have been dissuaded from studying Candida allergy because they were afraid of ruining their professional reputations and not getting their grants funded. As a result of the influence of this uninformed 1986 AAAI opinion paper, untold numbers of Candida sufferers have been denied necessary medical care and continue to suffer. Since 1986, when patients with symptoms of CHS contact allergists, they are refused skin testing for Candida allergy and treatment with shots of Candida allergen even though these tests and treatments have been proven effective in many controlled clinical studies (cited above).

The good news for patients is that allergists can now resume skin testing and injection immuno-therapy with Candida because the 2011 version of the renamed AAAAI website tells visitors not to rely upon any position statements of theirs more than five years old. Thus, without admitting they were wrong, this organization of allergists has essentially retracted its 1986 position state-ment denying the existence of the CHS.

The bad news is the Candida controversy continues. If you contact an allergist on your own, you will probably be denied testing and treatment for Candida allergy. That is why you need the backing and support of the M.D. who has been treating your yeast infections. Show this book to your doctor, and ask for a written referral to an allergist-immunologist summarizing your case and requesting that you be given scratch (prick) skin testing for Candida allergy and intradermal testing for Candida immunity.

Then, when you call the allergist's office for an appointment, explain that you have a written referral to be skin tested for Candida from your physician. If the allergist's receptionist says, *"Doctor does not test for Candida,"* go back to your physician and ask for another referral. Also call customer service at your health insurance company, file a complaint about the allergist in your network who denied you evidence-based medical care, and ask for a referral to an allergist who does test and treat Candida allergy.

It is medical malpractice for physicians to refuse to comply with referrals from other physicians requesting evidence-based medical care for their patients. This dereliction of professional duty in denying patients needed treatment violates a professional standard of care and causes injury to patients.

Conclusions of Step 5
Candida Allergy

If you suffer from chronic or recurrent episodes of candidiasis, obtain diagnostic skin testing for Candida allergy. Positive results justify immunotherapy. Since Candida allergy is a major con-tributing risk factor for recurrent Candida infections, testing and immunotherapy for Candida are essential for overcoming the candidiasis hypersensitivity syndrome.

The key to preventing allergic reactions is avoiding allergens. Overcoming the candidiasis hyper-sensitivity syndrome is accomplished by treating Candida infections with topical and systemic antifungals (Steps 2 and 3), and treating Candida allergy with anti-inflammatory drugs (Step 4) and subcutaneous injection immunotherapy (this Step 5). Additional preventive measures are discussed in Steps 6 to 10.

STEP 6

Avoid *All* Risk Factors

EVEN IF PEOPLE HAD FULL cooperation from their doctors, yeast infections would still be difficult to overcome because there are so many risk factors that predispose people to develop candidiasis. To prevent recurrences, you must first identify and then avoid *all* of your individual susceptibility factors. If some predisposing conditions are unavoidable, protect yourself against repeated attacks of candidiasis by following Steps 6 through 10.

The importance of identifying and avoiding your specific risk factors is exemplified by the following estimation of the future incidence of recurrent vulvovaginal candidiasis. Denning et al. (2018) warned that the current high prevalence of women with this disease will rise from 138 million to 158 million worldwide by 2030 unless better solutions are found and the quality of medical care is improved for affected women. These authors also estimated that the substantial suffering and loss of productivity caused by recurrent yeast disease would lead to an economic burden in high-income countries of from USD14 to 39 billion annually. So, read this Step 6 carefully to learn what your risk factors are and then read the rest of this ten-step program to learn how to prevent recurrences of yeast infections.

Red Flag Warning

Candidiasis is a red flag signaling a disturbance in the healthy, balanced state (*homeostasis*) of your body. Usually, there is no mystery about the cause. Most yeast infections are caused by antibacterial antibiotics.

But there are dozens of other contributing factors that predispose people to develop yeast infections. Some are quite elusive. Hence, you and your doctor must become detectives to identify your individual susceptibility factors. Then together you and your doctor can develop a plan for avoiding *all* of them. Initially, your doctor will evaluate your condition by:

- performing a physical examination
- taking a detailed medical history

- ordering diagnostic tests for Candida infection and allergies to Candida and other substances
- ruling out diabetes, HIV infection, low WBC counts, and other conditions known to predispose to candidiasis

The good news is that once your test results are in, your doctor will probably know the underlying causes of your yeast infections.

Risk Factors

There are, unfortunately, a large number of predisposing conditions that make people susceptible to develop yeast infections. Not only that, predisposing risk factors are also cumulative. The more risk factors you have, the greater the chance you will develop a yeast infection. Each time you are exposed to a risk factor for candidiasis, the number of yeasts in your body increases. You may not develop a yeast infection right away after the first exposure because there is a lag before yeasts start to grow. But the next time you are exposed to a risk factor, the number of yeasts on your skin or mucous membranes may increase past a threshold, and you will develop symptoms.

If you do develop a yeast infection and receive antifungal treatment, you cannot just forget about the episode after your symptoms resolve. Your body is in a different state after a yeast infection making you susceptible to recurrences. A reservoir of infection of latent yeasts remains inside your affected tissues (Chapter 1). Hence, you must identify *all* of your susceptibility factors in order to prevent recurrences. Susceptibility to yeast infections is determined by your genetic background and your individual predisposing conditions, which can include medical, hospital, physiological, disease, and transmissible risk factors.

Medical Risk Factors

Illnesses caused by physicians' treatments are called *iatrogenic* diseases. Physicians know that antibiotics cause candidiasis, yet they rarely provide antifungal protection for susceptible patients. Then, when patients develop yeast infections, many doctors refuse even to test for Candida infection, let alone treat it.

If you have had yeast infections in the past, you know that you are susceptible—by definition. For this reason, you should ask for antifungal protection whenever you are prescribed one of the following treatments known to cause candidiasis: antibacterial antibiotics, antacids, certain diabetes drugs, corticosteroids, and estrogen.

Antibacterial Antibiotics

The number one cause of yeast infections is antibiotic treatment. Antibiotics kill pathogenic bacteria, but inadvertently also kill friendly bacteria that inhibit yeast growth in our body. The following antibiotics frequently cause yeast infections: Flagyl (metronidazole), Cipro (ciprofloxacin), Achromycin (tetracycline), Keflex (cephalexin), Eryc (erythromycin), Bicillin (penicillin),

Zithromax (azithromycin), Augmentin (amoxicillin plus clavulanate), and Bactrim (trimethoprim sulfamethoxazole).

Augmentin causes a persistent increase in gastrointestinal colonization by yeasts (Samonis et al., 1994). Antibiotics are implicated in recurrent vulvovaginal candidiasis (Sheary et al., 2005). Penicillin increased the risk of new-onset vaginal yeast infections the most, followed by cephalosporins and Flagyl (Meyn and Hillier, 2013). Flagyl is one of the worst offenders because it kills the obligately anaerobic bacteria, which are the "really friendly bacteria."

Question: Do IV antibiotics induce intestinal yeast overgrowth as do oral antibiotics?

Answer: According to https://www.quora.com/Do-IV-antibiotics-spare-the-gut-microbiome, existing human data suggest that iv antibiotics tested so far (Piperacillin, Tazobactam, Ampicillin, Gentamicin, Cefazolin, Meropenem, Ciprofloxacin) do not spare gut microbiota. In other words, when the above antibiotics are administered intravenously, they cause disturbances in the normal intestinal flora just as when the antibiotics are given orally.

Recently, exciting findings were reported in a paper by Arat et al. (2015). A new antibiotic, Lanopepden (GSK1322322) does not alter gut microbiota in healthy people when administered IV. However, when GSK1322322 is administered in a combined intravenous plus oral regimen, significant decreases occurred in species of Firmicutes and Bacteroides and increases occurred in Beta proteobacteria, Gamma proteobacteria and Bifidobacteriaceae.

People worried about getting another yeast infection might decide to not take antibiotics prescribed by their doctor. In most cases, this decision is a mistake because antibiotics cure bacterial infections and save lives. Instead of refusing antibiotic treatment, ask your doctor for preventive antiyeast treatments to be used at the same time (Step 10).

Antacids

Many people take antacids for stomach pain. Unfortunately, some OTC antacids containing calcium carbonate release CO_2 gas, which might increase your stomach symptoms. Other OTC antacids, such as famotidine, are better for occasional heartburn, gas, and stomach pain. Prescription antacids for peptic ulcers are stronger, but they significantly lower the acidity (raise the pH), which promotes yeast growth. To make matters worse, peptic ulcers are caused by a bacterium called *Helicobacter pylori*. To treat peptic ulcers, people are prescribed a combined treatment with two antibiotics plus an antacid. This combination therapy is a triple whammy! It almost assures the development of yeast infections in susceptible people.

Certain Diabetes Drugs Cause Genital Yeast Infections

In 2013, the FDA approved the drug Invokana (canagliflozin) as an adjunct to diet and exercise for adults with type-2 diabetes mellitus. This is the first oral agent in a novel class of diabetes drugs known as sodium–glucose co-transporter-2 (SGLT-2) inhibitors. Farxiga (dapagliflozin) and Jardiance (empagliflozin) were approved in 2014. All three SGLT-2 inhibitors work by helping the kidneys remove glucose from the bloodstream and excrete it into the urine. The excess sugar in the urine promotes the growth of yeasts on the surfaces of genital tissues in women and men resulting in vaginal or penile yeast infections.

WARNING

Common side effects of SGLT-2 inhibitors may include a higher rate of genital mycotic infections in females and uncircumcised men. People with a history of recurrent mycotic genital infections require oral and/or topical antifungal treatment.

Safety Tip: If you have type-2 diabetes and a history of candidiasis, tell your doctor not to prescribe a SGLT-2 inhibitor for your diabetes condition. Try a different class of oral antihyperglycemic agent.

Corticosteroids

Corticosteroids are secreted by the adrenal cortex, and are used to treat inflammation, asthma, allergy, and autoimmunity. Corticosteroids function by suppressing the activity of WBCs. However, WBCs are an essential part of our immune system that fights yeast infections. Hence, it is predictable that systemic corticosteroids make people susceptible to yeast infections (Sheary et al., 2005).

Estrogen

Estrogen is secreted by the ovaries and controls reproduction. Estrogen also promotes the growth of vaginal tissue and stimulates glycogen production inside vaginal epithelial cells. Glycogen is broken down into glucose, which feeds the yeasts and leads to yeast vaginitis. The following observations support the fact that estrogen predisposes women to develop vaginal yeast infections.

- **Puberty and menopause:** The lowest incidences of yeast vaginitis occur in prepubescent girls (Dei et al., 2009) and postmenopausal women because they have the lowest estrogen levels.
- **Fertile years:** The frequency of vulvovaginal candidiasis is elevated during the childbearing years when vaginal tissues are estrogenized.
- **Ovulation:** Estrogen levels rise each month at ovulation and remain high until menstruation (Tyler and Woodall, 1982; page 31). Symptoms of yeast vaginitis typically arise after the 14th day of the menstrual cycle (Eckert et al., 1998; Ilkit and Guzel, 2011) and worsen during the two weeks before menstruation (*luteal phase*).
- **Pregnancy:** During pregnancy, estrogen levels are the highest, vaginal yeast colonization is higher (Leli et al., 2013), and the frequency of vaginal yeast infections is the highest (Tyler and Woodall, 1982; page 31).
- **Estrogen treatments:** Estrogen prescribed for birth control pills, stimulation of fertility, hormone replacement therapy for menopause, and inappropriate treatment of vulvodynia makes women more susceptible to vaginal yeast infections. Oriel et al. (1972) found that 32% of women taking an oral contraceptive harbored yeast in their vagina compared with 18% of those who were not. Sobel et al. (1998) found that high dose oral contraceptives

predispose to vulvovaginal candidiasis. Rosentul et al. (2009) and Fischer and Bradford (2011) found that estrogen replacement therapy for menopause increases a postmenopausal woman's susceptibility to yeast vaginitis. In addition to its effect on vaginal cells, estrogen also exerts a direct effect on Candida cells by stimulating growth (Zhang et al., 2000).

- **Progesterone treatments:** The long-acting injectable progestogen Depo-Provera substantially reduces a woman's susceptibility to recurrent vulvovaginal candidiasis (Dennerstein, 1986). The rationale for progesterone therapy is that it creates a state of relative estrogen deficiency (Sobel, 1992). The hormone progestin in Depo-Provera contraceptive shots depletes estrogen and reduces a woman's risk for yeast vaginitis (Meyn and Hillier, 2013).
- **Experimental animal studies:** Female laboratory mice cannot be infected vaginally with Candida unless they are pretreated with estrogen (Sobel et al., 1984; Saavedra et al., 1999; Rosati et al., 2020). Estrogen pretreatment suppresses T cell-mediated immunity allowing Candida inoculated into the mouse vagina to grow (Hamad et al., 2004; 2006).

Hospital Risk Factors

Illnesses that develop when people are treated in hospitals are called *nosocomial diseases*. Life-threatening, nosocomial disseminated candidiasis may develop when seriously ill people with very low WBC counts (*neutropenia*) are treated with intravenous feeding, urinary catheters, chemotherapy and radiation for cancer, or immunosuppressants for organ transplantation.

Physiological Conditions

Conditions or states of the body that lower immunity and predispose people to develop candidiasis include stress, age, and pregnancy.

- **Stress** at school, work, or home for prolong periods causes the adrenals to release more cortisol, which suppresses WBC activity and lowers immunity.
- **Newborns** frequently develop oral thrush because yeasts enter their mouth from the mother's vagina during birth, and newborns are more susceptible to candidiasis because their immune systems are immature.
- **Elderly** people develop oral thrush because the immune system declines with age.
- **Pregnant women** have a high rate of vaginal yeast infections because their elevated estrogen levels stimulate yeast growth. Pregnant women are also immunosuppressed because they have elevated levels of cortisol (Elenkov et al., 2001), which inhibits the mother's WBCs thereby preventing them from attacking the fetus. This immunosuppressed condition also predisposes pregnant women to develop yeast vaginitis and other infections.

Predisposing Diseases

Illnesses that increase a person's vulnerability to yeast infections include diabetes, HIV, other infections, allergy, chemical sensitivity, immune defects, iron overload as well as iron-deficiency anemia, nutritional deficiencies, and low stomach acidity.

Diabetes

Diabetes (*hyperglycemia*) develops when the pancreas does not produce enough insulin. It is diagnosed by high levels of hemoglobin A1c and glucose in the blood after overnight fasting. The glucose tolerance test (GTT) for diabetes requires you to drink a concentrated glucose solution, and then have blood samples drawn every 30 or 60 minutes for four hours. Because of the time involved, multiple needle sticks, and the fact that sugar promotes yeast growth thereby provoking symptoms, Candida sufferers wisely refuse to take the GTT. Candidiasis is prevented if diabetes is controlled by diet and treatment. A diet high in sugar is a risk factor for recurrent vulvovaginal candidiasis (Ringdahl, 2000).

Human Immunodeficiency Virus

HIV infection makes patients more susceptible to other infections because the virus kills WBCs that are necessary to fight infection. Often the first sign of HIV infection is chronic yeast infection of the esophagus or vagina. When HIV infection progresses to a more serious stage, it is called acquired immune deficiency syndrome (AIDS).

Everyone should know her or his HIV status. If you suffer from frequent yeast infections, get tested for HIV. If your test result is negative, rejoice! You can stop worrying and focus on identifying what risk factors are responsible for your Candida infection. If your test result is positive for HIV:

- obtain highly active antiretroviral therapy (HAART)
- obtain preventive treatments for AIDS-related infections such as Candida
- change your lifestyle to protect yourself from catching other infections
- follow preventive measures to avoid spreading HIV to other people

Nowadays, people who are HIV-positive are living longer, and have a lower incidence of candidiasis because of effective medical treatments and lifestyle changes. In a happy coincidence, antiviral medicines that inhibit the HIV protease also inhibit the Candida protease (Borg-von Zepelin et al., 1999; Braga-Silva and Santos, 2011). Thus, HAART not only treats HIV, it also helps prevent candidiasis!

Other Infections

Bacterial infections can make you susceptible to candidiasis in two ways. First, infections caused by bacteria are treated with antibiotics, which cause yeast infections. Second, other infections can weaken your immune system by destroying WBCs. After WBCs phagocytize and kill bacteria, the WBCs die and accumulate in tissues forming pus. Hence, fewer WBC warriors remain to fight Candida. This is called *immunosuppression of infection.*

Allergy

Candida allergy is a predisposing risk factor for Candida infections. Allergic reactions release histamine and other mediators of inflammation, which suppress your immune system by inhibiting neutrophil chemotaxis and T cell proliferation (Crandall, 1991a; download from www.yeastconsulting.com). Chronic candidiasis can lead to allergic diseases such as Candida asthma, and allergic bronchopulmonary candidiasis. If you have chronic or recurrent yeast infections, you should obtain Candida intradermal testing for Candida allergy and Candida immunity (Step 5).

Chemical Sensitivity

Vaginal contact with irritating chemicals such as chlorine in pools and spas, spermicides, deodorants, colored toilet paper, or vaginal lubricants produces inflammation, which can trigger yeast vaginitis. The inflammatory response brings more blood to the area, and blood contains glucose and nutrients, which promote yeast growth. In addition, histamine and other substances, released during inflammatory reactions, inhibit WBCs needed to fight yeast infections.

Immune Defects

People with congenital T cell defects are usually identified in childhood, and can develop *granulomatous candidiasis* (previously called *chronic mucocutaneous candidiasis*; CMCC). Inborn errors of immunity also make people susceptible to other infections and cancer. Defects in immunity acquired later in life are termed *idiopathic*, which means their cause is unknown. The culprits could be medications, infections, environmental toxins, chemicals, etc. People with otherwise normal immunity who develop chronic intestinal yeast infections often have WBC counts slightly lower than normal. For example, their value might be 3.6, whereas the normal range is 4 to 10 thousand/mm^3. Poor T cell-mediated immunity to Candida is detected by the intradermal test, and follow-up blood tests that measure T lymphocyte function.

Iron Overload and Iron-deficiency Anemia

There is a delicate balance between the concentration of iron in the blood and susceptibility to candidiasis. Too much or too little iron predisposes to yeast infections. Abnormally high concentrations of iron in blood (*hyperferremia*) can be caused by taking iron supplements, or by the disease *hemochromatosis*. People with iron overload develop candidiasis because iron stimulates yeast growth (Weinberg, 1999). An elevated blood iron level is also a risk factor for cardiomyopathy, cancer, other infections, arthritis, endocrine disorders, and sudden infant death syndrome (Weinberg, 2004). Therefore, don't take iron supplements unless you test positive for *iron-deficiency anemia*. Abnormally low concentrations of iron in blood also predisposes to candidiasis because WBCs need iron to fight infections.

Nutritional Deficiencies

People in developed countries generally eat well-balanced diets, and rarely develop nutritional deficiencies that make them susceptible to yeast infections.

- **Zinc deficiency** can develop in the elderly, alcoholics, and people with anorexia or malabsorption. Conflicting findings have been reported about zinc deficiency and candidiasis. Edman et al. (1986) reported that zinc deficiency was associated with recurrent vaginal candidiasis. But Böhler et al. (1994) found no correlation between zinc levels in blood and cervicovaginal secretions in recurrent vaginal candidiasis.
- **Biotin deficiency** in a woman with persistent vaginal candidiasis was due to a congenital lack of biotinidase, an enzyme that absorbs biotin from food. The defective gene occurs in 1 out of 123 people. After taking pharmacologic doses of biotin for three months, the woman's yeast symptoms resolved (Strom and Levine, 1998).
- **Malabsorption** occurs in people with HIV and intestinal infections or other inflammatory conditions of the intestine, and results in nutritional deficiencies.

Low Stomach Acidity

Low hydrochloric acid concentration in gastric juice due to *hypochlorhydria* or treatment with antacids predisposes people to develop yeast infections of the gastrointestinal tract.

Transmission

Transmission of Candida from mother-to-child, medical staff-to-patients, and fingers-to-genitals is discussed here, and between sexual partners in Step 7.

Mother-to-Child

Transfer of germs from mother-to-child is called *vertical transmission*. Pathogenic microbes can be transmitted to the fetus in utero, or to the newborn during birth and breastfeeding. If pregnant women are colonized or infected with Candida vaginally, they should receive vaginal antifungal treatment to prevent transmission of Candida to the newborn.

Medical Staff-to-Patients

Transfer of germs from person-to-person is called *horizontal transmission*. The spread of Candida from patients to hospital staff and then from hospital staff to other patients is called *nosocomial transmission*. It is especially dangerous for two reasons. First, strains of Candida from patients who have been treated long-term with antifungals are often resistant to one or more antifungals. Second, other hospitalized patients are often immunocompromised and, therefore, more susceptible to infections transferred from staff.

Precautions for avoiding the transmission of germs in hospitals are discussed at length in books about infection control. Personnel should follow sterile techniques referred to as *universal precautions*. Hand sanitizers reduce, but do not eliminate germs. The most important preventive measures are hand washing and putting on new gloves before examining the next patient.

Fingers-to-Genitals

Yeast vaginitis is rarely caused by the yeast *Saccharomyces cerevisiae*. But, in one case report, a woman was infected with the specific yeast strain used at her husband's pizza shop where she helped make the dough (Nyirjesy et al., 1995). To prevent transmission of germs, always wash your hands before preparing foods, eating, having sex, and **before** as well as **after** using the toilet!

Conclusions of Step 6
Avoid *All* Risk Factors

After reading the above list of risk factors for yeast infections, you might think you have reached the end. Not so! The next step discusses lifestyle practices that predispose you to develop genital candidiasis. To overcome yeast infections, you must work with your physician to identify *all* of your susceptibility factors. Together, you must devise strategies for avoiding risk factors and managing predisposing conditions that are unavoidable. Tips for preventing yeast infections are presented in the rest of this program (Steps 7 to 10).

STEP 7

Lifestyle Changes

THERE ARE COUNTLESS PITFALLS ALONG your path through life that can trigger yeast infections. We discussed medical, hospital, physiological, disease, and transmission risk factors in the last step. Here we discuss behavioral activities that can make you susceptible to genital yeast infections including irritating chemicals, personal hygiene practices, laundry care, clothing choices, physical habits, birth control methods, sexual practices, and environmental mold contamination.

Irritating Chemicals

People who suffer from superficial yeast infections often have multiple chemical sensitivities and allergies that produce inflammation. Avoiding contact with irritating chemicals and allergenic substances prevents inflammation that can lead to the development of yeast infections. Just think about the number of chemical products that contact your genitals every day. Then eliminate *all* of them from your lifestyle. *Less is better!*

Safety Tips for Men and Women

If you are chemically sensitive and prone to genital yeast infections, use products labeled "Fragrance Free." Beware of products labeled "Unscented" because they often contain strong masking fragrances. Don't use the following products on your genitals:

- fragrances, perfumes, or scents in laundry detergents and hygiene products
- dyes, colors, or inks in toilet paper and underwear
- antibacterial or disinfectant soaps
- cleansing wipes containing alcohol
- bubble baths, bath salts, and bath oils
- chlorine in pools, spas, and hot tubs
- cornstarch in body powder

Safety Tips for Women

Any chemical substance can irritate the delicate tissues of the female genital tract, and vaginal inflammation can lead to yeast vaginitis (Rosenberg et al., 1987). To keep your vagina healthy, avoid contact with the chemicals listed above and follow these suggestions.

Douching is not necessary. The vagina has natural fluid secretions that self-cleanse and maintain its delicate pH balance. All you need for good hygiene is to wash the external genital area with mild soap and rinse with warm water. If you wish to remove menstrual blood, semen, spermicides, lubricants, or residual medication from your vagina, douche with plain water only and no more than once a week. Commercial douche products containing dilute acetic acid are pH 4.5, which is the normal acidity of the vagina in women of childbearing age. You can prepare acetic acid douches at home by diluting one tablespoon of distilled white vinegar in a quart of water. Don't use disinfecting douches such as Betadine. Vaginal douching increases the rate of vaginal colonization by non-*albicans Candida* strains that are generally resistant to the standard dosage of Diflucan (fluconazole; Shaaban et al., 2015).

Vaginal antifungal creams and suppositories can cause vaginal inflammation in sensitive women. A vaginitis center reported that 15% of cases referred to their clinic were due to *irritant dermatitis* (Nyirjesy et al., 1997). You can avoid irritation caused by vaginal antifungals by asking your doctor to prescribe an oral systemic antifungal agent such as Diflucan (fluconazole) tablets. Don't use unmedicated vaginal products sold OTC. They just cover up symptoms temporarily, but do not cure the underlying problem.

Lubricants used with latex barrier contraceptives (condoms, diaphragm, and cervical cap) should be water-soluble. Vegetable oils cause latex contraceptives to deteriorate, but if you have unprotected intercourse with a monogamous partner, you can use vegetable oils for lubrication. Coconut oil used as a lubricant for intercourse also has antifungal activity and can ease vaginal dryness. Avoid personal lubricants containing parabens, glycol, or glycerin (glycerine, glycerol) because these chemicals can irritate sensitive vaginal tissues. Intimacy products that are unlikely to cause irritation include Astroglide, Blossom Organics, Good Clean Love, Hathor Aphrodisia Pure, K-Y Jelly, Replens, Slippery Stuff, Sliquid Sassy, Sylk, and Yes.

Flavored lotions used for oral sex are unlikely to cause genital irritation because they are safe enough to be swallowed. But flavored condoms and lubricants that contain sugars should not be used for vaginal sex because sugar feeds yeasts.

Warming or stimulating gels create mild genital irritation in order to stimulate sexual pleasure. But beware of these products! There is a narrow line between warming and burning!

Honey made by bees is touted as a natural cure for yeast vaginitis. Don't believe everything you read! Don't apply any product containing honey on your urogenital area because the sugar in honey is very concentrated and the high osmotic pressure sucks water out of your tissues. In addition, sugar feeds yeasts!

Sanitary products such as menstrual pads, tampons, and panty liners made out of unbleached cotton are better for sensitive women. According to the Endometriosis Association, sanitary products made from chlorine-bleached cotton may contain dioxin, which can lead to the development of endometriosis. You can purchase unbleached cotton feminine hygiene products from www.mercola.com. Beware of tampons made from extra absorbent synthetic fibers because they dry out the vaginal lining as well as predisposing women to develop toxic shock syndrome caused by *Staphylococcus aureus*. Don't use sprays, panty liners, sanitary pads, and tampons containing deodorants, fragrances, perfumes, or scents.

Personal Hygiene Practices

Overzealous cleansing of your private parts with harsh disinfectants or strong antibacterial soaps can cause irritation, making tissues susceptible to candidiasis. Harsh soaps also remove friendly bacteria, natural oils, and organic acids that protect against infection.

Conversely, poor personal hygiene also leads to genital infections. Keep your genitals free of inflammation and infection by following these good hygiene practices:

- Wash your genital area with mild soap and rinse with warm water.
- Men should wash carefully under the foreskin where germs hide.
- A hand-held shower head on the end of a hose is convenient for rinsing off.
- Women can do a quick rinse by sitting on the toilet and pouring a glass of water over their genital area while wiping with their hand. Alternatively, use a bidet or a sitz bath.
- Women should not try to remove the white secretion (*smegma*) from under the hood of the clitoris. This natural secretion protects against infection.
- After a bowel movement, women should wipe with toilet paper from front to back to avoid spreading germs from the anus to the vagina. Cleanse the anal area with toilet tissue moistened with water.
- Don't shave your pubic hair. Tiny microscopic cuts or nicks allow entry of yeasts or other germs that can cause skin infections.

Laundry Care

- Don't use laundry detergents containing enzymes, fragrances or dyes for towels and clothing that touches your genital area.
- Likewise, don't use fabric softener with towels and underpants.
- Presoak heavily soiled underwear in detergent and warm water, hand scrub the crotch area, and rinse before putting in the washing machine.
- Don't use chlorine bleach in the washing machine because irritating byproducts may remain in the cloth.

Don't microwave your underwear!

Contrary to advice you may have read, sterilizing freshly laundered underwear in the microwave does not prevent yeast infections, and the bad news is it can cause a fire in your microwave oven! Here's the backstory.

In 1988, Friedrich and Phillips published a study of microwave sterilization of Candida on underwear fabric. After their conclusion got into newspapers and magazines, desperate women suffering from chronic yeast vaginitis followed the misguided advice of these two scientists who recommended microwaving underwear. Several kitchen fires resulted because microwave energy causes elastic and nylon to heat up rapidly.

When I read about these fires, I contacted several news agencies to set the record straight. Peter Tormey at United Press International interviewed me, and wrote an article entitled "Warning: Panties Aren't Hot Pants" published by the *San Francisco Chronicle* on March 4, 1989. This UPI article explained that these kitchen fires underscored the misinformation about yeast infections. Dr. Phillips said her study was taken out of context. Actually, the original premise of her study was wrong. You do not contract vaginal yeast infections from your underwear. The converse is true. Your underwear is soiled with vaginal discharge containing yeasts. To achieve a cure, the intracellular reservoir of yeasts in vaginal tissue must be eradicated with long-term oral systemic plus vaginal antifungal therapy (Step 2).

Clothing Choices and Physical Habits

The buildup of heat and moisture at body sites promotes the development of yeast infections such as jock itch or yeast vaginitis. To help prevent the buildup of heat and moisture in the crotch area, follow these suggestions.

Safety Tips for Men and Women:
- After exercising, change out of sweaty leotards, bicycle shorts, jock straps, or wet bathing suits as soon as possible. Shower and put on clean, dry clothing.
- Don't sit for long periods. Take frequent breaks and walk around.
- Sit on an absorbent cotton towel placed over plastic or wool seat covers.
- If your genital area is inflamed, get medical attention.
- Ease a burning bottom by soaking in a cool water sitz bath, or sitting on an ice pack covered by a towel, or with your clothes on.
- Wear absorbent underwear made of white cotton, not synthetic fabrics such as nylon, elastic (Spandex) or polyester.
- Don't wear tight-fitting slacks, jeans, or tights.

Safety Tips for Women:
- Don't wear girdles or control panties that constrict the genitals.
- Wear knee-high hosiery instead of panty hose.
- If you do wear panty hose, make sure it has a cotton crotch. Don't wear panties under your panty hose. If you do, cut a hole in the crotch of the panty hose.
- Don't use panty liners, inside panties, inside panty hose, inside slacks—that's four layers. **Let your genitals breathe!** Frequent use of panty liners (Janković et al., 2010) and panty hose is associated with vulvovaginal candidiasis (Patel et al. 2004).

- Don't follow misguided advice to avoid wearing panties in an attempt to cure yeast vaginitis. You need underwear to catch the leaks!
- Wear nightgowns instead of pajamas while sleeping.

Birth Control Methods that Can Cause Yeast Vaginitis

Spermicides, the diaphragm, and estrogen-based birth control pills are popular contraceptives. Unfortunately, all of these birth control methods predispose women to develop vaginal yeast infections. Manufacturers sell them, and doctors recommend them, but no one warns women about their risk of developing yeast vaginitis if they use these products. Women have to discover this painful side effect on their own!

Spermicides

The most commonly used spermicide is nonoxynol-9, a nonionic detergent. It kills sperm by disrupting their cell membranes. Spermicides also kill vaginal cells. Cytotoxicity of nonoxynol-9 increases with exposure; 89% of cultured vaginal epithelial cells were killed within 48 hours (Hillier et al., 2005). Nonoxynol-9 kills vaginal epithelial cells by disrupting their cell membranes. Damage to vaginal tissues makes women more susceptible to yeast vaginitis (Rosenberg et al., 1987). Nonoxynol-9 also increases adhesion of Candida to epithelial cells in vitro (McGroarty et al., 1990). Recurrent vulvovaginal candidiasis is associated with spermicidal contraception (Ringdahl, 2000; Amouri et al., 2011).

Nonoxynol-9 also kills the normal bacterial flora in the vagina thereby making women more susceptible to bacterial cystitis (Reid et al., 1990; Fihn et al., 1996), as well as increasing susceptibility to sexually transmitted diseases (STDs; Gupta, 2005). The normal bacterial flora also provide protection against candidiasis. And you know what happens when you take antibiotics for bacterial infections. Yes, that's right—the same thing that happens when you use vaginal spermicides—another vaginal yeast infection!

Spermicides are sold as vaginal jellies, gels, creams, foams, tablets, pessaries, and sponges. Some condoms use spermicides as lubricants. New vaginal products are being developed that contain spermicides plus microbicides to prevent HIV transmission. Antiviral microbicides, together with spermicides, and other chemical components of vaginal gels destroy vaginal epithelial cell viability and integrity, and induce inflammation (Gali et al., 2010).

It is time for the medical profession to stop thinking that the vagina is an inert vessel into which can be inserted all sorts of noxious chemicals!

The Diaphragm

The diaphragm looks like the end of a rubber ball that has been sliced off. It is a round ring covered with a convex latex membrane. It is a barrier contraceptive that covers the cervix and blocks sperm from entering the uterus and traveling up the fallopian tubes to reach the egg.

The diaphragm is available in different sizes that must be fitted inside a woman's vagina by a qualified gynecological practitioner. Before having vaginal intercourse, the woman fills the bowl of the diaphragm with spermicidal jelly and inserts it into her vagina over the cervix.

> **WARNING**
>
> Don't use the diaphragm for birth control if either partner is allergic to latex. Even though the diaphragm is one of the most effective forms of contraception, it can cause problems for both partners. Spermicide used with the diaphragm is a risk factor for yeast vaginitis. Men can develop irritation on their penis due to friction from rubbing on the ring edge during intercourse. Women can develop bacterial cystitis due to the repeated striking of the diaphragm internally against the urinary bladder during intercourse. Then, of course, antibiotics given to cure the bladder infection lead to yeast vaginitis. Does this nightmare ever end? No, there's more!

Estrogen-containing Birth Control Pills

Oral contraceptives containing estrogen and/or progestin inhibit female fertility and protect against pregnancy. Birth control pills containing estrogen increase estrogen levels in vaginal tissues, making women more susceptible to vaginal yeast infections. Evidence that estrogen is a risk factor for yeast vaginitis is presented in Step 6.

Birth Control Methods that Do *Not* Cause Yeast Vaginitis

The following contraceptives do not predispose women to develop vaginal yeast infections: the male condom, the female condom, the cervical cap, progesterone-based oral contraceptives, and other birth control methods discussed below.

Male Condom

The male condom is a sheath that fits over an erect penis. It is usually made of latex. If either partner is allergic to latex, use male condoms made out of polyurethane or condoms made out of animal intestines (called skins). Other names for the male condom include a rubber, sheath, or prophylactic. It is a barrier contraceptive that protects women against pregnancy and exposure to dangerous substances in semen, and protects both partners against STDs.

If you are prone to yeast vaginitis, use unlubricated condoms because lubricated condoms use the spermicide nonoxynol-9 as the lubricant. For additional protection against pregnancy, you can put spermicide inside the condom tip. Doing this has two advantages. First, the spermicide will not contact the vagina, which is more sensitive to chemicals than is the skin on the penis. Second, spermicide inside the male condom increases the man's pleasure.

Female Condom

The female condom is a polyurethane sheath that fits inside the vagina with a closed ring at the end next to the cervix, and an open ring at the top that covers the vulvar area. It is a barrier contraceptive that protects women against pregnancy and exposure to dangerous substances in semen, and it protects both partners against STDs. The female condom has these additional advantages.

- It can be used if either sexual partner is allergic to latex.
- The outer ring of the female condom covers the entire vulvar area giving the woman added protection against contracting STDs during oral sex.
- Spermicide put inside the female condom provides added contraceptive protection while not irritating the vagina and at the same time increasing the man's pleasure.

Cervical Cap

The cervical cap is made of latex and is shaped like a Derby hat with a rounded crown and narrow brim. If either partner is allergic to latex, don't use the cervical cap for birth control. The cervical cap is a barrier contraceptive that fits over the cervix, as does the diaphragm. However, the cap is much smaller, and fits snugly over the cervix. Hence, it is not necessary to put spermicide inside, but some women do use spermicide as added protection against pregnancy.

Progesterone-based Contraceptives

Contraceptives containing the hormone progesterone include Norplant implants, Depo-Provera injections (medroxyprogesterone acetate), and the progesterone-only minipill (Micronor). They do not predispose to vaginal yeast infections because they do not contain estrogen. Progesterone works by thickening the cervical mucus, thereby preventing passage of sperm into the uterus. In rare instances when fertilization occurs, progesterone prevents implantation. When women switch their birth control method to Depo-Provera or the progesterone-only mini pill, they often experience a remission from recurrent vaginal yeast infections (Dennerstein, 1986). Depo-Provera has a very strong progestin, which depletes estrogen in the vaginal epithelium, and reduces a woman's risk for yeast vaginitis (Meyn and Hillier, 2013).

Other Contraceptives

Other birth control methods that do not predispose women to develop yeast vaginitis include sterilization of the woman (*tubal ligation*), sterilization of the man (*vasectomy*), the rhythm method (*fertility awareness*), and withdrawal (*coitus interruptus*).

Two groups of clinicians have reported higher incidences of vaginal Candida colonization or infection associated with the intrauterine device (IUD). However, these reports are unconfirmed. Therefore, the IUD is included here with other birth control methods that do not predispose women to develop yeast vaginitis.

Sexual Practices

Unprotected sex predisposes women to develop yeast vaginitis, and also exposes women to pregnancy, sexually transmitted infections, and dangerous substances in semen.

Sexually Transmitted Infections (STIs)

Sex spreads germs! We all know that we should follow safe sex practices to avoid contracting HIV, gonorrhea, syphilis, Chlamydia, Trichomonas, and other genital infections. Yet, despite scientific evidence for the spread of Candida by sexual contact, many doctors mistakenly say that candidiasis is not a STI. This confusion is caused by terminology.

The definition of a *sexually transmitted disease* (STD) is an infection caused by a pathogen **not normally present in the genital tract**. For example, if the bacterium, *Neisseria gonorrhoeae,* is detected in genital specimens, it is diagnostic for the infection, gonorrhea. Since **Candida is normally present on skin and mucous membranes**, genital candidiasis is not classified as an STD. Yet, **Candida is transmitted sexually** as shown by these facts.

- Sexual partners carry the same strains of *Candida albicans* (Shi et al., 2007).
- In a study of 100 cases of women with recurrent vulvovaginal candidiasis, Candida was found in semen specimens from *all* of their sexual partners (Gilpin, 1967). After six months of wearing a condom during intercourse, only 15% of the males had reverted to negative yeast cultures. This means that Candida colonization is stable.
- Candida is passed to your partner by oral, vaginal, and anal sex, as well as by contaminated fingers and objects such as sex toys.
- Having two or more male sexual partners increases a woman's risk of developing yeast vaginitis 5-fold (Meyn and Hillier, 2013).

If the woman has undiagnosed yeast vaginitis, and a couple has unprotected intercourse, the man can later develop a yeast infection on his penis. If the man has uncontrolled diabetes, his penile yeast infection can lead to Candida prostatitis. Then Candida in his semen is inoculated into his partner's vagina each time they have unprotected intercourse. If the woman is treated with antifungals, but the man is not, he can give the yeast infection back to the woman. In such cases, both partners should be treated with antifungals to prevent "sexual Ping-Pong." But, in general, the male partner of a women with yeast vaginitis is usually not treated with an antifungal unless he has symptoms of genital candidiasis.

Substances in Semen that Cause Yeast Vaginitis

Some women are allergic to proteins normally present in semen. Allergic reactions to seminal proteins can cause vaginal inflammation, or sometimes even anaphylaxis.

If the man is taking oral antibiotics or other medications that stimulate yeast overgrowth, these drugs in his semen can trigger yeast vaginitis in his partner.

Condoms prevent transmission of seminal proteins, allergens, drugs, as well as germs and sperms in semen to the vagina.

Relapse or Reinfection?

If you develop a yeast infection after sex, is it a relapse or reinfection? A *relapse* is caused by the same yeast strain inside your tissues that caused your previous infection. A *reinfection* is caused by a different yeast strain contracted from an outside source.

Determining whether a recurrence is due to a previous or a new yeast requires laboratory testing to culture and identify the yeast species. Because of the cost for such specialized testing, it is not performed routinely. Therefore, you need to do some detective work to identify your risk factors. Consider your recent sexual partners, lifestyle, and other factors such as recent predisposing medications, medical procedures, or conditions (Steps 6 and 7).

Safety Tips for Preventing STIs:

- Practice safe sex. Actually, the term "safer sex" is more accurate. Only uninfected partners provide absolute safety from STDs. If you are not in a monogamous relationship, always use a condom during sexual intercourse.
- Don't have unprotected sex if either partner has a genital infection.
- Use barrier protection to guard against transmitting germs during oral sex. Cover the vulva and clitoris with a latex dental dam during oral stimulation of the female (*cunnilingus*). If either partner is allergic to latex, use plastic wrap as protection when women are receiving oral sex. Cover the penis with a condom during oral stimulation of the male (*fellatio*). Mardh et al. (2003) found that recurrent vulvovaginal candidosis is associated with oral sex.
- Both partners should wash their hands and genitals before and after sexual activity.
- Wash sexual aids such as dildos and vibrators after each use.
- Don't participate in anal intercourse because it can cause health problems. If you do engage in anal sex, be sure to use a condom. Use a fresh condom before proceeding from anal to vaginal intercourse. Wash fingers, penis, and objects that have been in contact with the anus before touching the vaginal area.
- Women should not douche before sex because it removes natural lubrication.
- Women should urinate before lovemaking for the sake of comfort, and right after intercourse to flush germs out of her urethra in order to prevent a bladder infection.
- Men rarely develop bacterial cystitis after sex because germs from the vagina have a long distance to travel up the male urethra to reach the urinary bladder. *And that's the long and short of this discussion!*

Environmental Mold Contamination

If you suffer from frequent yeast infections, consider the possibility that you may be allergic to molds. Since moisture promotes the growth of molds, keep your home environment dry, both inside as well as outside. Don't use a humidifier. Repair leaks as soon as you discover them, and replace wet carpet and padding, furnishings, and building materials. Molds also lurk in wet soils of potted plants. Make your home and workplace *healthy oases, refuges, or safe habitats that are free of allergens and toxic chemicals.*

Conclusions of Step 7
Lifestyle Changes

With so many risk factors, it is easy to understand why yeast infections are so common. To overcome chronic or recurrent candidiasis, you must make a life-long commitment to avoid *all* predisposing conditions. Discuss your individual sensitivity factors with your doctor, and formulate a plan for avoiding them by modifying your lifestyle and medical-care protocol. If some predisposing conditions are unavoidable, obtain antifungal prophylaxis (Step 10). *Your recovery is in your hands.*

STEP 8

Candida Diet

YOU MAY HAVE READ DIETARY advice for yeast infections on the internet, in books, and/or magazine articles for the general public. Or you may have been given dietary advice for yeast infections by a health care professional. Most of this advice is too restrictive and not based on scientific research.

My dietary advice for Candida sufferers can be summarized in two simple sentences:

1. If you eat something, and it makes you sick, don't eat it again.

2. If most everything you eat makes you sick, you need to follow an individualized program of medical care and self-help for Candida.

Test <u>Before</u> Treating!

If you think you have an intestinal yeast overgrowth, obtain an accurate medical diagnosis first before starting a restrictive diet and taking antifungal supplements. Your self-treatment for candidiasis may lead to falsely negative test results for Candida if you are tested later.

Ask your doctor to order the diagnostic tests explained in Steps 1 and 5 that are appropriate for your case. If blood and stool tests are positive for intestinal yeast overgrowth, and skin tests are positive for allergies to Candida, foods, and environmental allergens, follow *all* ten steps in this program. If your symptoms improve on this program, your diagnosis of intestinal candidiasis is confirmed.

The Candida diet involves restricting sugars and complex carbohydrates, and avoiding foods and beverages containing yeasts and molds, as well as foods that gave positive reactions in scratch and blood tests for allergies, and foods that cause adverse reactions when eaten.

Restricting simple and complex carbohydrates if you have intestinal candidiasis is based on the idea that *every time you eat, your yeasts eat!* Yeasts require sugar for growth. Yeasts ferment sugar producing metabolites that make people sick. Most people with the yeast syndrome experience a worsening of their symptoms after eating sweets, fruits, or starchy foods. Worsening of intestinal, systemic, and mental symptoms after eating carbohydrates is caused by yeast products, as well as allergic reactions to Candida and food antigens. Worsening of symptoms after eating is termed *postprandial exacerbation of symptoms,* and is a diagnostic criterion for the yeast syndrome when considered together with laboratory test results.

Mental symptoms like brain fog that do not worsen after eating are probably unrelated to intestinal yeast overgrowth. If you cannot identify a trigger for your brain fog, I suggest that you see a psychologist. She or he might be able to diagnose your problem and suggest some helpful coping strategies for problems with thought processes.

Origin of the Low Carbohydrate, Yeast-free Diet

Dietary studies discussed below found that a sugar-free, yeast-free diet decreased symptoms of intestinal candidiasis and skin rashes caused by Candida and food yeasts.

In 1966, Holti reported that nystatin alone cured 27 out of 49 people with hives (*urticaria*), whereas 18 patients out of 49 required nystatin plus a yeast-free diet. James and Warin (1971) reported similar observations.

In his 1983 book, *The Missing Diagnosis*, C. Orian Truss, M.D., described an extremely low carbohydrate diet that produced successful outcomes for patients he had diagnosed with chronic Candida infection of the intestine. Truss advised Candida sufferers to limit their intake of simple and complex carbohydrates as well as yeasty foods while receiving antifungal therapy and immunotherapy for candidiasis.

In 1985, Bolivar and Bodey reviewed studies showing that a yeast-free diet produces clinical improvement in intestinal candidiasis.

Eaton (1991) is the only investigator who performed laboratory studies that measured the effect of a low carbohydrate diet on intestinal candidiasis. Eaton chose subjects for the study if they tested positive for blood alcohol production after consuming glucose. A total of 241 people with auto-brewery syndrome were formed into three treatment groups. After following a low carbohydrate diet for 8 to 18 weeks, they were retested for blood alcohol production:

- Out of 64 subjects on diet alone, 42% tested negative.
- Out of 149 subjects on diet + antifungals, 78% tested negative.
- Out of 28 subjects on diet + antibiotics, 7% tested negative.

Thus, restricting carbohydrates helps cure intestinal candidiasis, and adding antifungals to a low carbohydrate diet is even better, but treating with antibiotics is worse—as expected.

C. Orian Truss, M.D., funded a study of intestinal candidiasis and supplied the patients to an independent researcher, W.E. Dismukes, M.D. Dismukes and coworkers (1990) designed and carried out the protocol. Unfortunately, their study was poorly designed and executed (Chapter 6). So, Truss et al. (1992) carried out a follow-up study of the same women previously treated with oral nystatin in the Dismukes study. In the follow-up study, the women followed a comprehensive protocol of nystatin treatment, a yeast-free diet with only 80 grams of carbohydrate per day, and allergy shots of Candida extract. Truss's comprehensive protocol resulted in dramatic improvements in 28 symptoms (vaginal, systemic, and psychological). Truss included a reprint of his 1992 follow-up study in his 2009 book, *The Missing Diagnosis II.*

Santelmann et al. (2001) selected subjects for their study who had a favorable response to a diet that restricted sugar and yeasty foods. Subjects were then treated with either oral nystatin or a placebo and the improvement in symptoms was analyzed statistically. Their results were used to validate the Yeast Questionnaire in Table 3.

The Low Carbohydrate Diet

The rationale for the Candida diet, which restricts sugar and complex carbohydrates, is to limit yeast growth in the intestine and prevent symptoms caused by yeast fermentation. Limiting dietary sugar may also help to prevent recurrent vulvovaginal candidiasis (Ringdahl, 2000).

There is a lot of misinformation about the Candida diet on the internet, in websites and blogs, books, and magazine articles. Myths and misconceptions about the sugar-free, yeast-free diet are discussed in the following paragraphs.

Yeast infections are caused by eating sugars and complex carbohydrates.

FACT: Most yeast infections are caused by antibiotics and other medical treatments. Most people eat a diet comprised mainly of carbohydrates, yet there is no worldwide epidemic of yeast infections.

If you do not eat enough calories from carbohydrates, you will lose weight. Even though weight loss is good for people who are overweight, it is not good if you are at your normal weight or below. *You cannot cure yeast infections by starving yourself!*

Yeast infections are cured by restricting sugar and carbohydrates.

FACT: While it is true that symptoms may be reduced by restricting carbohydrates, *you cannot cure yeast infections by diet alone!*

The low carbohydrate diet is followed while being treated with antifungals at the same time. You need to follow all of the medical care and self-help guidelines in this ten-step program that are relevant to your case in order to overcome yeast infections and yeast allergies.

Sugar cravings are diagnostic of intestinal yeast overgrowth.

FACT: If you are restricting carbohydrates or haven't eaten for a while and you are hungry because your blood sugar level is low, you will naturally crave sweets whether or not you have an intestinal yeast overgrowth.

Instead of grabbing a candy bar, plan ahead and prepare healthy snacks such as string cheese, hardboiled eggs, nuts, seeds, cooked soybeans (*edamame*), raw vegetables, beef jerky, nut butter, and whole grain crackers.

The ideal diet for people without chronic candidiasis should consist mainly of complex carbohydrates from fruits, vegetables, and whole grains. These foods supply the calories needed for energy plus the fiber, vitamins, and minerals needed for good health.

If you have chronic candidiasis and are following the low carbohydrate diet, you have to increase your caloric intake by eating more protein and fat to avoid losing weight. However, a diet high in protein and fat is unhealthy.

- **Too much protein** puts a heavy burden on the kidneys and exacerbates gout and other disorders of nitrogen metabolism.
- **Too much fat** causes hardening of the arteries and leads to heart disease and stroke. You can decrease fat in your diet by not eating meat, and substituting nonfat cheese, tofu, and hard-boiled egg whites plus fish that are low in fat such as orange roughy, tuna, pollock, mahi mahi, cod, hake, haddock, sole and flounder.

Since individual metabolisms vary tremendously, your diet should be tailor-made to fit your reactions to specific foods.

Eliminate Sweets

The primary focus of the Candida diet should be on eliminating sugars (simple carbohydrates). Sweets are just hollow calories lacking in nutrients. Eating too much sugar can result in obesity, which contributes to the development of diabetes, heart disease, and stroke. For all these reasons, Candida sufferers should not consume: *table sugar, corn syrup, maple syrup, molasses, honey, agave syrup, candy, ice cream, soda pop, cookies, cake, muffins, donuts, pie, other sweet desserts, sweet wine, and alcoholic drinks mixed with sugary soda or juice.*

Cheating on your diet by eating a sweet occasionally is not going to ruin your recovery, but may provoke symptoms. If you have a bad reaction to the following nutritious, sugar-containing foods, don't eat them again until after you respond to antifungal therapy.

- **Milk** is a perfect food that contains all the required nutrients for growth and sustenance. However, milk contains the sugar lactose, which is broken down by the enzyme *lactase* into glucose and galactose, which feeds the yeasts in your intestine. People who are lactase-deficient develop intestinal gas, bloating, and diarrhea after drinking milk, but can drink lactase-treated milk. Milk also contains proteins such as casein that are common allergens.

- **"Forbidden Fruit:"** A healthy diet should include at least one serving of fruit a day, but sugar in fruit may make you sick if you have an overgrowth of yeast in your gut. Fruits that score low on the glycemic index include berries, grapefruits, lemons, limes, green bananas, and green apples. However, beware of grapefruit—it contains chemicals that inhibit enzymes needed to metabolize drugs. In addition, lemons, limes, and unripened fruits can cause tummy problems. Watch out for grapes, berries, dried fruits, and cantaloupes because they may have yeasts and molds on their surfaces.
- **Sweet vegetables** such as *peas, corn, carrots, sweet potatoes, yams, beets, onions, and tomatoes* should be included in a balanced diet, but they contain sugar that may provoke symptoms in people with intestinal candidiasis.

Artificial sweeteners can be substituted for sugar, but some people experience intestinal or neurological symptoms after ingesting them. The natural sweetener "Stevia" appears to be well tolerated.

Reduce, But Don't Eliminate, Complex Carbohydrates

Fruits, vegetables, and whole grains are essential for a balanced diet because they provide the fiber, vitamins, minerals, and energy that everyone needs to survive. You should eat at least one starchy food at each meal such as *legumes, nuts, pasta, potatoes, rice, seeds, tapioca pearls, winter squash, and whole grains.*

If you get sick after eating complex carbohydrates, you need medical treatment. If you eliminate all carbohydrates in an attempt to overcome yeast infections, you will lose weight, become constipated, be unhappy because you cannot eat your favorite foods, and wonder why you are still suffering from yeast infections. No mystery there! You cannot cure candidiasis by attempting to starve yeasts in the gut. Diet is only one step in this comprehensive ten-step program of medical care and self-help for Candida patients.

Many people with the yeast syndrome experience symptoms after eating the following grains: *wheat, rye, barley, and oats.* If these cause bothersome symptoms, you should get tested for gluten intolerance and celiac disease. If you test positive, discontinue eating *wheat, rye, barley, and oats,* and substitute gluten-free grains and seeds such as *amaranth, buckwheat, corn, hemp, millet, poppy, quinoa, rice, sesame, sunflower, sorghum, and teff.*

Legumes

Candida sufferers on a low carbohydrate diet often substitute legumes for meat because they have the mistaken idea that legumes are high in protein. In fact, legumes are high in carbohydrate (80%), low in protein (10%), and the rest is water, vitamins, minerals, and ash (nonfat dry solids). The phrase 'high in protein' only has meaning when legumes are compared to vegetables such as spinach or celery, which contain very little protein.

> **WARNING**
>
> Eating too many servings of legumes, vegetables, and whole grains is self-defeating because they can cause diarrhea, gas, and bloating—the same symptoms as produced by intestinal candidiasis!

The main gas-producing culprits in a vegetarian diet are:

- legumes such as beans, peas, lentils, chick peas, and peanuts
- vegetables in the genus Allium such as onions, garlics, shallots, chives, and leeks
- cruciferous vegetables such as cabbage, Brussels sprouts, cauliflower, and broccoli
- whole grains such as wheat, rye, barley, and oats

All of these foods contain a trisaccharide (*raffinose*) that is not digested in the small intestine. When raffinose travels to the large intestine, it is fermented by gas-producing bacteria.

Safety Tip: If you develop gas after eating these foods, take an OTC enzyme supplement that contains alpha-D-galactosidase (such as beano®). It digests raffinose in the small intestine, thereby preventing it from reaching the large intestine where the gas-producing bacteria live. If some gas accumulates in your bowel, OTC products containing simethicone (such as Gas-X®) might help to eliminate it.

The following nonstarchy vegetables are healthy but provide very few calories because they are comprised mainly of *cellulose*, which humans cannot digest: *artichokes, asparagus, bean sprouts, bok choy, broccoli, Brussels sprouts, cabbage, chard, cauliflower, celery, endive, garlic, kale, kohlrabi, leeks, lettuce, okra, parsnips, peppers, radishes, rutabagas, seaweed, spinach, string beans, summer squash, turnips, water chestnuts, watercress, zucchini.*

Ideally, you should eat five servings of fruits and vegetables every day. It is better to eat whole fruits and vegetables. If you prepare juice from fruits and vegetables, add the pulp back because it contains beneficial fiber. The rest of your calories should come from whole grains, protein, and fat. Eat normal size servings of *meat, fish, poultry, shellfish, eggs, cheese, butter, margarine, cream, and oils.*

If you suffer from constipation, you are not eating enough fruit, vegetables, and whole grains that provide fiber. Plums and prunes (dried plums) contain a lot of fiber plus a natural chemical similar to the laxative in Ex-Lax. Fiber supplements keep the stool soft and help you to have regular bowel movements.

Vegans

Strict vegetarians, called *vegans*, eat only plant products, with no foods from animal sources such as meat, fish, dairy, or eggs. Therefore, their diet is almost completely carbohydrate with very little protein and fat. Yet, vegans do not have a higher incidence of yeast infections. Therefore, eating carbohydrates does not cause yeast overgrowths.

Since the vegan diet (high carbohydrate) and the low carbohydrate Candida diet are diametrically opposed, you cannot follow both diets or you will starve! Use common sense. Eat a balanced diet while eliminating sweets. Your diet should be based on your individual reactions to foods. *One diet does not fit all!*

Helpful Hint: If you feel more energetic and clear-headed before meals, don't eat a carbohydrate meal before an important event. After several weeks or months of antifungal therapy, gradually add back more carbohydrates to your diet while avoiding foods that cause symptoms.

Feast without Yeast

The other half of the Candida diet is to avoid consuming yeasts and molds in foods and beverages. People suffering from chronic yeast infections tend to be allergic to body yeasts (Candida), food yeasts (Saccharomyces), and molds. Hence, most Candida patients experience adverse reactions after eating fermented foods and beverages. These reactions have resulted in many misconceptions about the Candida diet. These myths have appeared so often in books, magazines, and websites that they have become dogma. You must understand why these myths are wrong before you can devise a healing program that works for you. The following discussions debunk myths about the Candida diet and substitute factual information.

MYTH

Eating yeast-leavened bread causes yeast infections.

FACT: Baking kills yeasts in bread, and dead yeasts don't cause infections! Symptoms experienced after consuming bread could be due to:

- allergy to baker's yeast or wheat
- cross-reactions between anti-Candida antibodies and baker's yeast (*Saccharomyces cerevisiae*)
- gluten sensitivity or celiac disease
- carbohydrate, which feeds intestinal yeasts

FACT: Some symptoms of the yeast syndrome can be prevented by following a yeast-free diet eliminating:

- **Yeast-leavened baked goods:** *bread, sour dough, pizza, English muffins, bagels, croissants, and raised donuts.*
- **Yeast-fermented beverages:** *beer, wine, apple cider, and kefir.*
- **Yeast-fermented foods:** *apple cider vinegar, wine vinegar, rice vinegar, soy sauce, and red yeast rice.*
- **Yeast extract-flavored foods:** *soups, gravies, sauces, crackers, tortillas, and flat bread.*
- **Yeast-containing consumables:** *Marmite, brewer's yeast, B vitamins made from yeast, and probiotics containing yeast extract.*

- **Probiotic yeast:** *Saccharomyces boulardii, is really Saccharomyces cerevisiae, and should not be consumed.*
- **Moldy foods:** *mushrooms, bleu cheese, Roquefort, grapes, berries, dried fruits, cantaloupe, fruit juices, malt, sprouts, and skins of root vegetables (potatoes, carrots, and beets).*
- **Fermented foods contaminated by yeasts and molds:** *Camembert, brie, and other ripened cheeses, smoked meat, fish, and sausage, kefir, sauerkraut, kimchee, olives, and pickles.*

MYTH

Apple cider vinegar has antifungal activity (Martin and Rona, 1996).

FACT: I challenge anyone to provide scientific studies showing that this assertion is valid. Apple cider vinegar is prepared from apple juice, which is fermented by yeasts that convert the sugar into alcohol. Then the hard (alcoholic) apple cider is converted into apple cider vinegar by adding the bacterium, Acetobacter, which converts the alcohol to acetic acid. Apple cider vinegar contains residual yeast, mold, and bacterial antigens, which can cause allergic reactions in sensitive people. It does not contain antifungal activity.

If you are allergic to yeasts, you can prepare salad dressing with distilled white vinegar, which has had the yeast antigens removed, or you can use lemon juice on your salad.

MYTH

Alcohol feeds intestinal yeasts.

FACT: Digestion of alcohol as a carbon and energy source can only occur in the presence of oxygen and our intestinal contents are anaerobic. Alcohol is produced by yeast fermentation of sugar and is not consumed as a food source by yeasts growing under anaerobic conditions in the gut.

If you are allergic to yeasts, you can drink alcoholic beverages containing distilled liquors such as whiskey, bourbon, rum, vodka, or gin, which have had the yeast antigens removed.

WARNING

Don't drink alcohol while you are taking systemic antifungal drugs or other drugs that are metabolized in the liver. Alcohol inhibits liver enzymes needed to break down drugs and, consequently, drugs can accumulate in the blood to toxic levels.

Safety Tip: If you want to drink alcoholic beverages at night, don't take the systemic antifungal drug that morning. You can drink alcohol while taking nystatin because it is not absorbed into the bloodstream, so it never reaches the liver.

Take home message: Don't believe everything you read, especially on the internet. Look for reliable scientific documentation published in medical journals. If something sounds like nonsense, it probably is. Always challenge nonsense statements by saying, *"Show me the data!"*

Helpful Hints:

- Allergic reactions can occur to Saccharomyces yeasts, which are found in leavened baked goods, beer, wine, some fermented foods, and probiotics containing *S. boulardii*. The best way to prevent these allergic reactions is to avoid eating products containing yeasts. Yeast-free baked goods and foods are sold by specialty companies. Read labels to avoid buying products with added yeasts.
- Yeast allergies are treated with allergy shots in the same way that allergy to other substances is treated (Step 5). After receiving injection immunotherapy against Saccharomyces and Candida, plus antifungal therapy for about six months, you may be able to consume bread, beer, wine, and other yeast-containing foods without experiencing symptoms.
- Eat foods while they are fresh or freeze them to prevent growth of contaminating yeasts and molds during storage.
- The following dairy products are fermented by bacteria—not yeast: *cheddar cheese, Swiss cheese, yogurt, cottage cheese, sour cream, and cream cheese.* Therefore, they may not cause symptoms in yeast syndrome patients.
- If you are casein intolerant and cannot eat milk products, you might be able to eat *ricotta*, a type of cheese made from coagulated milk proteins (albumin and globulin), which remain in whey after cheese production removes the casein.

Avoid Other Food Allergens

Generally, people who are allergic to yeasts and molds are often also allergic to foods such as:

- **Dairy:** *milk, cheese, yogurt, and casein additives.*
- **Legumes:** *beans (green, lima, kidney, pinto, soy, edamame, tofu), peas, peanuts, chick peas, and lentils.*
- **Citrus:** *oranges, lemons, limes, grapefruits, and tangerines.*
- **Shellfish:** *shrimp, lobster, crayfish, crabs, clams, mussels, and oysters.*
- **Others:** *eggs, albumin additives, corn, wheat, and tree nuts.*

The reason people with an intestinal yeast overgrowth often become sensitized to many foods is due to the development of a leaky gut (Chapter 5). Partially digested food particles and Candida antigens leak through the intestinal wall into the bloodstream where antibodies are formed against these foods and Candida. As a result, yeast syndrome patients often must limit their diet to just a few items that do not cause problems. If they don't get their yeast overgrowth treated with anti-fungals, eventually they can become allergic to even those few foods.

When you discontinue eating a food, antibodies against that substance decrease over time. The next time you eat that food, you may not have a reaction. But if you start eating a lot of that food again, more antibodies will be synthesized against it, and symptoms will return. This is called *rebound allergy.* Since food allergies are moving targets that constantly change, you should rotate foods in your diet to avoid developing allergies. Eat a variety of foods as part of a balanced diet. *Variety is the spice of life!*

Adverse Food Reactions

Most allergic reactions to foods cause symptoms within minutes after eating, but some food-related symptoms are delayed for hours. Different reaction times are due to different immune mechanisms.

Immediate Food Allergies

Most people use the term food allergy to refer to any unpleasant symptom experienced after eating. But the scientific definition of food allergy is a reaction caused by IgE antibodies that occurs within 5 to 60 minutes after eating. Determining if an adverse food reaction is due to IgE antibodies requires diagnostic skin testing.

Symptoms of IgE-mediated food allergies include hives (*urticaria*), scaly and itchy rashes (*eczema*), red rashes, stomach pain, nausea, vomiting, diarrhea, eosinophilic gastroenteritis, redness, swelling of lips, tongue, and face, difficulty in swallowing, shortness of breath, difficulty in breathing, and wheezing (*asthma*). Severe allergic reactions to foods can be life threatening (*anaphylactic shock*) during which blood pressure suddenly drops, throat closes off, patient cannot breathe, and death can occur within minutes.

Each time you eat that same food, your symptoms worsen because the allergen induces the synthesis of more of that specific IgE antibody. Therefore, you should assiduously avoid eating any food that previously caused a severe reaction because the next time you eat that same food, you could go into anaphylactic shock.

Read labels on packaged foods. If you eat out in restaurants, you may unknowingly eat a food you are allergic to. So, carry an *EpiPen* auto-injector with you. This is a syringe filled with *epinephrine* (the hormone *adrenaline*). It has antihistamine activity, which constricts blood vessels, and raises your blood pressure. EpiPen syringes are available by prescription only. You should also wear a medical emergency bracelet listing your serious health conditions.

Delayed Immune Reactions to Foods

A variety of immunological mechanisms can produce delayed symptoms that occur much later after eating a food.

- *Late phase* food reactions that occur four to six hours after eating are caused by IgG$_4$ antibodies, or by WBCs called basophils (Gamboa et al., 1986).
- *Delayed hypersensitivity* reactions mediated by WBCs called T cells develop after one to two days.

Thus, different types of delayed food reactions can produce symptoms tomorrow to foods you ate yesterday!

Food Intolerances

Not all adverse food reactions are caused by immune reactions. Some are due to intolerances such as:

histamine toxicity, lactose intolerance, celiac disease or gluten intolerance, food additives (dyes, preservatives, flavorings, seasonings, artificial sweeteners, sulfite, monosodium glutamate, and hydrolyzed proteins), stimulants (caffeine in coffee and theophylline in tea), oxalate sensitivity, and food poisoning.

Some food intolerances produce the same symptoms as yeast infections and allergies. So, it takes good diagnostic detective work to identify the substances causing your symptoms.

Keep a Food and Symptom Diary

To help identify the culprits responsible for your adverse food reactions:

- Record everything you eat, the time you ate it, and the amount of each food.
- List all of your symptoms, the time they started, and how long they lasted.
- Make a note if anyone else got sick after eating the same food.
- Write down when your menstrual period started because intestinal and vaginal symptoms, plus migraines, depression, etc., tend to occur in the week prior to menstruation. Collectively, these symptoms are called *premenstrual syndrome.*

Patterns will emerge from your diary that allow you to identify foods that provoke symptoms. This information will help you design a diet appropriate for your case. The patient's history is the mainstay of diagnosing food allergies, and the elimination diet is the mainstay of treatment of food allergies (Halpern and Scott (1987). Eliminating a sensitizing food from your diet for six to 12 weeks will decrease antibodies against that allergen, and decrease symptoms if you eat that food again. The only permanent cure for food allergy is avoidance (Boyce et al., 2010).

Diagnostic Food Testing

These diagnostic tests will help you identify the foods causing you problems:

- Scratch (prick) tests for IgE allergies
- Intradermal tests for T cell-mediated hypersensitivity to foods
- Blood tests for IgG_4 antibodies against foods

However, keep in mind that these tests for immune reactions to foods can yield false-positive and false-negative results. They are just a starting point for identifying problem foods. The only true measure of test results is if they correlate with symptoms that develop after eating that particular food during a *food challenge* or *food provocation test.*

Follow these safety guidelines for food challenges (Arslan Lied, 2007):

- Perform a challenge with only one food at a time.
- Don't eat anything that previously caused a severe allergic reaction.
- Place food inside your lower lip and wait 30 minutes to see if you develop a rash on your cheek, edema of your lip, conjunctivitis, rhinitis, or a systemic reaction.
- If you have no immediate symptoms, swallow the food, and wait 15 minutes.

- If no symptoms occur, eat increasing larger portions of that one food over the ensuing hour, waiting 15 minutes in-between.
- Keep a written record of your reactions to food challenges.
- If you develop symptoms during a challenge, avoid that food in the future, and discuss the results with your physician.

═══════════════ Conclusions of Step 8 ═══════════════
Candida Diet

Before you start following the Candida diet, obtain diagnostic testing for intestinal candidiasis and food allergies. If your test results are positive for Candida overgrowth of the gut, treat with antifungals, anti-inflammatory medications, and immunotherapy, and follow the Candida diet by eliminating sweets, restricting complex carbohydrates, avoiding foods and beverages containing yeasts and molds, and avoiding foods you tested positive for in skin tests, blood tests, and food challenges. Identifying foods that cause you symptoms is difficult because adverse food reactions can be caused by many different mechanisms. Despite your necessary food restrictions, try to eat a balanced and varied diet.

STEP 9

Probiotics and Prebiotics

Definitions

Microbiome: The community of microorganisms living inside or on surfaces of the human body.

Dysbiosis: An imbalance in the gut flora caused by antibiotic therapy.

Probiotics: Supplements containing beneficial bacteria that help restore your normal intestinal flora.

Prebiotics: Supplements and foods containing complex carbohydrates that humans cannot digest, but beneficial bacteria can break down and utilize as a food source.

Bacterial Probiotics for Intestinal Disorders

The ideal probiotic contains two bacterial genera, Lactobacillus and Bifidobacterium. Within each of these genera, there are many species that are effective probiotics such as *Lactobacillus acidophilus* and *Bifidobacterium bifidus.* These probiotic bacteria produce lactic acid as well as cyclic dipeptides that have antifungal activity (Magnussona et al., 2003).

Both lactobacilli and bifidobacteria are essential for bowel health. These beneficial bacteria help to replace pathogenic bacteria, heal a leaky gut wall damaged by candidiasis, and are important for self-treating dysbiosis, bloating, and other intestinal symptoms.

Lactobacillus is active mainly in the small intestine whereas Bifidobacterium is active mainly in the large intestine (Gibson and Roberfroid, 1995). Lactobacillus produces lactic acid but no gas from sugar metabolism. In contrast, Bifidobacterium produces mainly butyric acid and gas during fermentation of fiber.

Now, think about this: Butyric acid, produced by Bifidobacterium, is the sole food (carbon and energy source) utilized by our *colonocytes,* the epithelial cells lining the colon. How did this symbiotic relationship evolve between our normal gut flora and cells lining our gut?

Probiotic bacteria are found in yogurt starter cultures, which contain *Lactobacillus acidophilus*, *L. bulgaricus*, and *Streptococcus lactis*. These bacteria release the enzyme lactase, which breaks down milk sugar (*lactose*) into galactose and glucose. Then these simple sugars are fermented by the bacteria producing lactic acid, which gives yogurt its tangy, sour taste. Not all the lactose is broken down, and the remaining lactose in the final product is listed as sugar on the label. After fermentation, the bacteria are still alive, and remain active because yogurt is not pasteurized. When you eat yogurt, these active bacteria can function as probiotics.

> **WARNING**
>
> Yogurt does not always prevent antibiotic-associated diarrhea (Conway et al., 2007). Broad-spectrum antibiotics such as Augmentin (amoxicillin plus clavulanate) produce a high rate of diarrhea (Turck et al., 2003). Likewise, eating yogurt or taking probiotic supplements may not prevent antibiotic-induced yeast infections.

Safety Tip: If you must take antibiotics and you have a history of yeast infections, take antifungals and probiotics together with the antibacterial drug to help prevent oral, intestinal, and vaginal candidiasis (Step 10).

Certain probiotic supplements are effective for specific diseases. The probiotic VSL#3® contains Bifidobacterium, Lactobacillus, and Streptococcus, and is widely prescribed by physicians to combat intestinal yeast overgrowth. It is also helpful for inflammatory bowel diseases such as Crohn's disease and ulcerative colitis (Jobin, 2010). The beneficial bacterial strain *Escherichia coli* Nissle 1917 is specifically effective against inflammatory bowel diseases (Guzy et al., 2008).

Probiotics are sold as tablets or capsules; liquid suspensions are available for people who cannot swallow pills. Most commercial probiotics are effective. Different brands contain various species. If you are not happy with your response to your current probiotic, finish the bottle and buy a different brand next time. By rotating supplements, you benefit from the health-promoting activities of a variety of probiotic bacterial strains. In the future, mixtures of many microbes, called *competitive exclusion cultures*, may become available for scientifically balancing the gut microflora.

Question: Patients frequently ask me how many colony-forming units of a probiotic supplement should they take every day?

Answer: I suggest they follow the instructions on the bottle. But keep in mind that the manufacturer wants to sell as many bottles of their probiotic as possible. So, often the instructions say to take several capsules a day. Without any quantitative studies, I think one capsule a day should be sufficient considering the fact that each contains billions of bacteria.

Most probiotic bacteria do not permanently colonize the intestine, but instead they pass through and are eliminated in the feces (Bouhnik et al., 1992). However, during their transit through the gastrointestinal tract, probiotic bacteria may make conditions in the intestines conducive for regrowth of anaerobic bacteria, which are the "really friendly" normal flora.

Health Promoting Activities of Normal Intestinal Flora

Lactobacillus is a *facultative anaerobe*, which means that it can grow in the presence or absence of oxygen. But it is also *microaerophilic*, which means it can tolerate only low levels of oxygen. Most species of Bifidobacterium are strict anaerobes, but some species are microaerophilic.

While probiotic bacteria are beneficial, the "really friendly" intestinal bacterial flora that normally inhibit the growth of pathogens are *obligate* or *strict anaerobes*, and are killed by oxygen (Kennedy and Volz, 1985a; 1985b). The predominant anaerobic bacteria in the gut are Bacteroides, Clostridium, Faecalibacterium, and Fusobacterium. They form a dense layer or *biofilm* in the mucus gel covering the intestinal mucosa, thereby preventing attachment of pathogens. This is called *colonization resistance*.

Biofilms are polymicrobial communities of beneficial bacteria that can also include Candida as well as pathogenic bacteria embedded in the extracellular matrix (Ganguly and Mitchell, 2011). When the friendly anaerobes are killed by antibiotics, pathogenic bacteria and yeasts can adhere directly to the intestinal epithelium, invade underlying tissue, and cause infections (Kennedy et al., 1987). Infection disrupts the permeability barrier function of the gut wall causing "leaky gut syndrome."

According to Gibson and Roberfroid (1995), anaerobic intestinal bacteria are crucial to our health because they:

- produce short-chain fatty acids (SCFAs) such as acetic, propionic, and butyric acids; and, importantly, butyric acid is the main energy source of colonocytes
- produce secondary bile acids that inhibit pathogens
- improve digestion and absorption of essential nutrients
- synthesize B vitamins and folic acid
- lower blood cholesterol and ammonia levels
- stimulate the immune system to attack malignant cells

Probiotic supplements do not contain obligately anaerobic bacteria because it is difficult to grow anaerobes in large fermentation vats in the absence of oxygen. However, researchers have successfully isolated anaerobic bacteria, and restored them in the intestines of animals (Van Immerseel et al., 2010). Therefore, it is likely that commercial production of obligately anaerobic probiotic bacteria will be feasible in the future.

Safety of Probiotics

Probiotic strains of lactobacilli and bifidobacteria have been proven safe and beneficial in a multitude of studies. Oral administration of these two lactic acid bacteria to 7,526 subjects between 1961 and 1998 did not result in any adverse side effects (Naidu et al., 1999). Safety of probiotic bacteria was reviewed by Hammerman et al. (2006) who concluded that:

- Lactobacilli and bifidobacteria normally occur in the healthy intestine, and in fermented foods.

- Lactobacillus bloodstream infections are rare and occur only in people with severe underlying illnesses. Antony et al. (1996) reviewed 53 cases over a 12-year period and found that the cases of Lactobacillus bacteremia were not caused by the ingested probiotic strain. DNA analysis of the bloodstream isolate accurately identified the source of infection.
- The negligible risk of systemic infection caused by probiotics should be weighed against the high risk of serious diseases, such as necrotizing enterocolitis, which is prevented by probiotic therapy.
- Overall, the proven benefits of probiotic therapy outweigh any potential dangers.

Clinical Conditions Prevented by Probiotics

Probiotics supplements have an extraordinarily large number of health benefits. Taking probiotics helps fortify your natural immunity to Candida (Payne, 2003) as shown by numerous controlled clinical trials (Schulze and Sonnenborn, 2009). Probiotics are also effective in treating and preventing a wide variety of other illnesses (Naidu et al., 1999). Floch and Montrose (2005) reviewed 185 studies and concluded that probiotics successfully treated 68 different medical conditions.

According to the *Cochrane Database of Systematic Reviews*, the following conditions respond favorably to probiotics: infectious diarrhea, eczema, necrotizing enterocolitis, allergic disease, food hypersensitivity, chemotherapy-related diarrhea, radiotherapy-related diarrhea, *Clostridium difficile* diarrhea, ulcerative colitis, bacterial vaginosis, colic in neonates and infants, pediatric antibiotic-induced diarrhea, Crohn's disease, chronic constipation, vulvovaginal candidiasis, and multi-resistant infections.

Vanderpool et al. (2008) explained that probiotic bacteria block pathogens by:

- producing inhibitory substances
- competing for adherence sites on the intestinal epithelium
- enhancing innate immunity
- reducing pathogen-induced inflammation
- promoting intestinal epithelial cell survival
- enhancing barrier function (decreasing leaky gut)
- regulating host cell signaling pathways with cytokines that mediate intestinal epithelial functions

Saccharomyces boulardii vs. *Candida albicans*: A Tale of Two Yeasts

The yeast, *Saccharomyces boulardii*, has been touted to have beneficial effects when used as a probiotic. I have not cited any reports promoting the use of Saccharomyces therapeutic agents against Candida infections because Saccharomyces plays a role in the pathogenesis of Candida infections and, for this reason, **Candida patients are advised to not consume foods and beverages containing yeasts and molds** (Step 8). So, read the warning and evidence below before purchasing a probiotic supplement.

> **WARNING**
>
> I advise against taking oral probiotics containing *S. boulardii* or *S. cerevisiae* if you have intestinal candidiasis. Even though these yeasts have been reported to produce beneficial effects in some diseases, the fact is that Saccharomyces yeasts are involved in the Candida disease process.

Here is the evidence.

- First of all, be aware that *Saccharomyces boulardii* is really *Saccharomyces cerevisiae* as determined by genotypic and proteomic analyses (Herbrecht and Nivoix, 2005).
- Since *S. boulardii* and *S. cerevisiae* are not normally part of our intestinal microbiome, taking these yeasts as probiotic supplements does not restore normal bacterial flora killed by antibiotics.
- Patients with chronic candidiasis tend to be allergic to Candida and other yeasts and molds. For this reason, **Candida patients are advised to not consume foods and beverages containing yeasts and molds**. Likewise, Candida sufferers should not take *S. boulardii* or *S. cerevisiae* probiotic yeasts because Saccharomyces yeasts might trigger allergic or other immune reactions.
- Studies cited in Step 8 reported that Candida patients can decrease their symptoms by not consuming foods and beverages containing yeasts.
- *S. boulardii* or *S. cerevisiae* taken as living probiotic yeasts might overgrow the intestine and start fermenting your dietary carbohydrates producing alcohol. As a result, you might develop the auto-brewery syndrome.
- People who are immunosuppressed because they have *neutropenia* (very low WBC counts of neutrophils) should not take *S. boulardii* or *S. cerevisiae* probiotics because they might develop Saccharomyces septicemia (Herbrecht and Nivoix, 2005).
- Testing for anti-*Saccharomyces cerevisiae* antibodies (ASCA) in blood is used in the diagnosis of Crohn's disease, an inflammatory bowel disease (Kaila et al., 2005).
- Even though the ASCA test detects antibodies to baker's yeast (*S. cerevisiae*) in the laboratory, the *immunogen, i.e.,* the antigen that stimulated the synthesis of ASCA in the body, is actually *C. albicans* **not** *S. cerevisiae* (Standaert-Vitse et al., 2006). Thus, ASCA are really anti-*Candida albicans* antibodies that cross-react with related yeasts. Based on this evidence, **people with Crohn's disease may actually have undiagnosed intestinal candidiasis!**

Safety Tips:

- Instead of taking probiotic yeast supplements containing *S. boulardii* or *S. cerevisiae*, you should take probiotic bacterial supplements containing Lactobacillus and Bifidobacterium. These two bacteria are normally present in the intestinal microflora and will help restore friendly bacteria killed by antibiotics.
- Instead of taking *S. boulardii* because it secretes capric acid, a natural antifungal (Murzyn et al., 2010), take dietary supplements of capric acid and caprylic acid to help suppress intestinal Candida growth (Jadhav et al., 2017).

- In addition to taking probiotic bacteria, you should also take pharmaceutical agents that have been shown to specifically inhibit or kill Candida in controlled clinical studies. This recommendation is based on the "magic bullet" theory of the 19th-century German Nobel laureate physician, Dr. Paul Ehrlich. He proposed using treatments that selectively target disease-causing organisms without harming the body. Prescription antifungals for yeast infections fit this recommendation. If you take oral antifungals to treat Candida yeasts, they will destroy probiotic yeasts as well. That's another reason not to take *S. boulardii!*

Prebiotics

If you developed intestinal yeast overgrowth after taking antibiotics, you can recolonize your intestine with "really friendly" anaerobic bacteria by taking oral probiotic supplements containing Lactobacillus species and Bifidobacterium species of bacteria. These lactic acid bacteria make the intestinal environment suitable for regrowth of obligate anaerobic bacteria. As discussed earlier, there are no commercially available obligately anaerobic probiotics because they would be killed by oxygen during the large-scale production processes.

Another way to recolonize your intestine with beneficial anaerobes is to take an oral *prebiotic* supplement that feeds anaerobic bacteria. *Prebiotics* are carbohydrates that humans cannot digest, but can be utilized by beneficial bacteria in the gastrointestinal tract. When prebiotics are taken together with probiotics, the combinations are called *synbiotics* because they act synergistically to promote intestinal health. Three examples of prebiotics are discussed below.

Fructooligosaccharides

Prebiotic supplements of *fructooligosaccharides* are short chains (*polymers*) of the fruit sugar *fructose* that occur naturally. FOS are indigestible and pass through the human digestive tract to the colon where they are digested by bifidobacteria. Bifidobacteria ferment FOS, producing beneficial short-chain fatty acids that feed our colonocytes. A disadvantage of taking FOS is that it results in the production of methane gas, which causes *flatulence.*

Fiber Supplements

Yet another way to recolonize your intestine with anaerobic bacteria is to take a prebiotic fiber supplement (such as Benefiber®) that nourishes the good bacteria. This fiber product contains dextrin, a short polymer of glucose produced by the breakdown of starch or glycogen. Dextrin is heat-treated to cause branching of the polymer molecule, which prevents our digestive tract from breaking it down and releasing sugar. Bifidobacteria can digest this fiber product, producing beneficial short-chain fatty acids that feed our colonocytes. Benefiber also keeps the stool soft, thereby preventing constipation.

Lactulose

Lactulose is a disaccharide composed of galactose and fructose that is produced commercially by isomerization of lactose. Lactulose is a nonabsorbable sugar used to treat constipation. Because it is not broken down by human digestive enzymes, it stays in the intestinal contents causing retention of water through osmosis leading to softer, easier-to-pass stool. Lactulose is also a prebiotic carbohydrate that stimulates the growth of healthy bacteria. Another benefit of lactulose is that it inhibits the growth of pathogenic bacteria. Lactulose is fermented in the colon by gut flora, such as bifidobacteria and lactobacilli, which produce short-chain fatty acids including lactic acid and acetic acid that stimulate peristalsis. A disadvantage of lactulose is that it produces methane and hydrogen gases that cause flatulence, abdominal bloating, and cramps.

All three of the above-mentioned prebiotics function to promote the growth of anaerobic bacteria, which produce SCFA that promote the growth of epithelial cells lining the colon. Even though prebiotic supplements help repopulate the intestine with friendly bacteria, a better way to promote the regrowth of intestinal anaerobes killed by antibiotics is to eat more fruits, vegetables, and whole grains as discussed next.

Eat More Fiber

Instead of buying expensive prebiotic supplements, it is better to eat foods high in fiber. Fruits, vegetables, and whole grains contain fiber and fructooligosaccharides, which promote the growth of obligately anaerobic bacteria that are the "really friendly" normal flora.

Many Candida patients experience constipation caused by intestinal yeast overgrowth, and then make this problem worse by following an overly restrictive Candida diet that prohibits eating carbohydrates by eliminating fruits, starchy vegetables, and whole grains. It is important to eat these food groups because they contain two essential types of fiber:

- *Soluble fiber* dissolves in water.
- *Insoluble fiber* does not dissolve in water.

Humans cannot digest either type of fiber. But anaerobic intestinal bacteria can ferment soluble fiber, producing beneficial short-chain fatty acids (SCFA), such as acetate, propionate, and butyrate. Insoluble fiber, also called roughage, is not digested by either humans or intestinal bacteria. But insoluble fiber is beneficial because it absorbs water and increases in bulk as it moves through the digestive system, thereby easing fecal elimination.

The following food sources of dietary fiber contain certain carbohydrates that are not digestible by humans, but are fermentable by intestinal bacteria:

- Raw oats, unrefined barley, yacón root, and whole grain breakfast cereals are classified as prebiotics.
- Oats and barley have high amounts of beta-glucans.
- Fruit and berries contain pectins.
- Seeds contain gums.
- Onions and Jerusalem artichokes are rich in inulin and fructooligosaccharides.
- Bananas and legumes contain resistant starch.
- Bananas, onions, garlic, leeks, asparagus, artichokes, barley, wheat, jicama, yacón, tomatoes, and almonds contain fructooligosaccharides.

Eat Oat Bran

Whole grains such as unrefined oats, rice, corn, wheat, barley, and millet contain digestible carbohydrates plus an indigestible outer coat called *bran*, which has a high content of oil, nutrients, and soluble fiber. Anaerobic bacteria in the colon break down bran producing beneficial SCFA. Bran is separated from grains during milling, and sold separately. Oat bran is inexpensive, can be added to baked goods, cooked breakfast cereals, and stirred into yogurt, soups, and gravies.

Butyric Acid Helps Heal "Leaky Gut Syndrome"

Butyric acid is one of the short-chain fatty acids produced by anaerobic bacteria during the breakdown of soluble fiber. It has many beneficial effects on intestinal health. Butyric acid promotes the growth of bifidobacteria and other beneficial anaerobes in the large intestine (Olesen and Gudmand-Høyer, 2000). Butyric acid is also the preferred food source for *colonocytes*, the epithelial cells that line the colon wall (Gibson and Roberfroid, 1995). By promoting the growth of colonocytes, butyric acid decreases the permeability of the intestinal epithelium by increasing the expression of tight junction proteins (Van Immerseel et al., 2010). In other words, butyric acid helps heal "leaky gut syndrome." Here's how.

After a Candida infection has been cured, the damaged intestinal wall needs to be repaired. Part of the healing process involves the rapid turnover of intestinal epithelial cells (*enterocytes*) during tissue regeneration. Intestinal integrity is maintained by the constant movement of new enterocytes along the extracellular matrix from the crypts to the villus tips (Wagner, 2005).

Butyric acid:

- feeds the "really friendly" anaerobic bacteria as well as colonocytes
- improves abdominal symptoms in Crohn's and inflammatory bowel diseases (Wachtershauser and Stein, 2000; Vernia et al., 2003; Hallert et al., 2003)
- controls transepithelial fluid transport
- ameliorates mucosal inflammation and oxidative status
- reinforces the epithelial defense barrier
- modulates visceral sensitivity and intestinal motility
- prevents colorectal cancer (Canani et al., 2011)

Just think about how this amazing symbiotic relationship evolved. Friendly anaerobic bacteria in our gut produce the main food source, butyric acid, for our colon cells! Without butyric acid, our colonocytes cannot function properly and undergo *autophagy* (self-digestion). Thus, the best way for you to restore anaerobic bacteria and overcome "leaky gut syndrome" is to add more fiber to your diet by eating more fruits, vegetables, and whole grains. Your mother was right!

You can also take butyric acid orally or use it as an enema. Calcium and magnesium butyrate supplements are sold OTC as enteric-coated capsules. Rectal enemas containing sodium butyrate require a doctor's prescription, but experience has shown that rectal administration of butyric acid is hampered by low patient compliance (Van Immerseel et al., 2010). Rectal suppositories containing sodium butyrate are also available.

Probiotics for Yeast Vaginitis

The data are clear from a multitude of studies that oral probiotics are helpful in treating and preventing intestinal candidiasis and other diseases. But can women prevent yeast vaginitis by taking oral probiotics, eating yogurt, or inserting probiotics or yogurt into their vagina? The following studies were performed to answer this question.

- In 1992, Hilton et al. reported that women who ate yogurt with active cultures of *Lactobacillus acidophilus* daily for six months showed a decreased incidence of vaginal yeast infections. The media hailed this report as an effective self-treatment. However, scientists criticized this study because it lacked a control group of women who did not eat yogurt, and it had very low statistical power because only a small number of women (13) completed the protocol.

- Fitzsimmons and Berry (1994) reported that lactobacilli inhibited the growth of *Candida albicans* in laboratory media.

- Williams et al. (2001) found that vaginal yeast infections can be prevented in women who had HIV with weekly intravaginal insertion of *Lactobacillus acidophilus* capsules or clotrimazole tablets.

- Reid et al. (2003) found that oral supplements containing lactic acid bacteria restored vaginal lactobacilli, and reduced vaginal colonization by pathogenic bacteria and yeasts.

- Van Kessel et al. (2003) reviewed the literature, and concluded that Lactobacillus in yogurt and probiotics show promise for treating yeast vaginitis and bacterial vaginosis.

- However, Pirotta et al. (2004) reported that Lactobacillus taken orally and inserted vaginally failed to prevent yeast vaginitis induced by antibiotics.

- Hamad et al. (2006) found that the presence of Lactobacillus in the reproductive tract of mice can suppress *C. albicans* growth.

- Falagas et al. (2006) reviewed the literature, and concluded that lactobacilli inhibit *Candida albicans* growth and adherence to vaginal epithelium. While some studies found that vulvovaginal candidiasis is associated with a low number of lactobacilli in the vagina, or the presence of H_2O_2-nonproducing vaginal lactobacilli, other studies did not support these findings. Even though some clinical trials support the effectiveness of lactobacilli administered either orally or intravaginally in preventing infection of the vagina by *C. albicans*, other clinical trials did not corroborate these findings.

- Carriero et al. (2007) found that vaginal insertion of capsules containing *Lactobacillus plantarum* P17630 in patients with Candida vaginitis may enhance the therapeutic efficacy of oral fluconazole, and may help to prevent future episodes of vulvovaginal candidiasis. But they cautioned that further work is warranted.

- Martinez et al. (2009a) found that probiotic strains of Lactobacillus inhibit the growth of *C. albicans* in laboratory cultures of vaginal epithelial cells. Martinez et al. (2009b) reported that treating vulvovaginal candidiasis with oral fluconazole plus probiotics was successful.

- However, Abad and Safdar (2009) reviewed many studies, and found no clear benefit of oral Lactobacillus for vaginal candidiasis.

- Reid et al. (2009) proposed that the positive effects of eating yogurt or taking oral probiotic supplements on vaginal microflora must be indirect, acting through immune modulation.
- Kovachev and Vatcheva-Dobrevska (2015) found that treating women who have vaginal yeast infections with 150 mg of fluconazole orally plus a single vaginal globule of fenticonazole (600 mg) on the same day followed by ten applications of a vaginal probiotic containing *Lactobacillus acidophilus*, *L. rhamnosus*, *Streptococcus thermophilus*, and *L. delbrueckii* subsp. *bulgaricus* worked better than treating with just antifungal medications. Probiotic vaginal suppository products are available online, but like most probiotics, they are not regulated by the FDA.
- Vladareanu et al. (2018) observed that *L. plantarum* P17630 taken orally as a probiotic supplement can survive in the gastrointestinal tract and colonize the vagina by cross-contamination from the rectum.

While most of these studies found that eating yogurt or taking oral probiotics containing Lactobacillus were safe and helpful in preventing vaginal infection by *C. albicans*, researchers point out that many of these studies had methodological faults. Furthermore, there is no scientific consensus about the safety and efficacy of inserting yogurt or Lactobacillus probiotics intravaginally to prevent vaginal yeast infections. If you are tempted to insert yogurt or Lactobacillus probiotics intravaginally, take heed that this self-treatment can result in vaginal Lactobacillus overgrowth.

Lactobacillus Vaginosis

Terminology

Vaginosis means an imbalance of normal flora.

Vaginitis means an infection by a pathogen.

According to these strict definitions, Lactobacillus vaginitis and Candida vaginitis should be referred to as Lactobacillus vaginosis and Candida vaginosis because lactobacilli and yeasts are normally present in the vagina. Despite this scientific distinction, the terms vaginosis and vaginitis are generally used interchangeably.

> **WARNING**
>
> Until definitive research studies have been published, I advise against putting yogurt or Lactobacillus probiotics into your vagina because these remedies may cause a vaginal overgrowth of Lactobacillus bacteria. This infection is called by various names including:
>
> - *Lactobacillus vaginosis*
> - *desquamative inflammatory vaginitis*
> - *cytolytic vaginitis* (Secor, 1992; Cerikcioglu and Beksac, 2004)
> - *vaginal lactobacillosis* (Horowitz et al., 1994; Paavonen, 1995)

Diagnosis of Lactobacillus Vaginosis

Cytolytic vaginosis may be misdiagnosed as yeast vaginitis (Cerikcioglu and Beksac, 2004) because their symptoms are similar. However, these two infections are easily distinguished by the following laboratory tests:

- Microscopy of vaginal smears from Lactobacillus vaginosis teem with long rod-shaped bacteria (*bacilli*) and dead vaginal cells.
- Measuring the pH of vaginal discharge with narrow range pH paper shows that lactobacilli inserted vaginally produce so much lactic acid that the vaginal pH can be lowered from the normal pH 4.5 to as low as 2.5. This pH value is 100 times more acidic than normal, and causes vaginal epithelial cells to burst (undergo *cytolysis*). Dead epithelial cells turn white, and slough or peel off the vaginal wall (*desquamation*), producing a white, cheesy or creamy vaginal discharge similar to that in yeast vaginitis.
- Culture of a vaginal swab on a special medium (Lactobacillus-MRS agar; www.anaerobesystems.com) promotes the growth of lactobacilli. It is an enriched selective medium intended for the isolation and cultivation of Lactobacillus found in clinical specimens and in dairy and food products. The basal medium consisting of peptones, yeast extract, and glucose is supplemented with sorbitan monooleate complex (a source for fatty acids) and magnesium to meet additional growth requirements. Sodium acetate and ammonium citrate are added to inhibit growth of gram-negative bacteria, oral flora, and fungi.
- Cytolytic vaginosis is often a cyclic condition (Secor, 1992), occurring more often during the two weeks before menstruation (*luteal phase*) when estrogen is highest. Estrogen stimulates vaginal epithelial cells to synthesize more glycogen (Tyler and Woodall, 1982; page 31). Glycogen is broken down by enzymes from lactobacilli and vaginal cells into glucose, which is fermented by lactobacilli to produce lactic acid. Yeast vaginitis is also cyclic for the same reason—estrogen stimulates glycogen formation in vaginal cells. Glycogen is broken down into glucose, which feeds the yeasts. Symptoms of both cytolytic vaginosis and yeast vaginitis improve during menstruation when estrogen is lowest, and the vaginal pH is raised by menstrual blood, which is about pH 7.

Additional Reasons for Not Putting Yogurt or Probiotics into Your Vagina:

- Your self-diagnosis of yeast vaginitis may be incorrect.
- Yogurt contains milk proteins (caseins, albumins, and globulins) that are potentially allergenic, and could cause vaginal inflammation in sensitive women.
- Yogurt contains other bacteria that are not normal inhabitants of the vagina, and could overgrow causing bacterial vaginitis.
- The lactobacilli in yogurt and oral probiotic supplements differ from the strain of *Lactobacillus acidophilus* normally found in the vagina (named *Doderlein's bacillus* after its discoverer). *Doderlein's bacillus* adheres to the vaginal wall and produces lactic acid, bacteriocins, hydrogen peroxide, and biosurfactants, all of which help control the growth of pathogens (Reid, 2001).

Treatment of Lactobacillus Vaginosis

If you are diagnosed with cytolytic vaginosis:

- Stop inserting probiotics or yogurt into your vagina.
- Neutralize the acidity by douching once or twice a week with a solution of one teaspoon of sodium bicarbonate powder in a pint of warm water (Secor, 1992).
- Monitor the effectiveness of bicarbonate douches with pH paper (nitrazine test paper) that measures pH values from 1 to 12. You can buy pH indicator paper online from laboratory and medical supply companies. But remember that the number of lactobacilli in the vagina is determined by your age and estrogen level (Chapter 2). Before puberty and after menopause, estrogen is low, the number of vaginal lactobacilli is low, and the normal pH is around 6.0. During the childbearing years when women are estrogenized and menstruating, the normal vaginal pH is around 4.5.

Safety Tips: Follow this home treatment with bicarbonate douches to get rid of excess vaginal lactobacilli and resist the idea of treating vaginal Lactobacillus overgrowth with antibiotics. Review the sequence of events that got you into this condition, and don't make the same mistakes again. For example, were you treated with antibiotics for a bacterial infection, and you developed yeast vaginitis? Did you treat yeast symptoms with an antifungal, and then you inserted yogurt or Lactobacillus probiotics intravaginally to prevent a recurrence of yeast vaginitis? This last event is where you went wrong. I advise women not to insert lactobacilli intravaginally, especially because many studies have shown that taking lactobacilli by mouth is safe and effective for restoring normal intestinal and vaginal flora.

If you want to learn whether you have the normal number of lactobacilli in your vagina consistent with your age and estrogen level, ask your gynecologist to measure the pH of your vaginal discharge and order these tests: vaginal swab cultures for lactobacilli and yeasts, or PCR tests for vaginal microbial DNA.

After presenting the above carefully researched and thought out scientific explanation, I am now going to go out on a limb and say: Instead of inserting foreign bacteria into your vagina, think of a way to promote the regrowth of your normal Doderlein's bacillus killed by antibiotics. Some websites and articles (Collins et al., 2018) have suggested that lactulose might be useful as an intravaginal prebiotic to promote the growth of lactobacilli in the vagina. But, to date, no controlled clinical studies of this home remedy have been published. Look for reports on vaginal prebiotics and probiotics appearing in the medical literature in the future.

Fecal Microbiota Transplantation

Since I just went out on a limb to write about an unproven self-care remedy for vaginitis, I might as well discuss another unproven treatment for intestinal Candida infection here called *fecal microbiota transplantation*. In this procedure, feces are transferred from a healthy donor into a patient's intestinal tract. The term *microbiota* includes the entire population of microorganisms that colonizes a particular location in the body. The term *microbiome* refers to the genetic makeup of the respective microbiota. Our microbiome is comprised of bacteria, fungi, protozoa, and viruses.

FMT was originally developed for treating life-threatening, toxigenic *Clostridium difficile* colitis. While FMT is a scientifically proven, life-saving therapy in *C. difficile* colitis, it has not been studied in the case of chronic Candida infection of the gut. Nevertheless, many patients with intestinal candidiasis have tried FMT after becoming desperate for a cure because they haven't improved after taking oral antifungals and probiotics for weeks or months—or even years!

Several patients who consulted with me about their chronic intestinal yeast infection condition told me they intended to carry out self-administered FMT, or have already done so. One client told me she traveled out of the country and paid out-of-pocket for a physician to perform FMT for her intestinal Candida condition. From what little feedback I received from patients, the results from FMT were disappointing for some Candida patients after they paid thousands of dollars for a procedure that was unproven for yeast infections. Other Candida patients experienced positive results from self-administered FMT.

So, let's discuss the protocols used for medically assisted and self-administered FMT, and consider some difficulties associated with this treatment when used "off label" for an unapproved condition such as intestinal candidiasis.

Pitfalls with FMT

1. **It is unlikely that transplanted donor bacteria would be able to colonize the gut of a recipient unless the stubborn Candida infection is eradicated first.**

   Any FMT protocol for intestinal candidiasis must stipulate that effective oral antifungal treatment must be given at a high enough dose for a long enough time to eliminate yeasts that are free in the lumen, attached to the intestinal biofilm slime layer, and growing intracellularly inside intestinal epithelial cells.

   Effective oral antifungal treatment must include long-term nonabsorbed nystatin plus fluconazole or another systemic antifungal administered at higher than standard dosage to eradicate dose-dependent yeasts until a stool culture is negative for Candida. Only then would space become available on the gut wall to allow transferred fecal bacteria to attach and colonize the intestine.

2. **The major point emphasized here in Step 9 is that *the "really friendly bacteria" in our intestinal tract that protect against Candida overgrowth are obligately anaerobic bacteria.***

   Therefore, it is essential that when a fecal specimen is collected from a donor, it must be protected from contact with air. Unfortunately, published FMT protocols start with putting feces into a blender with a sterile saline solution and rapidly mixing, which aerates the sample! That procedure assures that the obligate anaerobes in feces from healthy donors would be dead by the time they are implanted into the recipient Candida patient. This prediction was shown to be true by the work of Papanicolas et al. (2019) who found that homogenization of stool in ambient air reduced microbial viability to 19%, and resulted in up to 12-fold reductions in the abundance of important commensal taxa, including the highly butyrogenic species *Faecalibacterium prausnitzii, Subdoligranulum variable,* and *Eubacterium hallii.*

Currently, no commercial probiotic supplement is available that contains obligately anaerobic bacteria because they would be killed by oxygen in fermentation vats during large scale production. The lactic acid bacteria in commercially available probiotics include species of Lactobacillus and Bifidobacterium, which grow under anaerobic conditions, but are microaerophilic and can tolerate low levels of oxygen.

The ideal specimen for FMT should contain several species of obligately anaerobic bacteria that have been isolated, purified, and identified under anaerobic conditions. Examples of ideal bacteria for FMT might be representative species of Bacteroidetes (*Bacteroides thetaiotamicron*) and clostridial Firmicutes (*Blautia producta*) because they were found to eliminate Candida from the GI tract in animal studies (Lopez-Medina and Koh, 2016). Interestingly, while *Bacteroides thetaiotamicron* promoted Candida reduction, *Bacteroides fragilis* had no effect on Candida colonization.

In the current absence of pure cultures of ideal probiotic anaerobes that inhibit Candida colonization in the gut, the easiest way to prepare a specimen for FMT would be to allow a stool specimen to remain in its formed state after collection, and then insert chunks into gelatin capsules. In this way, bacteria in the center of the fecal sample would be protected from contact with air. The recipient should swallow a couple of freshly encapsulated feces after meals three times a day.

Anaerobically prepared stool for FMT was compared to aerobically processed stool in a study of ulcerative colitis patients by Costello et al. (2019) in a randomized, double-blind, clinical trial. Remission occurred in 32% of patients receiving anaerobic preparations compared with 9% of those who received aerobic preparations. Thus, anaerobic processing of specimens for FMT has been found to improve microbial viability.

3. **A danger associated with self-administered FMT is that the donor may be carrying pathogenic microorganisms to which the donor is immune but the recipient is susceptible.**

The consensus among infectious disease professionals is that the FMT donor should be a healthy household member, preferably a blood relative or spouse, who presumably shares a similar gut microbiome. In medically assisted FMT, the donor's feces and blood should be screened for pathogens by performing these tests:

- **Microscopy of stool** for ova, parasites, and Giardia
- **Culture, sensitivity, and PCR of stool** for Candida, and enteric bacterial pathogens
- **Serology of blood** for complete blood count with manual differential, plus comprehensive metabolic panel, and viruses (HIV1 and HIV2, hepatitis A, B, and C, and CMV), and syphilis

While microscopy of donor stool will reveal some parasites, special laboratory media are needed to select for growth of yeasts and bacteria, and antibody testing is needed for viruses. Initial diagnostic testing of the recipient should be based on her/his risk factors and medical history. Testing of the recipient and donor may not be covered by your health insurance, and will cost $1,000 or more.

4. **In addition to screening tests, there are inclusion and exclusion factors that scientists and physicians must consider in designing a protocol for a controlled clinical study of FMT to treat chronic intestinal candidiasis. For example:**

Some medically assisted FMT protocols call for pretreatment of the Candida patient with strong antibacterial antibiotics to clear away the recipient's gut bacteria allowing space for the incoming donor bacteria to attach. Most Candida patients view this pretreatment with horror since treatment with antibiotics is why they developed intestinal candidiasis in the first place!

A step that should be included in any FMT protocol is that patients need to be instructed on how to provide the proper gut environment that will preserve the implanted donor bacteria and allow them to thrive. The many helpful hints offered here in Step 9 will help promote the growth of newly transferred friendly microbiome.

Note: Before you contemplate using FMT for your intestinal yeast problem, read the Protocol for Nystatin Enemas to Treat Intestinal Candidiasis and the rest of the information about anti-fungal treatments in Step 2.

Conclusions of Step 9
Probiotics and Prebiotics

Oral probiotics containing Lactobacillus and Bifidobacterium are safe and effective if taken by mouth to treat and prevent numerous diseases resulting from antibiotic disruption of the normal intestinal flora. Oral probiotics containing Saccharomyces should be avoided since yeasts are involved in the candidiasis disease process. That is why the Candida diet warns against consuming foods and beverages containing yeasts and molds. Women are advised against inserting probiotics or yogurt intravaginally since lactic acid-producing bacteria can cause the vaginal pH to drop below the normal pH of 4.5. While supplements, diet, and probiotics may ameliorate some intestinal symptoms, they may not result in a permanent cure. In most cases, oral antifungal prescription drugs are needed for long-term daily treatment of candidiasis followed by weekly prophylactic antifungal maintenance as discussed next in Step 10.

STEP 10

Antifungal Prophylaxis

ONCE YOU HAVE HAD A yeast infection, you know that you are susceptible to Candida overgrowth—by definition. So, in the future, if your physician prescribes a medication known to cause yeast infections, such as antibiotics or other drugs discussed in Step 6, ask for preventive antiyeast medicine to be used *at the same time.*

Prevention Is Better Than Cure

Epidemiologists estimate for every $1 spent on vaccinations and other preventive treatments, $4 are saved because people will not have to be treated for that disease. The savings in terms of preventing suffering cannot be calculated in terms of dollars.

However, before physicians can develop protocols to prevent yeast infections, they must first acknowledge the inadvertent iatrogenesis caused by certain medical treatments. Even though the concept of prevention is self-evident, it is unfortunately not standard of care.

Take home message: Ask for antifungal prophylaxis when you are prescribed a medication that causes yeast infections. Be assertive. *Don't suffer in silence any longer!*

Preventive Protocols

There are no standard protocols for preventing yeast infections in people with a history of yeast infections. Therefore, physicians must design preventive treatments to fit each individual patient. Doctors must use their best clinical judgment based on past successes with preventing candidiasis in other susceptible patients. Guidelines for antifungal prophylaxis can be concurrent or intermittent.

Concurrent Antifungal Prophylaxis

If you are taking a medication that causes yeast infections, use an antifungal *at the same time* as explained in these examples.

- After taking a puff from a steroid inhaler for asthma, rinse out your mouth with water, and then swish and swallow a dose of nystatin suspension to prevent oral thrush.
- When taking an oral systemic antibacterial antibiotic or other systemic drug that predisposes to candidiasis, there are two alternative protocols you can use to prevent yeast infections from developing. The first is to use antifungals that are not absorbed into the bloodstream so they will not interact with systemic drugs. For example, use intravaginal capsules of boric acid powder to prevent vaginal infections (Reichman et al., 2009), and/or take oral nystatin powder or suspension to prevent intestinal candidiasis.
- The second protocol to use to prevent yeast infections from developing when taking an oral systemic drug that predisposes to candidiasis is to take a systemic antifungal agent every second or third day to avoid drug interactions. Since systemic antibiotics and systemic antifungals are broken down by the same detoxification enzymes in the liver, concentrations of both drugs can increase to toxic levels if both are taken together every day.
- Alternatively, you can choose an antibiotic + antifungal combination that does not interact with cytochrome P450 (CYP) liver enzymes. Drug combinations that compete for the same cytochrome proteins are listed on this website by Preissner et al. (2010): http://bioinformatics.charite.de/supercyp/index.php?site=drug_interaction_checker. For example, since Diflucan (fluconazole) and Cipro (ciprofloxacin) both utilize CYP-1A2 and 3A4 liver enzymes, choose an antibiotic from this website that does not interact with Diflucan, such as Avelox (moxifloxacin).

Intermittent Maintenance or Suppression

Researchers have developed various antifungal protection protocols for people who experience repeated yeast infections. Instead of just treating each new episode as it occurs, these studies found that providing maintenance antifungal therapy on an intermittent schedule is effective in suppressing yeast growth.

Sobel (1985) treated women suffering from recurrent vulvovaginal candidiasis with 400 mg of ketoconazole daily for two weeks, followed by intermittent prophylactic ketoconazole 400 mg a day for five days each month for three menstrual cycles.

Ringdahl (2000) stated that long-term maintenance therapy is warranted because many women experience recurrences of yeast vaginitis after antifungal treatment is discontinued. Women are more likely to comply with antifungal prophylaxis if it is administered orally rather than vaginally.

Williams et al. (2001) suggest that most suppression regimens treat for one day each week; others treat daily for one week out of each month.

Donders et al. (2008) emphasized the importance of individualizing treatment for each woman rather than adhering to a fixed regimen. Women who harbored non-*albicans Candida* vaginally relapsed more often and needed a higher dose of a systemic antifungal agent for suppression.

Vazquez and Bronze (2011) recommended Diflucan (fluconazole) 150 mg weekly for six months for recurrent vulvovaginal candidiasis after initial control of relapse.

Rosa et al. (2012) found that maintenance with one oral fluconazole tablet (150 mg) a week for six months prevented recurrences of vulvovaginal candidiasis **if** the yeast was susceptible to fluconazole.

Take home messages:

- After yeast symptoms resolve with antifungal treatment, switch from daily treatment to weekly maintenance to suppress yeast growth and prevent future recurrences.
- Weekly suppression can be followed if you have just completed a course of a drug that predisposes people to develop candidiasis, or if you have a chronic disease condition that makes you susceptible to yeast infections.
- If your recurrent yeast vaginitis is estrogen-dependent, and you get another vaginal yeast infection every month during the two weeks between ovulation and menstruation, follow monthly cyclic prophylaxis by using oral plus vaginal antifungals daily for 3 to 7 days at midcycle each month for six months.
- Since non-*albicans Candida* species tend to be dose dependent (resistant to low dosages and sensitive to high dosages), these infections require a higher dose of a systemic antifungal agent for both treatment and suppression protocols. Guidelines for dosages of older antifungals, newer more effective antifungals, or synergistic combinations of antifungals are provided in Step 2.

Durable Power of Attorney for Health Care

If you have a history of repeated yeast infection, explain your susceptibility to candidiasis in your Durable Power of Attorney for Health Care. Ask your health care advocate to request prophylactic antifungals if you are given treatments that predispose to candidiasis. A DPAHC indicates your wishes in case you are unable to speak for yourself. Give copies to your physician and your advocate (spouse, child, relative, or friend).

Conclusions of Step 10
Antifungal Prophylaxis

The key to preventing yeast infections is avoiding *all* risk factors and using antifungal prophylaxis when some predisposing conditions are unavoidable. Instead of waiting—in dread—for your next yeast infection, launch a preemptive strike against Candida. Obtain antifungal prophylaxis and follow the other medical care and self-help guidelines in this ten-step program. *You **can** conquer Candida!*

PART III

Literature Cited

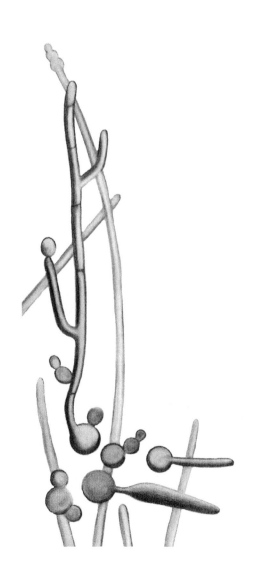

AAAAI. 2011a. www.aaaai.org/members/academy_statements/position_statements/ps35.asp.

AAAAI. 2011b. www.aaaai.org/media/statistics/allergy-statistics.asp.

AAAI. 1986. Candidiasis Hypersensitivity Syndrome. Position Statement by the Executive Committee of the American Academy of Allergy and Immunology. *Journal of Allergy and Clinical Immunology* 78:271-2. (Note: This organization subsequently changed their name to American Academy of Allergy, Asthma, and Immunology. www.aaaai.org).

Abad CL, Safdar N. 2009. The role of lactobacillus probiotics in the treatment or prevention of urogenital infections--a systematic review. *Journal of Chemotherapy* 21:243-52.

Akiyama K. 2000. The role of fungal allergy in bronchial asthma. *Japanese Journal of Medical Mycology* 41:149-55.

Akiyama K, Mathison DA, Riker JB, Greenberger PA, Patterson R. 1984. Allergic bronchopulmonary candidiasis. *Chest* 85:699-701.

Alexander JG. 1969. Tetracycline and nystatin. *British Medical Journal* 2:251.

Alexander JG. 1975. Allergy in the gastrointestinal tract. *Lancet* 2:1264.

Alexander JW, Boyce ST, Babcock GF, Gianotti L, Peck MD, Dunn DL, Pyles T, Childress CP, Ash SK. 1990. The process of microbial translocation. *Annals of Surgery* 212:496-512.

Alexander RB, Brady F, Ponniah S. 1997. Autoimmune prostatitis: evidence of T cell reactivity with normal prostatic proteins. *Urology* 50:893-9.

AMA. 1987. In Vivo Diagnostic testing and immunotherapy for allergy. Position statement by the Council on Scientific Affairs of the American Medical Association. *JAMA* 258:1505-8.

Amouri I, Sellami H, Borji N, Abbes S, Sellami A, Cheikhrouhou F, Maazoun L, Khaled S, Khrouf S, Boujelben Y, Ayadi A. 2011. Epidemiological survey of vulvovaginal candidosis in Sfax, Tunisia. *Mycoses* 54: e499-505.

Anderson MR, Klink K, Cohrssen A. 2004. Evaluation of vaginal complaints. *JAMA* 291:1368-79.

Antico A, Pagani M, Vescovi PP, Bonadonna P, Senna G. 2011. Food-specific IgG$_4$ lack diagnostic value in adult patients with chronic urticaria and other suspected allergy skin symptoms. *International Archives of Allergy and Immunology* 155:52-6.

Antony SJ, Stratton CW, Dummer JS. 1996. Lactobacillus bacteremia: description of the clinical course in adult patients without endocarditis. *Clinical Infectious Diseases* 23:773-8.

Arat S, Spivak A, Van Horn S, Thomas E, Traini C, Sathe G, Livi GP, Ingraham K, Jones L, Aubart K, Holmes DJ, Naderer O, James R. Brown JR. 2015. *Antimicrobial Agents and Chemotherapy* 59:1182-92.

Aridogan IA, Izol V, Ilkit M. 2011. Superficial fungal infections of the male genitalia: a review. *Critical Reviews in Microbiology* 37:237-44.

Arslan Lied G. 2007. Gastrointestinal food hypersensitivity: Symptoms, diagnosis and provocation tests. *Turkish Journal of Gastroenterology* 18:5-13.

Ashman RB, Ott AK. 1989. Autoimmunity as a factor in recurrent vulvovaginal candidosis and the minor vestibular gland syndrome. *Journal of Reproductive Medicine* 34:264-6.

Atkins RC. 1997. *Dr. Atkins' New Diet Revolution*, Avon Books, New York.

Axelsen NH. 1976. Analysis of human Candida precipitins by quantitative immunoelectrophoresis: a model for analysis of complex microbial antigen-antibody systems. *Scandinavian Journal of Immunology* 5:177-90.

Bachmann GA, Rosen R, Arnold LD, Burd I, Rhoads GG, Leiblum SR, Avis N. 2006a. Chronic vulvar and other gynecologic pain: prevalence and characteristics in a self-reported survey. *Journal of Reproductive Medicine* 51:3-9.

Bachmann GA, Rosen R, Pinn VW, Utian WH, Ayers C, Basson R, Binik YM, Brown C, Foster DC, Gibbons JM Jr, Goldstein I, Graziottin A, Haefner HK, Harlow BL, Spadt SK, Leiblum SR, Masheb RM, Reed BD, Sobel JD, Veasley C, Wesselmann U, Witkin SS. 2006b. Vulvodynia: a state-of-the-art consensus on definitions, diagnosis and management. *Journal of Reproductive Medicine* 51:447-56.

Bacigalupo A, Van Lint M, Frassoni F, Podestà M, Marmont A, Colombo L. 1983. Mepartricin: a new antifungal agent for the treatment of disseminated candida infections in the immunocompromised host. *Acta Haematologica* 69:409–3.

Baggish MS, Sze EH, Johnson R. 1997. Urinary oxalate excretion and its role in vulvar pain syndrome. *American Journal of Obstetrics and Gynecology* 177:507-11.

Barclay GR, McKenzie H, Pennington J, Parratt D, Pennington CR. 1992. The effect of dietary yeast on the activity of stable chronic Crohn's disease. *Scandinavian Journal of Gastroenterology* 27:196-200.

Barrett S. 2005. Dubious "yeast allergies." www.quackwatch.org/01QuackeryRelatedTopics/candida.html.

Barrie SA. 1986. Comprehensive digestive stool analysis. In: Pizzorno JE, Murray MT, eds. *A Textbook of Natural Medicine*. Seattle: JBC Press: II: CDSA-1-4.

Bartie KL, Williams DW, Wilson MJ, Potts AJ, Lewis MA. 2001. PCR fingerprinting of *Candida albicans* associated with chronic hyperplastic candidosis and other oral conditions. *Journal of Clinical Microbiology* 39:4066-75.

Bauman DS, Hagglund HE. 1991. Correlation between polysystem chronic complaints and an enzyme immunoassay with antigens of *Candida albicans*. *Journal of Advancement in Medicine* 4:5-19.

Baykushev R, Ouzounova-Raykova V, Stoykova V, Mitov I. 2014. Reliable microbiological diagnosis of vulvovaginal candidiasis. *Akush Ginekol (Sofiia)* 53:17-20.

Bazin S, Bouchard C, Brisson J, Morin C, Meisels A, Fortier M. 1994. Vulvar vestibulitis syndrome: an exploratory case-control study. *Obstetrics and Gynecology* 83:47–50.

Benitez LL, Carver PL. 2019. Adverse effects associated with long-term administration of azole antifungal agents. *Drugs* 79:833-53.

Bennett JW, Klich M. 2003. Mycotoxins. *Clinical Microbiology Reviews* 16:497–516.

Bennett JE. 1990. Searching for the yeast connection. *New England Journal of Medicine* 323:1766-7.

Berglund AL, Nigaard L, Rylander E. 2002. Vulvar pain, sexual behavior and genital infections in a young population: A pilot study. *Acta Obstetricia et Gynecologica Scandinavica* 81:738-742.

Bilo HJ. 2006. Susceptibility to infection in patients with diabetes mellitus. *Nederlands tijdschrift voor geneeskunde* 150:533-4.

Blackwell JM, Jamieson SE, Burgner D. 2009. HLA and infectious diseases. *Clinical Microbiology Reviews* 22:370-85.

Bodey G, Sobel J. 1993. Lower gastrointestinal candidiasis. In: *Candidiasis: Pathogenesis, Diagnosis and Treatment*, edited by Bodey G. Raven Press, New York. pp. 205-23.

Böhler K, Meisinger V, Klade H, Reinthaller A. 1994. Zinc levels of serum and cervicovaginal secretion in recurrent vulvovaginal candidiasis. *Genitourinary Medicine* 70:308-10.

Bohm-Starke N, Hilliges M, Falconer C, Rylander E. 1998. Increased Intraepithelial Innervation in Women with Vulvar Vestibulitis Syndrome. *Gynecologic and Obstetric Investigation* 46:256-60.

Bolivar R, Bodey GP. 1985. Candidiasis of the gastrointestinal tract. In: *Candidiasis*, Bodey G.P. and Fainstein V., Editors. Raven Press, New York. pp. 181-201.

Borg-von Zepelin M, Meyer I, Thomssen R, Würzner R, Sanglard D, Telenti A, Monod M. 1999. HIV-Protease inhibitors reduce cell adherence of *Candida albicans* strains by inhibition of yeast secreted aspartic proteases. *Journal of Investigative Dermatology* 113:747–51.

Bornstein J, Goldschmid N, Sabo E. 2004. Hyperinnervation and mast cell activation may be used as histopathologic diagnostic criteria for vulvar vestibulitis. *Gynecologic and Obstetric Investigation* 58:171-8.

Boselli F, Petrella E, Campedelli A, Muzi M, Rullo V, Ascione L, Papa R, Saponati G. 2012. Efficacy and tolerability of fitostimoline (vaginal cream, ovules, and vaginal washing) and of benzydamine hydrochloride (tantum rosa vaginal cream and vaginal washing) in the topical treatment of symptoms of bacterial vaginosis. *International Scholarly Research Network Obstetrics and Gynecology* 2012:183403.

Bouchard C, Brisson J, Fortier M, Morin C, Blanchette C. 2002. Use of oral contraceptive pills and vulvar vestibulitis: a case-control study. *American Journal of Epidemiology* 156:254-61.

Bouhnik Y, Pochart P, Marteau P, Arlet G, Goderei I, Rambaud JC. 1992. Fecal recovery in humans of viable Bifidobacterium sp. ingested in fermented milk. *Gastroenterology* 102:875-8.

Boyce JA, Assa'ad A, Burks AW, Jones SM, Sampson HA, Wood RA, Plaut M, Cooper SF, Fenton MJ, Arshad SH, Bahna SL, Beck LA, Byrd-Bredbenner C, Camargo CA Jr, Eichenfield L, Furuta GT, Hanifin JM, Jones C, Kraft M, Levy BD, Lieberman P, Luccioli S, McCall KM, Schneider LC, Simon RA, Simons FE, Teach SJ, Yawn BP, Schwaninger JM. 2010. Guidelines for the diagnosis and management of food allergy in the United States: report of the NIAID-sponsored expert panel. *Journal of Allergy and Clinical Immunology* 126:S1-S58.

Brabander JOW, Blank F, Butas CA. 1957. Intestinal moniliasis in adults. *Canadian Medical Association Journal* 77:478-83.

Braga-Silva LA, Santos AL. 2011. Aspartic protease inhibitors as potential anti-*Candida albicans* drugs: impacts on fungal biology, virulence and pathogenesis. *Current Medicinal Chemistry* 18:2401-19.

Bressler R. 2006. Grapefruit juice and drug interactions. Exploring mechanisms of this interaction and potential toxicity for certain drugs. *Geriatrics*. 61:12-8.

Broughton A, Lanson S. 1997. Increased intestinal permeability and reduced leucocyte phagocytosis in patients with chronic unresponsive *Candida* overgrowth. *Journal of Advancement in Medicine* 10:187-94.

Bunting JR, DerBalian G, Guilford FT, et al. 1988. Human serum immunoglobulin G, A, M levels in low grade chronic candidiasis. *Journal of Advancement in Medicine* 1:12-30.

Campbell DG. 1983. The Ordeal of 'Poor Old Charlie,' Drinkless Drunk. *Los Angeles Times*, January 4.

Canadian Paediatric Society. 1988. Candidiasis: current misconceptions. *Canadian Medical Association Journal* 139:728-30.

Canani RB, Costanzo MD, Leone L, Pedata M, Meli R, Calignano A. 2011. Potential beneficial effects of butyrate in intestinal and extraintestinal diseases. *World Journal of Gastroenterology* 17:1519-28.

Carriero C, Lezzi V, Mancini T, Selvaggi L. 2007. Vaginal capsules of *Lactobacillus plantarum* P17630 for prevention of relapse of Candida vulvovaginitis: an Italian multicentre observational study. *International Journal of Probiotics and Prebiotics* 2:155-162.

Caselli M, Trevisani L, Bighi S, Aleotti A, Balboni PG, Gaiani R, Bovolenta MR, Stabellini G. 1988. Dead fecal yeasts and chronic diarrhea. *Digestion* 41:142-8.

Cateau E, Cognee AS, Tran TC, Vallade E, Garcia M, Belaz S, Kauffmann-Lacroix C, Rodier MH. 2012. Impact of yeast-bacteria coinfection on the detection of Candida sp. in an automated blood culture system. *Diagnostic Microbiology and Infectious Disease* 72:328-31.

Cauwenbergh G. 1989. Safety aspects of ketoconazole, the most commonly used systemic antifungal. *Mycoses* 32:59-63.

Centers for Disease Control. 2008. Candidiasis disease listing. www.cdc.gov/nczved/dfbmd/ disease_listing/candidiasis_gi.html

Cerikcioglu N, Beksac MS. 2004. Cytolytic vaginosis: misdiagnosed as candidal vaginitis. *Infectious Diseases in Obstetrics and Gynecology* 12:13-6.

Chai LY, Netea MG, Vonk AG, Kullberg BJ. 2009. Fungal strategies for overcoming host innate immune response. *Medical Mycology* 47:227-36.

Chaim W. 1997. Fungal vaginitis caused by non-*albicans* species. *American Journal of Obstetrics and Gynecology* 177:485–6.

Chaim W, Meriwether C, Gonik B, Qureshi F, Sobel JD. 1996. Vulvar vestibulitis subjects undergoing surgical intervention: a descriptive analysis and histopathological correlates. *European Journal of Obstetrics, Gynecology, and Reproductive Biology* 68:165-8.

Chattaway FW, Odds FC, Barlow AJE. 1971. An examination of the production of hydrolytic enzymes and toxins by pathogenic strains of *Candida albicans*. *Journal of General Microbiology* 67:255-63.

Chiu A, Kelly K, Thomason J, Otte T, Mullins D, Fink J. 1999. Recurrent vaginitis as a manifestation of inhaled latex allergy. *Allergy* 54:184-6.

Ciclitira PJ, Johnson MW, Dewar DH, Ellis HJ. 2005. The pathogenesis of coeliac disease. *Molecular Aspects of Medicine* 26:421-58.

Cleary TG. 1985. Chronic mucocutaneous candidiasis. In: *Candidiasis*, Bodey G.P. and Fainstein V., Editors. Raven Press, New York. pp. 181-201.

Clemons KV, Calich VL, Burger E, Filler SG, Grazziutti M, Murphy J, Roilides E, Campa A, Dias MR, Edwards JE Jr, Fu Y, Fernandes-Bordignon G, Ibrahim A, Katsifa H, Lamaignere CG, Meloni-Bruneri LH, Rex J, Savary CA, Xidieh C. 2000. Pathogenesis I: Interactions of host cells and fungi. *Medical Mycology* 38:99-111.

Cochrane Database of Systematic Reviews. www.cochrane.org/search/site/probiotics.

Cohen JM, Fagin AP, Hariton E, Niska JR, Pierce MW, et al. 2012. Therapeutic intervention for chronic prostatitis/chronic pelvic pain syndrome (CP/CPPS): A systematic review and meta-analysis. PLoS ONE 7:e41941.

Collins SL, McMillan A, Seney S, van der Veer C, Kort R, Sumarah MW, Reid G. 2018. Promising prebiotic candidate established by evaluation of lactitol, lactulose, raffinose, and oligofructose for maintenance of a Lactobacillus-dominated vaginal microbiota. *Applied Environmental Microbiology* 84:e02200-17.

Conway S, Hart A, Clark A, Harvey I. 2007. Does eating yogurt prevent antibiotic-associated diarrhea? A placebo-controlled randomised controlled trial in general practice. *British Journal of General Practice* 57:953-9.

Costa-de-Oliveira S, Miranda IM, Ricardo E, Silva-Dias A, Rodrigues AG, Pina-Vaz C. 2012. Effective reversion of fluconazole resistance by ibuprofen in an animal model. Abstract presented at the *22nd European Congress of Clinical Microbiology and Infectious Diseases* (ECCMID). Clinical and therapeutic developments in fungal infection.

Costello SP, Hughes PA, Waters O, Bryant RV, Vincent AD, Blatchford P, Katsikeros R, Makanyanga J, Campaniello MA, Mavrangelos C, Rosewarne CP, Bickley C, Peters C, Schoeman MN, Conlon MA, Roberts-Thomson IC, Andrews JM. 2019. Effect of fecal microbiota transplantation on 8-week remission in patients with ulcerative colitis: A randomized clinical trial. JAMA 321:156-64.

Crandall M. 1991a. Allergic predisposition in recurrent vulvovaginal candidiasis. *Journal of Advancement in Medicine* 4:21-38. Download from www.yeastconsulting.com.

Crandall M. 1991b. A controlled trial of nystatin for the candidiasis hypersensitivity syndrome, Letter to the editor, *New England Journal of Medicine.* 324:1593-4.

Crandall M. 2004. The pathogenetic significance of intestinal candida colonization. Letter to the editor. *International Journal of Hygiene and Environmental Health* 207:79-81.

Crandall M. 2008. Yeast infections, candida allergy, and vulvodynia. www.empowher.com/news/2008/10/03/dr-marjorie-crandall-yeast-infections-candida-allergy-and-vulvodynia.

Crandall M, Nelson A, Sustarsic D. 1988. An EIA for *Candida albicans* proteinase. *Abstracts of the Annual Meeting of the American Society for Microbiology* F-42.

Crayton JW, Winger EE, Rippon J. 1989. Anti-Candida antibody levels in polysymptomatic patients (self-published). Reprints: Edward E. Winger, M.D., Immunodiagnostic Laboratories, P.O. Box 5755, San Leandro, CA 94577.

Crook WG. 1983. *The Yeast Connection*, Professional Books, Jackson, Tennessee.

Crook WG. 1991. A controlled trial of nystatin for the candidiasis hypersensitivity syndrome, Letter to the editor, *New England Journal of Medicine* 324:1592.

Crook WG. 1995. *The Yeast Connection and the Woman*, Professional Books, Inc., Jackson, Tennessee. Survey online: www.yeastconnection.com; click on "Dr. Crook's Famous Yeast Evaluation Questionnaire" to download yeastfullsurv.pdf.

Crutcher N, Rosenberg EW, Belew PW, Skinner RB Jr, Eaglstein NF, Baker SM. 1984. Oral nystatin in the treatment of psoriasis. *Archives of Dermatology* 120:435-6.

Cutler JE, Friedman L, Milner KC. 1972. Biological and chemical characterization of toxic substances from *Candida albicans*. *Infection and Immunity* 6:616-27.

Czeizel AE, Kazy Z, Puhó E. 2003. A population-based case-control teratological study of oral nystatin treatment during pregnancy. *Scandinavian Journal of Infectious Diseases* 35:830-5.

Darroch CJ, Barnes RM, Dawson J. 1999. Circulating antibodies to *Saccharomyces cerevisiae* (bakers'/brewers' yeast) in gastrointestinal disease. *Journal of Clinical Pathology* 52:47-53.

das Neves J, Pinto E, Teixeira B, Dias G, Rocha P, Cunha T, Santos B, Amaral MH, Bahia MF. 2008. Local treatment of vulvovaginal candidosis. General and practical considerations. *Drugs* 68:1787-802.

Davies JNP. 1985. Correspondence: Endogenous production of alcohol in humans. *Journal of the Forensic Science Society* 25:299.

Davis MR, Nguyen Minh-Vu H, Donnelley MA, and Thompson III GR. 2019. Tolerability of long-term fluconazole therapy. *Journal of Antimicrobial Chemotherapy* 74:768–771.

Day T, Borbolla Foster A, Phillips S, Pagano R, Dyall-Smith D, Scurry J, Garland SM. 2016. Can routine histopathology distinguish between vulvar cutaneous candidosis and dermatophytosis? *Journal of Lower Genital Tract Disease* 20:267–71.

De Rose AF, Gallo F, Giglio M, Carmignani G. 2004. Role of mepartricin in category III chronic nonbacterial prostatitis/chronic pelvic pain syndrome: a randomized prospective placebo-controlled trial. *Urology* 63:13-6.

Dei M, Di Maggio F, Di Paolo G, Bruni V. 2010. Vulvovaginitis in childhood. *Best Practice & Research. Clinical Obstetrics & Gynaecology* 24:129-37.

Delia P, Sansotta G, Donato V, Messina G, Frosina P, Pergolizzi S, De Renzis C. 2002. Prophylaxis of diarrhoea in patients submitted to radiotherapeutic treatment on pelvic district: personal experience. *Digestive and Liver Disease* 34:S84-86.

Dennerstein, GJ. 1968. Cytology of the vulva. *Journal of Obstetrics and Gynaecology of the British Empire* 75:603-9.

Dennerstein, GJ. 1986. Depo-Provera in the treatment of recurrent vulvovaginal candidiasis. *Journal of Reproductive Medicine* 31:801-3.

Dennerstein GJ, Ellis DH. 2001. Oestrogen, glycogen and vaginal candidiasis. *Australian & New Zealand Journal of Obstetrics & Gynaecology* 41:326-8.

Denning DW, Kneale M, Sobel JD, Rautemaa-Richardson R. 2018. Global burden of recurrent vulvovaginal candidiasis: a systematic review. *The Lancet Infectious Diseases*, published online August 2, http://dx.doi.org/10.1016/S1473-3099(18)30103-8.

Dismukes WE, Wade JS, Lee JY, Dockery BK, Hain JD. 1990. A randomized, double-blind trial of nystatin therapy for the candidiasis hypersensitivity syndrome. *New England Journal of Medicine* 323:1717-23.

Dismukes WE, Lee JY. 1991. A controlled trial of nystatin for the candidiasis hypersensitivity syndrome. Reply to letters to the editor. *New England Journal of Medicine* 324:1594.

Dixon PN, Warin RP, English MP. 1969. Role of *Candida albicans* infection in napkin rashes. *British Medical Journal* 2:23-27.

Doctor Fungus. 2007. The official website of the mycoses study group. www.doctorfungus.org.

Dodd CL, Greenspan D, Katz MH, Westenhouse JL, Feigal DW, Greenspan JS. 1991. Oral candidiasis in HIV infection: pseudomembranous and erythematous candidiasis show similar rates of progression to AIDS. *AIDS* 5:1339–43.

Donders G, Bellen G, Byttebier G, Verguts L, Hinoul P, Walckiers R, Stalpaert M, Vereecken A, Van Eldere J. 2008. Individualized decreasing-dose maintenance fluconazole regimen for recurrent vulvovaginal candidiasis (ReCiDiF trial). *American Journal of Obstetrics and Gynecology* 199:613. e1-9.

Donders GG, Marconi C, Bellen G. 2010. Easiness of use and validity testing of VS-Sense device for detection of abnormal vaginal flora and bacterial vaginosis. *Infectious Diseases in Obstetrics and Gynecology* 2010:1-7.

Dorrell L, Edwards A. 2002. Vulvovaginitis due to fluconazole resistant *Candida albicans* following self treatment with non-prescribed triazoles. *Sexually Transmitted Infections* 78:308-9.

Dupuis A, Tournier N, Le Moal G, Venisse N. 2009. Preparation and stability of voriconazole eye drop solution. *Antimicrobial Agents and Chemotherapy* 53:798-9.

Dybowski B. 2013. Antifungal azoles - new antidote for chronic pelvic pain? *Central European Journal of Urology* 66:200-1.

Eaton KK. 1991. Gut fermentation: a reappraisal of an old clinical condition with diagnostic tests and management: discussion paper. *Journal of the Royal Society of Medicine* 84:669-71.

Eckert LO, Hawse SE, Stevens CE, Koutsky LA, Eschenbach DA, Holmes KK. 1998. Vulvovaginal candidiasis: clinical manifestations, risk factors, management algorithm. *Obstetrics and Gynecology* 92:757–65.

Edenberg HJ. 2007. The genetics of alcohol metabolism: role of alcohol dehydrogenase and aldehyde dehydrogenase variants. *Alcohol Research & Health* 30:5-13.

Edge G, Pepys J. 1980. Antibodies in different immunoglobulin classes to *Candida albicans* in allergic respiratory disease. *Clinical Allergy* 10:47-58.

Edman J, Sobel JD, Taylor ML. 1986. Zinc status in women with recurrent vulvovaginal candidiasis. *American Journal of Obstetrics and Gynecology* 155:1082-5.

Edwards JE Jr. 1988a. "The Yeast Connection" interviewed on a Lifetime Medical Television program, Physicians Journal Update.

Edwards JE Jr. 1988b. Systemic symptoms from Candida in the gut: real or imaginary? *Bulletin of the New York Academy of Medicine* 64:544-9. Draft position statement of the Infectious Diseases Society of America.

Edwards JE Jr, Gaither TA, O'Shea JJ, Rotrosen D, Lawley TJ, Wright SA, Frank MM, Green I. 1986. Expression of specific binding sites on Candida with functional and antigenic characteristics of human complement receptors. *Journal of Immunology* 137:3577-83.

Edwards JE Jr, Schwartz MM, Schmidt CS, Sobel JD, Nyirjesy P, Schodel F, Marchus E, Lizakowski M, DeMontigny EA, Hoeg J, Holmberg T, Cooke MT, Hoover K, Edwards L, Jacobs M, Sussman S, Augenbraun M, Drusano M, Yeaman MR, Ibrahim AS, Filler SG, Hennessey JP. 2018. A fungal immunotherapeutic vaccine (NDV-3A) for treatment of recurrent vulvovaginal candidiasis—A phase 2 randomized, double-blind, placebo-controlled trial. *Clinical Infectious Diseases* 66:1928–1936, https://doi.org/10.1093/cid/ciy185.

Edwards S. 1996. Balanitis and balanoposthitis: a review. *Genitourinary Medicine* 72:155-9.

Ehrlich SD. 2009. *Lactobacillus acidophilus*. www.umm.edu/altmed/articles/lactobacillus-acidophilus-000310.htm.

Ehrström S, Kornfeld D, Rylander E. 2007. Perceived stress in women with recurrent vulvovaginal candidiasis. *Journal of Psychosomatic Obstetrics & Gynecology* 28:169-76.

Ekgren JS. 2000. Vulvovaginitis treated with anticholinergics. *Gastroenterology International* 13:72.

El-Din SS, Reynolds MT, Ashbee HR, Barton RC, Evans EG. 2001. An investigation into the pathogenesis of vulvo-vaginal candidosis. *Sexually Transmitted Infections* 77:179-83.

Elenkov IJ, Wilder RL, Bakalov VK, Link AA, Dimitrov MA, Fisher S, Crane M, Kanik KS, Chrousos GP. 2001. IL-12, TNF-alpha, and hormonal changes during late pregnancy and early postpartum: implications for autoimmune disease activity during these times. *Journal of Clinical Endocrinology and Metabolism* 86:4933-8.

Eras P, Goldstein MJ, Sherlock P. 1972. Candida infection of the gastrointestinal tract. *Medicine* 51:367-79.

Ereaux LP, Craig GE. 1949. The oral administration of undecylenic acid in the treatment of psoriasis. *Canadian Medical Association Journal* 61:361-4.

Fail PA, Chapin RE, Price CJ, Heindel JJ. 1998. General, reproductive, developmental, and endocrine toxicity of boronated compounds. *Reproductive Toxicology* 12:1–18.

Falagas ME, Betsi GI, Athanasiou S. 2006. Probiotics for prevention of recurrent vulvovaginal candidiasis: a review. *Journal of Antimicrobial Chemotherapy* 58:266-272.

Farage MA, Miller KW, Summers PR, Sobel JD, Ledger WJ. 2010. Chronic pain of the vulva without dermatologic manifestations: distinguishing among a spectrum of clinical disorders. *Clinical Medicine Insights: Women's Health* 3:1–13. (www.la-press.com/ chronic-pain-of-the-vulva-without-dermatologic-manifestations-distingu-a1821).

Farmer MA, Taylor AM, Bailey AL, Tuttle AH, MacIntyre LC, Milagrosa ZE, Crissman HP, Bennett GJ, Ribeiro-da-Silva A, Binik YM, Mogil JS. 2011. Repeated vulvovaginal fungal infections cause persistent pain in a mouse model of vulvodynia. *Science Translational Medicine* 3:101ra91.

Fem-VTM. (www.fem-v.com; www.synovahealthcare.com).

Fernández L, Langa S, Martín V, Maldonado A, Jiménez E, Martín R, Rodríguez JM. 2013. The human milk microbiota: origin and potential roles in health and disease. *Pharmacological Research* 69:1-10. doi: 10.1016/j.phrs.2012.09.001. Epub 2012 Sep 10.

Ferris DG, Dekle C, Litaker MS. 1996. Women's use of over-the-counter antifungal medications for gynecologic symptoms. *Journal of Family Practice* 42:595-600.

Ferwerda B, Ferwerda G, Plantinga TS, Willment JA, van Spriel AB, Venselaar H, Elbers CC, Johnson MD, Cambi A, Huysamen C, Jacobs L, Jansen T, Verheijen K, Masthoff L, Morré SA, Vriend G, Williams DL, Perfect JR, Joosten LA, Wijmenga C, van der Meer JW, Adema GJ, Kullberg BJ, Brown GD, Netea MG. 2009. Human dectin-1 deficiency and mucocutaneous fungal infections. *New England Journal of Medicine* 361:1760-7.

Fidel PL Jr. 2005. Immunity in vaginal candidiasis. *Current Opinion in Infectious Diseases* 18:107–11.

Fidel PL Jr, Vazquez JA, Sobel JD. 1999. *Candida glabrata*: review of epidemiology, pathogenesis, and clinical disease with comparison to *C. albicans*. Clinical Microbiology Reviews 12: 80–96.

Fidel PL Jr, Huffnagle GB (Editors). 2005. *Fungal Immunology: From an Organ Perspective*, Springer-Verlag, Düsseldorf, Germany.

Fihn SD, Boyko EJ, Normand EH, Chen CL, Grafton JR, Hunt M, Yarbro P, Scholes D, Stergachis A. 1996. Association between use of spermicide-coated condoms and *Escherichia coli* urinary tract infection in young women. *American Journal of Epidemiology* 144:512-20.

Filler SG, Sheppard DC. 2006. Fungal invasion of normally non-phagocytic host cells. *PLoS Pathogens* 2:e129.

Fischer G, Bradford J. 2011. Vulvovaginal candidiasis in postmenopausal women: the role of hormone replacement therapy. *Journal of Lower Genital Tract Disease* 15:263-7.

Fischer G. 2014. Coping with chronic vulvovaginal candidiasis. *Medicine Today* 15:33-40.

Fitzsimmons N, Berry DR. 1994. Inhibition of *Candida albicans* by *Lactobacillus acidophilus*: evidence for the involvement of a peroxidase system. *Microbios* 80:125-33.

Floch M, Montrose DC. 2005. Use of probiotics in humans: an analysis of the literature. *Gastroenterology Clinics of North America* 34:547-70.

Fong IW. 1992. The value of treating the sexual partners of women with recurrent vaginal candidiasis with ketoconazole. *Genitourinary Medicine* 68:174-6.

Foster DC, Piekarz KH, Murant TI, LaPoint R, Haidaris CG, Phipps RP. 2007. Enhanced synthesis of proinflammatory cytokines by vulvar vestibular fibroblasts: Implications for vulvar vestibulitis. *American Journal of Obstetrics and Gynecology* 196:346. 341e1-346e8.

Fridkin SK. 2005. The changing face of fungal infections in health care settings. *Clinical Infectious Diseases* 41:1455-60.

Friedrich EG Jr. 1983. The vulvar vestibule. *Journal of Reproductive Medicine* 28:773-7.

Friedrich EG Jr. 1987. Vulvar vestibulitis syndrome. *Journal of Reproductive Medicine* 32:110-4.

Friedrich EG Jr, Phillips LE. 1988. Microwave sterilization of *Candida* on underwear fabric. *Journal of Reproductive Medicine* 33:421-2.

Fungal Research Trust. www.fungalresearchtrust.org.

Gali Y, Delezay O, Brouwers J, Addad N, Augustijns P, Bourlet T, Hamzeh-Cognasse H, Ariën KK, Pozzetto B, Vanham G. 2010. In vitro evaluation of viability, integrity, and inflammation in genital epithelia upon exposure to pharmaceutical excipients and candidate microbicides. *Antimicrobial Agents and Chemotherapy* 54:5105-14.

Galland L. 1985. Nutrition and Candidiasis. *Journal of Orthomolecular Psychiatry* 14:50-60.

Gamboa PM, Tabard A, Wong E, Oehling A. 1986. IgG$_4$ characteristics and its role in allergic diseases. *Allergologia et immunopathologia* 14:155-63.

Ganguly S, Mitchell AP. 2011. Mucosal biofilms of *Candida albicans. Current Opinion in Microbiology* 14:380–85.

García-Tamayo J, Castillo G, Martínez AJ. 1982. Human genital candidiasis: histochemistry, scanning and transmission electron microscopy. *Acta Cytologica* 26:7-14.

Garner RE, Childress AM, Human LG, Domer JE. 1990. Characterization of *Candida albicans* mannan-induced, mannan-specific delayed hypersensitivity suppressor cells. *Infection and Immunity* 58:2613-20.

Gaur SK, Frick K, Dandolu V. 2009. A cost effectiveness analysis of rapid yeast detection kits. *Womens Health Issues.* Nov 25.

Geertinger P, Bodenhoff J, Helweg-Larsen K, Lund A. 1982. Endogenous alcohol production by intestinal fermentation in sudden infant death. *International Journal of Legal Medicine* 89:167-72.

Gentles JC, La Touche CJ. 1969. Yeasts as human and animal pathogens, pp. 107-182, In: Volume 1, *The Yeasts: Biology of Yeasts*, A.H. Rose, and J.S. Harrison, editors, Academic Press, London.

Ghannoum MA, Elewski B. 1999. Successful treatment of fluconazole-resistant oropharyngeal candidiasis by a combination of fluconazole and terbinafine. *Clinical and Diagnostic Laboratory Immunology* 6:921–3.

Ghodke Y, Joshi K, Chopra A, Patwardhan B. 2005. HLA and disease. *European Journal of Epidemiology* 20:475-88.

Gibson GR, Roberfroid MB. 1995. Dietary modulation of the human colonic microbiota: introducing the concept of prebiotics. *Journal of Nutrition* 125:1401-12.

Gilpin CA. 1967. Resistant monilial vaginitis: the male aspect. *Journal of the Florida Medical Association* 54:337-8.

Giraldo PC, Babula O, Gonçalves AK, Linhares IM, Amaral RL, Ledger WJ, Witkin SS. 2007. Mannose-binding lectin gene polymorphism, vulvovaginal candidiasis, and bacterial vaginosis. *Obstetrics and Gynecology* 109:1123–8.

Glazer HI. 2000. Dysesthetic vulvodynia. Long-term follow-up after treatment with surface electromyography-assisted pelvic floor muscle rehabilitation. *Journal of Reproductive Medicine* 45:798-802.

Goetsch MF. 1991. Vulvar vestibulitis: prevalence and historic features in a general gynecologic practice population. *American Journal of Obstetrics and Gynecology* 164:1609-16.

Goldman DL, Huffnagle GB. 2009. Potential contribution of fungal infection and colonization to the development of allergy. *Medical Mycology* 47:445-56.

Goldstein AT, Thaçi D, Luger T. 2009. Topical calcineurin inhibitors for the treatment of vulvar dermatoses. *European Journal of Obstetrics, Gynecology, and Reproductive Biology* 146:22-9.

Goswami D, Goswami R, Banerjee U, Dadhwal V, Miglani S, Lattif AA, Kochupillai N. 2006. Pattern of Candida species isolated from patients with diabetes mellitus and vulvovaginal candidiasis and their response to single dose oral fluconazole therapy. *Journal of Infection* 52:111-7.

Greer N.D. 2003. Voriconazole: the newest triazole antifungal agent. *Proceedings of the Baylor University Medical Center* 16:241–8.

Gumowski P, Lech B, Chaves I, Girard JP. 1987. Chronic asthma and rhinitis due to *Candida albicans*, Epidermophyton, and Trichophyton. *Annals of Allergy* 59:48–51.

Gunderson SM, Hoffman H, Ernst EJ, Pfaller MA, Klepser ME. 2000. In vitro pharmacodynamic characteristics of nystatin including time-kill and postantifungal effect. *Antimicrobial Agents and Chemotherapy* 44:2887-90.

Gunsalus KTW, Tornberg-Belanger SN, Matthan NR, Lichtenstein AH, Kumamoto CA. 2015. Manipulation of host diet to reduce gastrointestinal colonization by the opportunistic pathogen *Candida albicans*. *mSphere* 1:e00020-15. doi:10.1128/ mSphere.00020-15.

Gupta G. 2005. Microbicidal spermicide or spermicidal microbicide? *European Journal of Contraception & Reproductive Health Care* 10:212-8.

Guzel AB, Ilkit M, Akar T, Burgut R, Demir SC. 2011a. Evaluation of risk factors in patients with vulvovaginal candidiasis and the value of chromID Candida agar versus CHROMagar Candida for recovery and presumptive identification of vaginal yeast species. *Critical Reviews in Microbiology* 49:16-25.

Guzel AB, Ilkit M, Burgut R, Urunsak IF, Ozgunen FT. 2011b. An evaluation of risk factors in pregnant women with Candida vaginitis and the diagnostic value of simultaneous vaginal and rectal sampling. *Mycopathologia* 172:25-36.

Guzy C, Paclik D, Schirbel A, Sonnenborn U, Wiedenmann B, Sturm A. 2008. The probiotic Escherichia coli strain Nissle 1917 induces γδ T cell apoptosis via caspase- and FasL-dependent pathways. *International Immunology* 20:829-40.

Gygax SE, Vermitsky JP, Chadwick SG, Self MJ, Zimmerman JA, Mordechai E, Adelson ME, Trama JP. 2008. Antifungal resistance of *Candida glabrata* vaginal isolates and development of a quantitative reverse transcription-PCR-based azole susceptibility assay. *Antimicrobial Agents and Chemotherapy* 52:3424-6.

Haas A, Stiehm ER. 1986. The "yeast connection" meets chronic mucocutaneous candidiasis. *New England Journal of Medicine* 314:854-5.

Haefner HK, Collins ME, Davis GD, Edwards L, Foster DC, Hartmann ED, Kaufman RH, Lynch PJ, Margesson LJ, Moyal-Barracco M, Piper CK, Reed BD, Stewart EG, Wilkinson EJ. 2005. The vulvodynia guideline. *Journal of Lower Genital Tract Disease* 9:40-51.

Hagglund HE. 1984. *Why do I feel so bad (When the doctor says I'm O.K.)?* IED Press, Oklahoma City, Oklahoma.

Hallert C, Björck I, Nyman M, Pousette A, Grännö C, Svensson H. 2003. Increasing fecal butyrate in ulcerative colitis patients by diet: controlled pilot study. *Inflammatory Bowel Diseases* 9:116-21.

Halpern GM, Scott JR. 1987. Non-IgE antibody mediated mechanisms in food allergy. *Annals of Allergy* 58:14-27.

Hamad M, Abu-Elteen KH, Ghaleb M. 2004. Estrogen-dependent induction of persistent vaginal candidosis in naïve mice. *Mycoses* 47:304-9.

Hamad M, Muta'eb E, Abu-Shaqra Q, Fraij A, Abu-Elteen K, and Yasin SR. 2006. Utility of the oestrogen-dependent vaginal candidosis murine model in evaluating the efficacy of various therapies against vaginal *Candida albicans* infection. *Mycoses* 49:104-8.

Hamilton-Miller. 1999. Too many unreliable probiotic products on the market. *Public Health and Nutrition* 2:223-9.

Hammerman C, Bin-Nun A, Kaplan M. 2006. Safety of probiotics: comparison of two popular strains. *BMJ* 333:1006-8.

Harlow BL, Stewart EG. 2003. A population-based assessment of chronic unexplained vulvar pain: have we underestimated the prevalence of vulvodynia? *Journal of the American Medical Women's Association* 58:82-8.

Harlow BL, Wei He, Nguyen RHN. 2009. Allergic reactions and risk of vulvodynia. *Annals of Epidemiology* 19:771-7.

Hatakka K, Savilahti E, Ponka A, Meurman JH, Poussa T, Nase L, Saxelin M, Korpela R. 2001. Effect of long term consumption of probiotic milk on infection in children attending day care centres: double blind, randomised trial. *British Medical Journal* 322:1-5.

Havlickova B, Czaika VA, Friedrich M. 2008. Epidemiological trends in skin mycoses worldwide. *Mycoses* 51:2–15.

Hector RF, Davidson AP, Johnson SM. 2005. Comparison of susceptibility of fungal isolates to lufenuron and nikkomycin Z alone or in combination with itraconazole. *American Journal of Veterinary Research* 66:1090-3.

Herbrecht R, Nivoix Y. 2005. *Saccharomyces cerevisiae* fungemia: an adverse effect of *Saccharomyces boulardii* probiotic administration. *Clinical Infectious Diseases* 40:1635–7.

Hillier SL. 2013. Yeast infection four times as likely with penicillin use. Abstract presented at the *Annual Meeting of the Infectious Diseases Society for Obstetrics and Gynecology.*

Hillier SL, Moench T, Shattock R, Black R, Reichelderfer P, Veronese F. 2005. In vitro and in vivo: the story of nonoxynol 9. *Journal of Acquired Immune Deficiency Syndromes* 39:1-8.

Hilton E, Isenberg HD, Alperstein P. 1992. Ingestion of yogurt containing *Lactobacillus acidophilus* as prophylaxis for candidal vaginitis. *Annals of Internal Medicine* 116:353-7.

Hoffstetter SE, Barr S, LeFevre C, Leong FC, Leet T. 2008. Self-reported yeast symptoms compared with clinical wet mount analysis and vaginal yeast culture in a specialty clinic setting. *Journal of Reproductive Medicine* 53:402-6.

Holti G. 1966. Candida allergy. In: Winner HI, Hurley R, eds. *Symposium on Candida Infections.* E&S Livingstone, Edinburgh and London. pages 74-81.

Homei A, Worboys M. 2013. *Fungal Disease in Britain and the United States 1850–2000.* Palgrave Macmillan, Basingstoke, UK.

Hong E, Dixit S, Fidel PL, Bradford J, Fischer G. 2014. Vulvovaginal candidiasis as a chronic disease: diagnostic criteria and definition. *Journal of Lower Genital Tract Disease* 18:31-8.

Hopwood V, Evans EGV, Carney JA. 1985. A comparison of methods for the detection of Candida antigens: evaluation of a new latex reagent. *Journal of Immunological Methods* 80:199-210.

Horowitz BJ. 1986. Topical flucytosine therapy for chronic recurrent *Candida tropicalis* infections. *Journal of Reproductive Medicine* 31:821-4.

Horowitz BJ, Mårdh PA, Nagy E, Rank EL. 1994. Vaginal lactobacillosis. *American Journal of Obstetrics and Gynecology* 170:857-61.

Hosen H. 1988. Chronic asthma and rhinitis due to *Candida albicans. Annals of Allergy* 60:272-3.

Hospenthal DR, Beckius ML, Floyd KL, Horvath LL, Murray CK. 2006. Presumptive identification of Candida species other than *C. albicans, C. krusei*, and *C. tropicalis* with the chromogenic medium CHROMagar Candida. *Annals of Clinical Microbiology and Antimicrobials* 5:1-5.

Hunnisett A, Howard J, Davies S. 1990. Gut fermentation (or the 'auto-brewery') syndrome: a new clinical test with initial observations and discussion of clinical and biochemical implications. *Journal of Nutritional and Environmental Medicine* 1:33-8.

Iavazzo C, Gkegkes ID, Zarkada IM, Falagas ME. 2011. Boric acid for recurrent vulvovaginal candidiasis: the clinical evidence. *Journal of Women's Health* 20:1245-55.

Ilkit M, Guzel AB. 2011. The epidemiology, pathogenesis, and diagnosis of vulvovaginal candidosis: A mycological perspective. *Critical Reviews in Microbiology* 37:250-61.

Ilkit M, Durdu M, Karakas M. 2012. Cutaneous id reactions: a comprehensive review of clinical manifestations, epidemiology, etiology, and management. *Critical Reviews in Microbiology* 38:191-202.

Indudhara R, Singh SK, Vaidyanathan S, Banerjee CK. 1992. Isolated invasive candidal prostatitis. *Urologia Internationalis* 48:362-4.

Iwata K, Uchida K, Endo H. 1967. 'Canditoxin', a new toxic substance isolated from a strain of *Candida albicans*. 1. Relationship between strains and virulence and conditions for toxin substance production. *Medicine and Biology* 74:345–350; 351–355; 75:192–195; 77:159–164; 83:283–286 (in Japan).

Iwata K. 1977. Toxins produced by *Candida albicans*. *Contributions to Microbiology and Immunology* 4:77-85.

Iwata K. 1978. Fungal toxins as a parasitic factor responsible for the establishment of fungal infections. *Mycopathologia* 65:141-54.

Jadhav A, Mortale S, Halbandge S, Jangid P, Patil R, Gade W, Kharat K, Karuppayil SM. 2017. The dietary food components capric acid and caprylic acid inhibit virulence factors in *Candida albicans* through multitargeting. *Journal of Medicinal Food* 20:1083-1090.

Jaeger M, Plantinga TS, Joosten LA, Kullberg BJ, Netea MG. 2013. Genetic basis for recurrent vulvo-vaginal candidiasis. *Current Infectious Disease Reports* 15:136-42.

James J, Warin RP. 1971. An assessment of the role of *Candida albicans* and food yeasts in chronic urticaria. *British Journal of Dermatology* 84:227-37.

Janković S, Bojović D, Vukadinović D, Daglar E, Janković M, Laudanović D, Lukić V, Misković V, Potpara Z, Projović I, Cokanović V, Petrović N, Folić M, Savić V. 2010. Risk factors for recurrent vulvovaginal candidiasis. *Vojnosanitetski Pregled. Military-Medical and Pharmaceutical Review* 67:819–24.

Jobin C. 2010. Probiotics and ileitis: could augmentation of TNF/NFκB activity be the answer? *Gut Microbes* 1:196-9.

Johnson MD, MacDougall C, Ostrosky-Zeichner L, Perfect JR, Rex JH. 2004. Combination antifungal therapy. *Antimicrobial Agents and Chemotherapy* 48:693-715.

Jost T, Lacroix C, Braegger CP, Rochat F, Chassard C. 2014. Vertical mother-neonate transfer of maternal gut bacteria via breastfeeding. *Environmental Microbiology* 16:2891-904. doi: 10.1111/1462-2920.12238.

Jouault T, Sarazin A, Martinez-Esparza M, Fradin C, Sendid B, Poulain D. 2009. Host responses to a versatile commensal: PAMPs and PRRs interplay leading to tolerance or infection by *Candida albicans*. *Cellular Microbiology* 11:1007-15.

Kahn BS, Tatro C, Parsons CL, Willems JJ. 2009. Prevalence of interstitial cystitis in vulvodynia patients detected by bladder potassium sensitivity. *Journal of Sexual Medicine* 7:996-1002.

Kaila B, Orr K, Bernstein CN. 2005. The anti-*Saccharomyces cerevisiae* antibody assay in a province-wide practice: accurate in identifying cases of Crohn's disease and predicting inflammatory disease. *The Canadian Journal of Gastroenterology* 19:717–721.

Kaji H, Asanumaa Y, Yaharaa O, Shibuea H, Hisamuraa M, Saitoa N, Kawakamia Y, Muraoa M. 1984. Commentary: Intragastrointestinal alcohol fermentation syndrome: Report of two cases and review of the literature. *Journal of the Forensic Science Society* 24:461-71.

Kalkanci A, Guzel AB, Khalil II, Aydin M, Ilkit M, Kustimur S. 2012. Yeast vaginitis during pregnancy: susceptibility testing of 13 antifungal drugs and boric acid and the detection of four virulence factors. *Medical Mycology* 50:585-93.

Kallmyer T. 2011. https://www.thecandidadiet.com/alcohol-and-candida/.

Kane JG, Chretien JH, Caragus VF. 1976. Diarrhea caused by Candida. *Lancet* 1: 335-6.

Katz DH. 1978. The allergic phenotype: Manifestation of "allergic breakthrough" and imbalance in normal "damping" of IgE antibody production. *Immunological Reviews* 41:77-108.

Kauppila S, Kotila V, Knuuti E, Väre PO, Vittaniemi P, Nissi R. 2010. The effect of topical pimecrolimus on inflammatory infiltrate in vulvar lichen sclerosus. *American Journal of Obstetrics and Gynecology* 202:181.e1-4.

Keeney E.L. 1951. Candida asthma. *Annals of Internal Medicine* 34:223-6.

Kennedy MJ, Volz PA. 1985a. Effect of various antibiotics on gastrointestinal colonization and dissemination by *Candida albicans. Sabouraudia* 23:265-73.

Kennedy MJ, Volz PA. 1985b. Ecology of *Candida albicans* gut colonization: inhibition of Candida adhesion, colonization, and dissemination from the gastrointestinal tract by bacterial antagonism. *Infection and Immunity* 49:654-63.

Kennedy MJ, Volz PA, Edwards CA, Yancey RJ. 1987. Mechanisms of association of *Candida albicans* with intestinal mucosa. *Journal of Medical Microbiology* 24:333-41.

Khosravi AR, Bandghorai AN, Moazzeni M, Shokri H, Mansouri P, Mahmoudi M. 2009. Evaluation of *Candida albicans* allergens reactive with specific IgE in asthma and atopic eczema patients. *Mycoses* 52:326-33.

Kirkpatrick CH. 1989. Chronic mucocutaneous candidiasis. *European Journal of Clinical Microbiology & Infectious Diseases* 8:448-56.

Knight TE, Shikuma CY, Knight J. 1991. Ketoconazole-induced fulminant hepatitis necessitating liver transplantation. *Journal of the American Academy of Dermatology* 25:398-400.

Koivikko A, Kalimo K, Nieminen E, Viander M. 1988. Relationship of immediate and delayed hypersensitivity to nasopharyngeal and intestinal growth of *Candida albicans* in allergic subjects. *Allergy* 43:201-5.

Kosalec I, Puel O, Delaforge M, Kopjar N, Antolovic R, Jelic D, Matica B, Galtier P, Pepeljnjak S. 2008. Isolation and cytotoxicity of low-molecular-weight metabolites of *Candida albicans. Frontiers in Bioscience* 13:6893-904.

Kotb AF, Ismail AM, Sharafeldeen M, Elsayed EY. 2013. Chronic prostatitis/chronic pelvic pain syndrome: the role of an antifungal regimen. *Central European Journal of Urology* 66:196-9.

Kovachev SM, Vatcheva-Dobrevska RS. 2015. Local probiotic therapy for vaginal *Candida albicans* infections. *Probiotics and Antimicrobial Proteins* 7:38–44.

Kozinn PJ, Taschdjian CL. 1962. Enteric candidiasis. Diagnosis and clinical considerations. *Pediatrics* 30:71-85.

Krause W, Matheis H, Wulf K. 1969. Fungemia and funguria after oral administration of *Candida albicans*. *Lancet* 1:598-9.

Kroker GF. 1987. Chronic candidiasis and allergy. In: *Food Allergy and Intolerance*, J. Brostoff, S.J. Challacombe (Editors), Baillière Tindall, London, pp. 850-872.

Kroker GF. 2011a. Research bibliography of sublingual immunotherapy publications. www.lacrosseallergy.com/Benefits/ScientificEvidence/default.aspx.

Kroker GF. 2011b. 30 Years of SLIT: Learning through experience. Clinical pearls for your practice. www.renaissanceallergist.com/new-powerpoint-presentations.

Kumamoto CA. 2011. Inflammation and gastrointestinal Candida colonization. *Current Opinion in Microbiology* 14:386-91.

Kumar S, Bansal A, Chakrabarti A, Singhi S. 2013. Evaluation of efficacy of probiotics in prevention of Candida colonization in a PICU—A randomized controlled trial. *Critical Care Medicine* 41:565–572. doi: 10.1097/CCM.0b013e31826a409c.

Kupfahl C, Ruppert T, Dietz A, Geginat G, Hof H. 2007. Candida species fail to produce the immunosuppressive secondary metabolite gliotoxin in vitro. *FEMS Yeast Research* 7:986-92.

Lacour M, Zunder T, Huber R, Sander A, Daschner F, Frank U. 2002. The pathogenetic significance of intestinal *Candida* colonization – a systematic review from an interdisciplinary and environmental medical point of view. *International Journal of Hygiene and Environmental Health* 205:257-68.

Lanson S. 1997. Immune complexes to *Candida* mannan: an objective marker of *Candida* overgrowth. *Journal of Advancement in Medicine* 10:179-86.

Larsen S, Bendtzen K, Nielsen OH. 2010. Extraintestinal manifestations of inflammatory bowel disease: epidemiology, diagnosis, and management. *Annals of Medicine* 42:97-114.

Larson JM, Sehnert KW. 1992. *Alcoholism - The Biochemical Connection*. Villard Books, a division of Random House, New York.

Lass-Flörl C, Dierich MP, Fuchs D, Semenitz E, Ledochowski M. 2001. Antifungal activity against *Candida* species of the selective serotonin-reuptake inhibitor, sertraline. *Clinical Infectious Diseases* 33:e135-6.

Ledger WJ, Witkin SS. 1991. A controlled trial of nystatin for the candidiasis hypersensitivity syndrome, Letter to the editor, *New England Journal of Medicine* 324:1593.

Lee MJ. 1995. Parasites, yeasts and bacteria in health and disease. *Journal of Advancement in Medicine* 8:121-30.

Lehmann PF, Reiss E. 1980. Comparison by ELISA of serum anti-*Candida albicans* mannan IgG levels of a normal population and in diseased patients. *Mycopathologia* 70:89-93.

Leli C, Mencacci A, Meucci M, Bietolini C, Vitali M, Farinelli S, D'alò F, Bombaci JC, Perito S, Bistoni F. 2013. Association of pregnancy and Candida vaginal colonization in women with or without symptoms of vulvovaginitis. *Minerva Ginecologica* 65:303-9.

Lewis JH, Zimmerman HJ, Benson GD, Ishak KG. 1984. Hepatic injury associated with ketoconazole therapy. Analysis of 33 cases. *Gastroenterology*; 86:503-13.

Lewis K. 2010. Persister cells. *Annual Review of Microbiology* 64:357-72.

Lewith GT, Chopra S, Radcliffe MJ, Abraham N, Prescott P, Howarth PH. 2007. Elevation of Candida IgG antibodies in patients with medically unexplained symptoms. *Journal of Alternative and Complementary Medicine* 13:1129-33.

Li Q, Wang C, Tang C, He Q, Li N, Li J. 2013. Dysbiosis of gut fungal microbiota is associated with mucosal inflammation in Crohn's Disease. *Journal of Clinical Gastroenterology* November 29.

Lin XL, Li Z, Zuo XL. 2011. Study on the relationship between vaginal and intestinal candida in patients with vulvovaginal candidiasis. [Article in Chinese] *Zhonghua Fu Chan Ke Za Zhi* 46:496-500.

Lipsky MS, Taylor C. 1996. The use of over-the-counter antifungal vaginitis preparations by college students. *Family Medicine* 28:493-5.

Lisboa C, Santos A, Azevedo F, Pina-Vaz C, Rodrigues AG. 2010. Direct impression on agar surface as a diagnostic sampling procedure for Candida balanitis. *Sexually Transmitted Infections* 86:32–5.

Lopez-Medina E, Koh AY. 2016. The complexities of bacterial-fungal interactions in the mammalian gastrointestinal tract. *Microbial Cell* 3:191-5.

Lord RS, Burdette CK, Bralley JA. 2004. Urinary markers of yeast overgrowth. *Integrative Medicine* 3:24-9.

Lotery HE, McClure N, Galask RP. 2004. Vulvodynia. *Lancet* 363:1058-60.

MacNeill C, Weisz J, Carey JC. 2003. Clinical resistance of recurrent *Candida albicans* vulvovaginitis to fluconazole in the presence and absence of in vitro resistance. *Journal of Reproductive Medicine* 48:63-8.

Magnussona J, Ströma K, Roosa S, Sjögrenb J, Schnürera J. 2003. Broad and complex antifungal activity among environmental isolates of lactic acid bacteria. *FEMS Microbiology Letters* 219:129–35.

Magri V, Cariani L, Bonamore R, Restelli A, Garlaschi MC, Trinchieri A. 2005. Microscopic and microbiological findings for evaluation of chronic prostatitis. *Archivio Italiano di Urologia, Andrologia* 77:135-8.

Mahon WA, De Gregorio M. 1985. Benzydamine: a critical review of clinical data. *International Journal of Tissue Reactions* 7:229–35.

Mann MS, Kaufman RH, Brown Jr, D, Adam E. 1992. Vulvar vestibulitis; significant clinical variables and treatment outcome. *Obstetrics and Gynecology* 79:122-5.

Marchaim D, Lemanek L, Bheemreddy S, Kaye KS, Sobel JD. 2012. Fluconazole-resistant *Candida albicans* vulvovaginitis. *Obstetrics and Gynecology* 120:1407-14.

Mårdh PA, Colleen S. 1975. Search for uro-genital tract infections in patients with symptoms of prostatitis. Studies on aerobic and strictly anaerobic bacteria, mycoplasmas, fungi, trichomonads and viruses. *Scandinavian Journal of Urology and Nephrology* 9:8-16.

Mårdh PA, Novikova N, Stukalova E. 2003. Colonisation of extragenital sites by candida in women with recurrent vulvovaginal candidosis. *BJOG* 110:934–7.

Mårdh PA, Novikova N, Witkin SS, Korneeva I, Rodriques AR. 2003. Detection of Candida by polymerase chain reaction vs. microscopy and culture in women diagnosed as recurrent vulvovaginal cases. *International Journal of STD & AIDS* 14:753-6.

Martin JM, Rona ZP. 1996. *Complete Candida Yeast Guidebook.* Rocklin, California: Prima Health Publishing, pp. 90-1.

Martinez RC, Seney SL, Summers KL, Nomizo A, De Martinis EC, Reid G. 2009a. Effect of *Lactobacillus rhamnosus* GR-1 and *Lactobacillus reuteri* RC-14 on the ability of *Candida albicans* to infect cells and induce inflammation. *Microbiology and Immunology* 53:487-95.

Martinez RCR, Franceschini SA, Patta MC, Quintana SM, Candido RC, Ferreira JC, De Martinis ECP, Reid G. 2009b. Improved treatment of vulvovaginal candidiasis with fluconazole plus probiotic Lactobacillus rhamnosus GR-1 and Lactobacillus reuteri RC-14. *Letters in Applied Microbiology* 48:269–74.

Mathur S, Melchers JT III, Ades EW, Williamson HO, Fudenberg HH. 1980. Anti-ovarian and anti-lymphocyte antibodies in patients with chronic vaginal candidiasis. *Journal of Reproductive Immunology* 2:247-62.

Mayer CL, Diamond RD, Edwards JE Jr. 1990. Recognition of binding sites on *Candida albicans* by monoclonal antibodies to human leukocyte antigens. *Infection and Immunity* 58:3765-9.

McGroarty JA, Soboh F, Bruce AW, Reid G. 1990. The spermicidal compound nonoxynol-9 increases adhesion of Candida species to human epithelial cells in vitro. *Infection and Immunity* 58:2005–7.

McKay M. 1993. Dysesthetic ("essential") vulvodynia. treatment with amitriptyline. *Journal of Reproductive Medicine* 38:9-13.

Medical Economics Co. *Physicians' Desk Reference.* Montvale, NJ. www.PDR.net.

Mendling W, Brasch J. 2012. Guideline vulvovaginal candidosis (2010) of the German Society for Gynecology and Obstetrics, the Working Group for Infections and Infectimmunology in Gynecology and Obstetrics, the German Society of Dermatology, the Board of German Dermatologists and the German Speaking Mycological Society. *Mycoses* 55:1-13.

Merck Manual for Health Care Professionals. www.merckmanuals.com/professional/ immunology_allergic_disorders/immunodeficiency_disorders/chronic_mucocutaneous_candidiasis.html.

Meyn L, Hillier SL. 2013. Relationship of class-specific antibiotic use and hormonal contraception to developing symptomatic vulvovaginal candidiasis. A11, *Abstracts of the Annual Meeting of the Infectious Disease Society of Obstetrics and Gynecology*, August 8-10, Santa Ana Pueblo, New Mexico.

Michael C, Bierbach U, Frenzel K, Lange T, Basara N, Niederwieser D, Mauz-Körholz C, Preiss R. 2010. Voriconazole pharmacokinetics and safety in immunocompromised children compared to adult patients. *Antimicrobial Agents and Chemotherapy* 54:3225-32.

Milani M, Iacobelli P. 2012. Vaginal use of Ibuprofen isobutanolammonium (ginenorm): efficacy, tolerability, and pharmacokinetic data: a review of available data. *International Scholarly Research Network Obstetrics and Gynecology* 2012: 673131.

Mølgaard-Nielsen D, Pasternak B, Hviid A. 2013. Use of oral fluconazole during pregnancy and the risk of birth defects. *New England Journal of Medicine* 369:830-9.

Montes LF, Wilborn WH. 1985. Fungus-host relationship in candidiasis. A brief review. *Archives of Dermatology* 121:119-24.

Moosa MY, Sobel JD, Elhalis H, Du W, Akins RA. 2004. Fungicidal activity of fluconazole against *Candida albicans* in a synthetic vagina-simulative medium. *Antimicrobial Agents and Chemotherapy* 48:161–7.

Moraes PS, de Lima Goiaba S, Taketomi EA. 2000. *Candida albicans* allergen immunotherapy in recurrent vaginal candidiasis. *Journal of Investigational Allergology & Clinical Immunology* 10:305-9.

Moyes DL, Wilson D, Richardson JP, Mogavero S, Tang SX, Wernecke J, Höfs S, Gratacap RL, Robbins J, Runglall M, Murciano C, Blagojevic M, Thavaraj S, Förster TM, Hebecker B, Kasper L, Vizcay G, Iancu SI, Kichik N, Häder A, Kurzai O, Luo T, Krüger T, Kniemeyer O, Cota E, Bader O, Wheeler RT, Gutsmann T, Hube B, Naglik JR. 2016. Candidalysin is a fungal peptide toxin critical for mucosal infection. *Nature* 532:64-68.

Mullin GE, Swift KM, Lipski L, Turnbull LK, Rampertab SD. 2010. Testing for food reactions: the good, the bad, and the ugly. *Nutrition in Clinical Practice* 25:192-8.

Munoz M, Estes G, Kilpatrick M, Di Salvo A, Virella G. 1980. Purification of cytoplasmic antigens from the mycelial phase of *Candida albicans*: possible advantages of its use in Candida serology. *Mycopathologia* 72:47-53.

Murzyn A, Krasowska A, Stefanowicz P, Dziadkowiec D, Łukaszewicz M. 2010. Capric acid secreted by *S. boulardii* inhibits *C. albicans* filamentous growth, adhesion and biofilm formation. *PLoS One* 5: e12050.

Mukherjee PK, Sendid B, Hoarau G, Colombel JF, Poulain D, Ghannoum MA. 2015. Mycobiota in gastrointestinal diseases. *Nature Reviews Gastroenterology & Hepatology* 12:77-87.

Naidu AS, Bidlack WR, Clemens RA. 1999. Probiotic spectra of lactic acid bacteria (LAB). *Critical Reviews in Food Science and Nutrition* 39:13-126.

Neves NA, Carvalho LP, De Oliveira MA, Giraldo PC, Bacellar O, Cruz AA, Carvalho EM. 2005a. Association between atopy and recurrent vaginal candidiasis. *Clinical and Experimental Immunology* 142:167-71.

Neves NA, Carvalho LP, Lopes AC, Cruz A, Carvalho EM. 2005b. Successful treatment of refractory recurrent vaginal candidiasis with cetirizine plus fluconazole. *Journal of Lower Genital Tract Disease* 9:167-70.

Nguyen MH, Yu CY. 1998. Voriconazole against fluconazole-susceptible and resistant candida isolates: in-vitro efficacy compared with that of itraconazole and ketoconazole. *Journal of Antimicrobial Chemotherapy* 42:253-6.

Nguyen RH, Swanson D, Harlow BL. 2009. Urogenital infections in relation to the occurrence of vulvodynia. *Journal of Reproductive Medicine* 54:385-92.

Nieuwenhuizen WF, Pieters RH, Knippels LM, Jansen MC, Koppelman SJ. 2003. Is *Candida albicans* a trigger in the onset of coeliac disease? *Lancet* 361:2152-4.

Nose Y, Komori K, Inouye H, Nomura K, Yamamura M, Tsuji K. 1980. Relationship between HLA-D and in vitro and in vivo responsiveness to Candida allergen. *Clinical and Experimental Immunology* 40:345-50.

Nose Y, Komori K, Inouye H, Nomura K, Yamamura M, Tsuji K. 1981. Role of macrophages in T lymphocyte response to Candida allergen in man with special reference to HLA-D and DR. *Clinical and Experimental Immunology* 45:152-7.

Noverr MC, Noggle RM, Toews GB, Huffnagle GB. 2004. Role of antibiotics and fungal microbiota in driving pulmonary allergic responses. *Infection and Immunity* 72:4996-5003.

Nyilasi I, Kocsubé S, Krizsán K, Galgóczy L, Pesti M, Papp T, Vágvölgyi C. 2010. In vitro synergistic interactions of the effects of various statins and azoles against some clinically important fungi. *FEMS Microbiology Letters* 307:175-84.

Nyirjesy P. 2000. Vulvar vestibulitis syndrome: a post-infectious entity? *Current Infectious Disease Reports* 2:531-5.

Nyirjesy P. 2008. Superficial dyspareunia and vulvar vestibulitis. *Global Library of Women's Medicine* 10053. www.glowm.com.

Nyirjesy P, Halpern M. 1995. Medical management of vulvar vestibulitis: results of a sequential treatment plan. *Infectious Diseases in Obstetrics and Gynecology* 3:193-7.

Nyirjesy P, Weitz MV, Grody MHT, Lorber B. 1997. Over-the-counter and alternative medicines in the treatment of chronic vaginal symptoms. *Obstetrics and Gynecology* 90:50-3.

Nyirjesy P, Seeney SM, Grody MH, Jordan CA, Buckley HR. 1995. Chronic fungal vaginitis: the value of cultures. *American Journal of Obstetrics and Gynecology* 173:820-3.

Nyirjesy P, Sobel JD, Weitz MV, Leaman DJ, Small MJ, Gelone SP. 2001. Cromolyn cream for recalcitrant idiopathic vulvar vestibulitis: results of a placebo controlled study. *Sexually Transmitted Infections* 77:53-7.

Nyirjesy P, Vazquez JA, Ufberg DD, Sobel JD, Boikov DA, Buckley HR. 1995. *Saccharomyces cerevisiae* vaginitis: transmission from yeast used in baking. *Obstetrics & Gynecology* 86:326-9.

Odds FC. 1979. *Candida and Candidosis: A Review and Bibliography*, University Park Press, Baltimore. pp. 109, 112, 118, 203.

Odds FC. 1988. *Candida and Candidosis: A Review and Bibliography*, 2nd edition, Baillière Tindall, London.

Olesen M, Gudmand-Høyer E. 2000. Efficacy, safety, and tolerability of fructooligosaccharides in the treatment of irritable bowel syndrome. *American Journal of Clinical Nutrition* 72:1570–5.

Olivares M, Díaz-Ropero MP, Martín R, Rodríguez JM, Xaus J. 2006. Antimicrobial potential of four Lactobacillus strains isolated from breast milk. *Journal of Applied Microbiology* 101:72-9.

Oriel JD, Partridge BM, Denny MJ, Coleman JC. 1972. Genital yeast infections. *British Medical Journal* 4:761–4.

Paavonen J. 1995. Vulvodynia - a complex syndrome of vulvar pain. *Acta Obstetricia et Gynecologica Scandinavica* 74:243-7.

Pagano R. 2007. Value of colposcopy in the diagnosis of candidiasis in patients with vulvodynia. *Journal of Reproductive Medicine* 52:31-4.

Paillaud E, Merlier I, Dupeyron C, Scherman E, Poupon J, Bories PN. 2004. Oral candidiasis and nutritional deficiencies in elderly hospitalised patients. *British Journal of Nutrition* 92:861-7.

Palma-Carlos AG, Palma-Carlos ML, Costa AC. 2002. Candida and allergy. *Allergie et Immunologie* 34:322-4.

Panizo MM, Reviákina V, Dolande M, Selgrad S. 2009. Candida spp. in vitro susceptibility profile to four antifungal agents. Resistance surveillance study in Venezuelan strains. *Medical Mycology* 47:137-43.

Papanicolas LE, Choo JM, Wang Y, Leong LEX, Costello SP, Gordon DL, Wesselingh SL, Rogers GB. 2019. Bacterial viability in faecal transplants: Which bacteria survive? *EBioMedicine* 41:509–16.

Pappas PG, Kauffman CA, Andes D, Benjamin DK Jr, Calandra TF, Edwards JE Jr, Filler SG, Fisher JF, Kullberg B-J, Ostrosky-Zeichner L, Reboli AC, Rex JH, Walsh TJ, Sobel JD. 2009. Clinical practice guidelines for the management of candidiasis: 2009 update by the Infectious Diseases Society of America. *Clinical Infectious Diseases* 48:503–35.

Patel DA, Gillespie B, Sobel JD, Leaman D, Nyirjesy P, Weitz MV, Foxman B. 2004. Risk factors for recurrent vulvovaginal candidiasis in women receiving maintenance antifungal therapy: results of a prospective cohort study. *American Journal of Obstetrics and Gynecology* 190:644-53.

Payne S, Gibson G, Wynne A, Hudspith B, Brostoff J, Tuohy K. 2003. In vitro studies on colonization resistance of the human gut microbiota to *Candida albicans* and the effects of tetracycline and *Lactobacillus plantarum* LPK. *Current Issues in Intestinal Microbiology* 4:1-8.

Peckham BM, Maki DG, Patterson JJ, Hafez GR. 1986. Focal vulvitis: a characteristic syndrome and cause of dyspareunia. Features, natural history, and management. *American Journal of Obstetrics and Gynecology* 154:855-64.

Pepys J, Faux JA, McCarthy DS, Hargreave FE. 1968. *Candida albicans* precipitins in respiratory disease in man. *Journal of Allergy* 41:305-18.

Pepys J. 1984. Skin tests. *British Journal of Hospital Medicine* 32:120, 122, 124.

Petersen CD, Lundvall L, Kristensen E, Giraldi A. 2008. Vulvodynia. Definition, diagnosis and treatment. *Acta Obstetricia et Gynecologica Scandinavica* 87:893-901.

Pfizer. http://media.pfizer.com/files/products/uspi_diflucan.pdf; www.pfizer.com/products/rx/prescription.jsp.

Phillips N, Bachmann G. 2010. Vulvodynia: An often-overlooked cause of dyspareunia in the menopausal population. *Menopausal Medicine* 18:S1, S3-S5. www.srm-ejournal.com/pdf%2FMed0%2FMenMed0510_vulvodynia.pdf.

Pina-Vaz C, Sansonetty F, Rodrigues AG, Martinez-De-Oliveira J, Fonseca AF, Mårdh PA. 2000. Antifungal activity of ibuprofen alone and in combination with fluconazole against Candida species. *Journal of Medical Microbiology* 49:831-40.

Pirotta MV, Gunn JM, Chondros P. 2003. "Not thrush again!" Women's experience of post-antibiotic vulvovaginitis. *Medical Journal of Australia* 179:43-6.

Pirotta M, Gunn J, Chondros P, Grover S, O'Malley P, Hurley S, Garland S. 2004. Effect of lactobacillus in preventing post-antibiotic vulvovaginal candidiasis: a randomised controlled trial. *BMJ* 329:548.

Prayson RA, Stoler MH, Hart WR. 1995. Vulvar vestibulitis. *American Journal of Surgical Pathology* 19:154-60.

Preissner S, Kroll K, Dunkel M, Senger C, Goldsobel G, Kuzman D, Güenther S, Winnenburg R, Schroeder M, Preissner R. 2010. SuperCYP: a comprehensive database on cytochrome P450 enzymes including a tool for analysis of CYP-drug interactions. *Nucleic Acids Research* 38:D237-43.

Pyka RE, Wilkinson EJ, Friedrich EG Jr, Croker BP. 1988. The histopathology of vulvar vestibulitis syndrome. *International Journal of Gynecological Pathology* 7:249-57.

Rainey MM, Korostyshevsky D, Lee S, Perlstein EO. 2010. The antidepressant sertraline targets intracellular vesiculogenic membranes in yeast. *Genetics* 185:1221-33.

Ramirez De Knott HM, McCormick TS, Do SO, Goodman W, Ghannoum MA, Cooper KD, Nedorost ST. 2005. Cutaneous hypersensitivity to *Candida albicans* in idiopathic vulvodynia. *Contact Dermatitis* 53:214–8.

Rappleye CA, Goldman WE. 2008. Fungal stealth technology. *Trends in Immunology* 29:18-24.

Ray D, Goswami R, Banerjee U, Dadhwal V, Goswami D, Mandal P, Sreenivas V, Kochupillai N. 2007. Prevalence of *Candida glabrata* and its response to boric acid vaginal suppositories in comparison with oral fluconazole in patients with diabetes and vulvovaginal candidiasis. *Diabetes Care* 30:312-7.

Reed BD, Crawford S, Couper M, Cave C, Haefner HK. 2004. Pain at the vulvar vestibule: a Web-based survey. *Journal of Lower Genital Tract Disease* 8:48-57.

Reed BD, Harlow SD, Sen A, Legocki LJ, Edwards RM, Arato N, Haefner HK. 2012. Prevalence and demographic characteristics of vulvodynia in a population-based sample. *American Journal of Obstetrics and Gynecology* 206:170.e1-9.

Reichman O, Akins R, Sobel JD. 2009 Boric acid addition to suppressive antimicrobial therapy for recurrent bacterial vaginosis. *Sexually Transmitted Diseases* 36:732-4.

Reid G. 2001. Probiotic agents to protect the urogenital tract against infection. *American Journal of Clinical Nutrition* 73:437S-43S.

Reid G, Dols J, Miller W. 2009. Targeting the vaginal microbiota with probiotics as a means to counteract infections. *Current Opinion in Clinical Nutrition and Metabolic Care* 12:583-7.

Reid G, Bruce AW, McGroarty JA, Cheng KJ, Costerton JW. 1990. Is there a role for lactobacilli in prevention of urogenital and intestinal infections? *Clinical Microbiology Reviews* 3:335-44.

Reid G, Charbonneau D, Erb J, Kochanowski B, Beuerman D, Poehner R, Bruce AW. 2003. Oral use of *Lactobacillus rhamnosus* GR-1 and *L. fermentum* RC-14 significantly alters vaginal flora: randomized, placebo-controlled trial in 64 healthy women. *FEMS Immunology and Medical Microbiology* 35:131-4.

Renfro L, Feder HM, Lane TJ, Manu P, Matthews DA. 1989. Yeast connection among 100 patients with chronic fatigue. *American Journal of Medicine* 86:165-8.

Ridley CM. 1998. Vulvodynia. Theory and management. *Dermatologic Clinics* 16:775-8, xiii.

Rigg D, Miller MM, Metzger WJ. 1990. Recurrent allergic vulvovaginitis: treatment with *Candida albicans* allergen immunotherapy. *American Journal of Obstetrics and Gynecology* 162:332-6.

Ringdahl EN. 2000. Treatment of recurrent vulvovaginal candidiasis. *American Family Physician* 61:3306-12; 3317.

Riordan AM, Hunter JO, Cowan RE, Crampton JR, Davidson AR, Dickinson RJ, Dronfield MW, Fellows IW, Hishon S, Kerrigan GN, et al. 1993. Treatment of active Crohn's disease by exclusion diet: East Anglian multicentre controlled trial. *Lancet* 342:1131-4.

Robinett RW. 1968. Asthma due to *Candida albicans*. *University of Michigan Medical Center Journal*. 34:12-5.

Romani L, Puccetti P. 2007. Controlling pathogenic inflammation to fungi. *Expert Review of Anti-infective Therapy* 5:1007-17.

Romani L, Zelante T, De Luca A, Fallarino F, Puccetti P. 2008. IL-17 and therapeutic kynurenines in pathogenic inflammation to fungi. *Journal of Immunology* 180:5157-62.

Romeo MG, Romeo DM, Trovato L, Oliveri S, Palermo F, Cota F, Betta P. 2011. Role of probiotics in the prevention of the enteric colonization by Candida in preterm newborns: incidence of late-onset sepsis and neurological outcome. *Journal of Perinatology* 31:63–9.

Rosa MI, Silva BR, Pires PS, Silva FR, Silva NC, Silva FR, Souza SL, Madeira K, Panatto AP, Medeiros LR. 2013. Weekly fluconazole therapy for recurrent vulvovaginal candidiasis: a systematic review and meta-analysis. *European Journal of Obstetrics, Gynecology, and Reproductive Biology* 167:132-6.

Rosati D, Bruno M, Jaeger M, Oever J ten, Netea MG. 2020. Recurrent vulvovaginal candidiasis: an immunological perspective. *Microorganisms* 8:144.

Rosenberg EW, Noah PW, Skinner RB Jr. 1994. Microorganisms and psoriasis. *Journal of the National Medical Association* 86:305-10.

Rosenberg MJ, Rojanapithayakorn W, Feldblum PJ, Higgins JE. 1987. Effect of the contraceptive sponge on chlamydial infection, gonorrhea, and candidiasis. A comparative clinical trial. *JAMA* 257:2308-12.

Rosentul D, Delsing C, Joosten LAB, van der Meer JWM, Kullberg BJ and Netea MG. 2009. Polymorphism in innate immunity genes and susceptibility to recurrent vulvovaginal candidiasis. *Journal de Mycologie Médicale* 19:191-6.

Ruiz-Sánchez D, Calderón-Romero L, Sánchez-Vega JT, Tay J. 2002. Intestinal candidiasis. A clinical report and comments about this opportunistic pathology. *Mycopathologia* 156:9-11.

Ryder NS, Wagner S, Leitner I. 1998. In vitro activities of terbinafine against cutaneous isolates of *Candida albicans* and other pathogenic yeasts. *Antimicrobial Agents and Chemotherapy* 42:1057-61.

Samonis G, Gikas A, Toloudis P, Maraki S, Vrentzos G, Tselentis Y, Tsaparas N, Bodey G. 1994. Prospective study of the impact of broad-spectrum antibiotics on the yeast flora of the human gut. *European Journal of Clinical Microbiology & Infectious Diseases* 13:665-7.

San José B, Baskaran Z, Serrano L, Bilbao I, Sordo B, Bustinza A, Castaño M, Baza B, Sautua S, Rodriguez E. 2012. Hospital formulations for the treatment of non-albicans vulvovaginitis. *European Journal of Hospital Pharmacy* 19:142.

Santelmann H, Lærum E, Rønnevig J, Fagertun HE. 2001. Effectiveness of nystatin in polysymptomatic patients. A randomized, double-blind trial with nystatin versus placebo in general practice. *Family Practice* 18:258-65. Download PDF from: www.candidaallergy.com/us/article.asp.

Santelmann H, Howard JM. 2005. Yeast metabolic products, yeast antigens and yeasts as possible triggers for irritable bowel syndrome. *European Journal of Gastroenterology & Hepatology* 17:21-6.

Sarma A, Foxman B, Bayirli B, Haefner H, Sobel JD. 1999. Epidemiology of vulvar vestibulitis syndrome: an exploratory case-control study. *Sexually Transmitted Infections* 75:320-6.

Savino F, Cordisco L, Tarasco V, Palumeri E, Calabrese R, Oggero R, Roos S, Matteuzzi D. 2010. *Lactobacillus reuteri* DSM 17938 in infantile colic: a randomized, double-blind, placebo-controlled trial. *Pediatrics* 126:e526-33.

Savolainen J, Lammintausta K, Kalimo K, Viander M. 1993. *Candida albicans* and atopic dermatitis. *Clinical and Experimental Allergy* 23:332-9.

Schaffer T, Müller S, Flogerzi B, Seibold-Schmid B, Schoepfer AM, Seibold F. 2007. Anti-*Saccharomyces cerevisiae* mannan antibodies (ASCA) of Crohn's patients crossreact with mannan from other yeast strains, and murine ASCA IgM can be experimentally induced with *Candida albicans*. *Inflammatory Bowel Diseases* 13:1339-46.

Scheinfeld N. 2003. The role of gabapentin in treating diseases with cutaneous manifestations and pain. *International Journal of Dermatology* 42:491-5.

Schnell JD. 1982a. Investigations into the pathoaetiology and diagnosis of vaginal mycoses. *Chemotherapy* 28: Suppl 1:14-21.

Schnell JD. 1982b. Epidemiology and the prevention of peripartal mycoses. *Chemotherapy* 28:66-72.

Schnell JD, Voigt WH. 1976. Are yeasts in vaginal smears intracellular or extracellular? *Acta Cytologica* 20:343-6.

Schulze J, Sonnenborn U. 2009. Yeasts in the gut: from commensals to infectious agents. *Deutsches Ärzteblatt International* 106:837-42.

Schwiertz A, Taras D, Rusch K, Rusch V. 2006. Throwing the dice for the diagnosis of vaginal complaints? *Annals of Clinical Microbiology and Antimicrobials* 5:4.

Secor RM. 1992. Cytolytic vaginosis: a common cause of cyclic vulvovaginitis. *Nurse Practitioner Forum* 3:145-8.

Secor RM, Fertitta L. 1992. Vulvar vestibulitis syndrome. *Nurse Practitioner Forum* 3:161-8.

Seebacher C. 1996. Mycophobia—a new disease? *Mycoses* 39:30-2.

Seelig MS. 1966. Mechanisms by which antibiotics increase the incidence and severity of candidiasis and alter the immunological defenses. *Bacteriological Reviews* 30:442–59.

Segal BH, Leto TL, Gallin JI, Malech HL, Holland SM. 2000. Genetic, biochemical, and clinical features of chronic granulomatous disease. *Medicine* 79:170-200.

Sehnert KW, Struve JK, Komoto TS, Fosse M. 1990. An evaluation of self-administered questionnaires as an aid in diagnosis of Candida-related-complex. *Journal of Advancement in Medicine* 3:93-101.

Sehnert KW, Mathews-Larson J. 1991. Candida-related complex (CRC), a complicating factor in treatment and diagnostic screening for alcoholics: A pilot study of 213 patients. *International Journal of Biosocial & Medical Research* 13:67-76.

Semmelweis IP. 1847. Hochst wichtige Erfahrungen uber die Aetiologie der in Gebaranstalten epidemischen Puerperalfieber. *Ztschr. d. K. K. Gesellsch. d. Aerzte in Wien* 242; 1849, v, 64.

Sepah T. 1998. Is it really a yeast infection? *Ms. Magazine.* January/February, p. 38.

Shaaban OM, Abbas AM, Moharram AM, Farhan MM, Hassanen IH. 2015. Does vaginal douching affect the type of candidal vulvovaginal infection? *Medical Mycology* 53:817-27.

Shah DT, Glover DD, Larsen B. 1995. In situ mycotoxin production by *Candida albicans* in women with vaginitis. *Gynecologic and Obstetric Investigation* 39:67-9.

Shahid Z, Sobel JD. 2009. Reduced fluconazole susceptibility of *Candida albicans* isolates in women with recurrent vulvovaginal candidiasis: effects of long-term fluconazole therapy. *Diagnostic Microbiology and Infectious Disease* 64:354-6.

Shakib F. 1987. The role of IgG$_4$ in food allergy, pp. 898-906, In: *Food Allergy and Intolerance*, J. Brostoff, S.J. Challacombe (Editors), Baillière Tindall, London.

Shakib F. 1988. Clinical relevance of food-specific IgG$_4$ antibodies. *New England and Regional Allergy Proceedings* 9:63-6.

Shaw W, Kassen E, Chaves E. 1995. Increased urinary excretion of analogs of Krebs cycle metabolites and arabinose in two brothers with autistic features. *Clinical Chemistry* 41:1094-104.

Shaw W, Kassen E, Chaves E. 2000. Assessment of antifungal drug therapy in autism by measurement of suspected microbial metabolites in urine with gas chromatography-mass spectrometry. *Clinical Practice in Alternative Medicine* 1:15-26.

Sheary B, Dayan L. 2005. Clinical practice. Recurrent vulvovaginal candidiasis. *Australian Family Physician* 34:147–50.

Shi WM, Mei XY, Gao F, Huo KK, Shen LL, Qin HH, Wu ZW, Zheng J. 2007. Analysis of genital *Candida albicans* infection by rapid microsatellite markers genotyping. *Chinese Medical Journal* 120:975-80.

Simon-Nobbe B, Denk U, Pöll V, Rid R, Breitenbach M. 2008. The spectrum of fungal allergy. *International Archives of Allergy and Immunology* 145:58-86.

Smeekens SP, van de Veerdonk FL, Kullberg BJ, Netea MG. 2013. Genetic susceptibility to Candida infections. *EMBO Molecular Medicine* 5:1–9.

Smith EM, Ritchie JM, Galask R, Pugh EE, Jia J, Ricks-McGillan J. 2002. Case-control study of vulvar vestibulitis risk associated with genital infections. *Infectious Diseases in Obstetrics and Gynecology* 10:193-202.

Sobel JD. 1985. Management of recurrent vulvovaginal candidiasis with intermittent ketoconazole prophylaxis. *Obstetrics and Gynecology* 65:435-40.

Sobel JD. 1992. Pathogenesis and treatment of recurrent vulvovaginal candidiasis. *Clinical Infectious Diseases* 14 (Supplement 1):S148–S153.

Sobel JD. 2007. Vulvovaginal candidosis. *Lancet* 369:1961-71.

Sobel JD, Chaim W. 1997. Treatment of *Torulopsis glabrata* vaginitis: a retrospective review of boric acid therapy. *Clinical Infectious Diseases* 24:649–52.

Sobel JD, Muller G, Buckley HR. 1984. Critical role of germ tube formation in the pathogenesis of candidal vaginitis. *Infection and Immunity* 44:576-80.

Sobel JD, Chaim W, Nagappan V, Leaman D. 2003. Treatment of vaginitis caused by *Candida glabrata*: use of topical boric acid and flucytosine. *American Journal of Obstetrics and Gynecology* 189:1297- 300.

Sobel JD, Faro S, Force RW, Foxman B, Ledger WJ, Nyirjesy PR, Reed BD, Summers PR. 1998. Vulvovaginal candidiasis: epidemiologic, diagnostic, and therapeutic considerations. *American Journal of Obstetrics and Gynecology* 178:203–11.

Sobel JD, Wiesenfeld HC, Martens M, Danna P, Hooton TM, Rompalo A, Sperling M, Livengood C 3rd, Horowitz B, Von Thron J, Edwards L, Panzer H, Chu TC. 2004. Maintenance fluconazole therapy for recurrent vulvovaginal candidiasis. *New England Journal of Medicine* 351:876-83.

Sobel JD, Nyirjesy P, Kessary H, Ferris DG. 2009. Use of the VS-Sense swab in diagnosing vulvovaginitis. *Journal of Womens Health* 18:1467-70.

Sorey W. 2009. Diagnosis: Dermatophytid reaction (Id reaction). Commentary. *Clinical Pediatrics* 48:335.

Spadt SK, Fariello JY, Safaeian P. 2007. Renewing relationships: treating sexual pain in women. *Advance for Nurse Practitioners* 15:39-42. nurse-practitioners.advanceweb.com/Article/Renewing-Relationships-1.aspx.

Spinillo A, Capuzzo E, Gulminetti R, Marone P, Colonna L, Piazzi G. 1997. Prevalence of and risk factors for fungal vaginitis caused by non-albicans species. *American Journal of Obstetrics and Gynecology* 176:138-41.

Staab JF, Bahn YS, Tai CH, Cook PF, Sundstrom P. 2004. Expression of transglutaminase substrate activity on *Candida albicans* germ tubes through a coiled, disulfide-bonded N-terminal domain of Hwp1 requires C-terminal glycosylphosphatidylinositol modification. *Journal of Biological Chemistry* 24:40737-47.

Standaert-Vitse A, Jouault T, Vandewalle P, Mille C, Seddik M, Sendid B, Mallet JM, Colombel JF, Poulain D. 2006. *Candida albicans* is an immunogen for anti-*Saccharomyces cerevisiae* antibody markers of Crohn's disease. *Gastroenterology* 130:1764-75.

Stapel SO, Asero R, Ballmer-Weber BK, Knol EF, Strobel S, Vieths S, Kleine-Tebbe J. 2008. Testing for IgG_4 against foods is not recommended as a diagnostic tool: EAACI Task Force Report. *Allergy* 63:793-6.

Steel HC, Tintinger GR, Anderson R. 2008. Comparison of the anti-inflammatory activities of imidazole antimycotics in relation to molecular structure. *Chemical Biology and Drug Design* 72:225-8.

Steinberg AC, Oyama IA, Rejba AE, Kellogg-Spadt S, Whitmore KE. 2005. Capsaicin for the treatment of vulvar vestibulitis. *American Journal of Obstetrics & Gynecology* 192:1549-53.

Stricker BH, Blok AP, Bronkhorst FB, Van Parys GE, Desmet VJ. 1986. Ketoconazole-associated hepatic injury. A clinicopathological study of 55 cases. *Journal of Hepatology* 3:399-406.

Strom CM, Levine EM. 1998. Chronic vaginal candidiasis responsive to biotin therapy in a carrier of biotinidase deficiency. *Obstetrics and Gynecology* 92:644-6.

Sun S, Li Y, Guo Q, Shi C, Yu J, Ma L. 2008. In vitro interactions between tacrolimus and azoles against *Candida albicans* determined by different methods. *Antimicrobial Agents and Chemotherapy* 52:409-17.

Sutton JT, Bachmann GA, Arnold LD, Rhoads GG, Rosen RC. 2008. Assessment of vulvodynia symptoms in a sample of U.S. women: a follow-up national incidence survey. *Journal of Women's Health (Larchmt.)* 17:1285-92.

Tanizaki Y, Kitani H, Okazaki M, Mifune T, Mitsunobu F. 1992. Humoral and cellular immunity to *Candida albicans* in patients with bronchial asthma. *Internal Medicine* 31:766-9.

Tchoudomirova K, Mardh PA, Hellberg D. 2001. Vaginal microbiological flora, and behavioural and clinical findings in women with vulvar pain. *BJOG* 108:451-5.

Tormey P. 1989. "Warning: Panties Aren't Hot Pants." United Press International in *San Francisco Chronicle*, March 4.

Trowbridge JP, Walker M. 1986. *The Yeast Syndrome*, Bantam Books, New York.

Truss CO. 1978. Tissue injury induced by *Candida albicans*: mental and neurologic manifestations. *Journal of Orthomolecular Psychiatry* 7:17-37.

Truss CO. 1980. Restoration of immunologic competence to *Candida albicans*. *Journal of Orthomolecular Psychiatry* 9:287-301.

Truss CO. 1981. The role of *Candida albicans* in human illness. *Journal of Orthomolecular Psychiatry* 10:228-38.

Truss CO. 1983. *The Missing Diagnosis*, P.O. Box 26508, Birmingham, Alabama 35226. pp. 35-7.

Truss CO. 1984. Metabolic abnormalities in patients with chronic candidiasis: the acetaldehyde hypothesis. *Journal of Orthomolecular Psychiatry* 13:66-93.

Truss CO. 2009. *The Missing Diagnosis II*, P.O. Box 26508, Birmingham, Alabama 35226.

Truss CO, Truss CV, Cutler RB, et al. 1991. A controlled trial of nystatin for the candidiasis hypersensitivity syndrome. Letter to the editor. *New England Journal of Medicine* 324:1592-3.

Truss CO, Truss CV, Cutler RB. 1992. Generalized symptoms in women with chronic yeast vaginitis: treatment with nystatin, diet and immunotherapy versus nystatin alone. *Journal of Advancement in Medicine* 5:139-75.

Turck D, Bernet JP, Marx J, Kempf H, Giard P, Walbaum O, Lacombe A, Rembert F, Toursel F, Bernasconi P, Gottrand F, McFarland LV, Bloch K. 2003. Incidence and risk factors of oral antibiotic-associated diarrhea in an outpatient pediatric population. *Journal of Pediatric Gastroenterology and Nutrition* 37:22–6.

Tyler SL, Woodall GM. 1982. *Female Health and Gynecology: Across the Lifespan*. Robert J. Brady Co., A Prentice-Hall Publishing and Communications Co., Bowie, Maryland.

Tympanidis P. 2003. Increased innervation of the vulval vestibule in patients with vulvodynia. *British Journal of Dermatology* 148:1021-7.

University of Michigan Health System. 2008. Selected Herb-Drug Interactions. www.med.umich.edu/1libr/aha/umherb01.htm.

Vagisil Screening Kit®. www.vagisilkit.com/kit2/index.shtml.

van Burik JH, Magee PT. 2001. Aspects of fungal pathogenesis in humans. *Annual Review of Microbiology* 55:743-72.

van de Veerdonk FL, Netea MG, Joosten LA, van der Meer JW, Kullberg BJ. 2010. Novel strategies for the prevention and treatment of Candida infections: the potential of immunotherapy. *FEMS Microbiology Reviews* 34:1063-75.

Van Immerseel F, Ducatelle R, De Vos M, Boon N, Van De Wiele T, Verbeke K, Rutgeerts P, Sas B, Louis P, Flint HJ. 2010. Butyric acid-producing anaerobic bacteria as a novel probiotic treatment approach for inflammatory bowel disease. *Journal of Medical Microbiology* 59:141-3.

Van Kessel K, Assefi N, Marrazzo J, Eckert L. 2003. Common complementary and alternative therapies for yeast vaginitis and bacterial vaginosis: a systematic review. *Obstetrical & Gynecological Survey* 58:351-8.

van Slyke KK, Michel VP, Rein MF. 1981. Treatment of vulvovaginal candidiasis with boric acid powder. *American Journal of Obstetrics and Gynecology* 141:145–8.

Vanderpool C, Yan F, Polk DB. 2008. Mechanisms of probiotic action: Implications for therapeutic applications in inflammatory bowel diseases. *Inflammatory Bowel Diseases* 14:1585-96.

Vazquez JA. 2003. Combination antifungal therapy against Candida species: the new frontier-are we there yet? *Medical Mycology* 41:355-68.

Vazquez JA, Bronze MS. 2011. Candidiasis organism-specific therapy. http://emedicine.medscape.com/article/2012015-overview.

Vazquez JA, Sobel JD, Demitriou R, Vaishampayan J, Lynch M, Zervos MJ. 1994. Karyotyping of *Candida albicans* isolates obtained longitudinally in women with recurrent vulvovaginal candidiasis. *Journal of Infectious Diseases* 170:1566-9.

Ventolini G, Barhan S, Duke J. 2009. Vulvodynia, a step-wise therapeutic prospective cohort study. *Journal of Obstetrics and Gynaecology* 29:648-50.

Vernia P, Annese V, Bresci G, d'Albasio G, D'Incà R, Giaccari S, Ingrosso M, Mansi C, Riegler G, Valpiani D, Caprilli R. 2003. Topical butyrate improves efficacy of 5-ASA in refractory distal ulcerative colitis: results of a multicentre trial. *European Journal of Clinical Investigation* 33:244-8.

Vladareanu R, Mihu D, Mitran M, Mehedintu C, Boiangiu A, Manolache M, Vladareanu S. 2018. New evidence on oral *L. plantarum* P17630 product in women with history of recurrent vulvovaginal candidiasis (RVVC): a randomized double-blind placebo-controlled study. *European Review for Medical and Pharmacological Sciences* 22:262-7.

Vojdani A, Rahimian P, Kalhor H, Mordechai E. 1996. Immunological cross reactivity between *Candida albicans* and human tissue. *Journal of Clinical and Laboratory Immunology* 48:1-15.

Wachtershauser A, Stein J. 2000. Rationale for the luminal provision of butyrate in intestinal diseases. *European Journal of Nutrition* 39:164–71.

Wagner RD. 2005. Innate and adaptive immunity against *Candida* species infections in the gastrointestinal tract, pp. 303-22, In: *Fungal Immunology: From an Organ Perspective*, P.L. Fidel, Jr., G.B. Huffnagle (Editors), Springer-Verlag, New York.

Waksman BH. 1979. Cellular hypersensitivity and immunity: Conceptual changes in last decade. *Cellular Immunology* 42:155-69.

Walker LA, Munro CA, de Bruijn I, Lenardon MD, McKinnon A, Gow NA. 2008. Stimulation of chitin synthesis rescues *Candida albicans* from echinocandins. *PLoS Pathogens* 4: e1000040.

Wasan KM, Wasan EK, Gershkovich P, Zhu X, Tidwell RR, Werbovetz KA, Clement JG, Thornton SJ. 2009. Highly Effective oral amphotericin B formulation against murine visceral leishmaniasis. *Journal of Infectious Diseases* 200:357–60.

Watson CJ, Grando D, Fairley CK, Chondros P, Garland SM, Myers SP, Pirotta M. 2014. The effects of oral garlic on vaginal candida colony counts: a randomised placebo controlled double-blind trial. *BJOG* 121:498–506.

Watson MC, Grimshaw JM, Bond CM, Mollison J, Ludbrook A. 2002. Oral versus intra-vaginal imidazole and triazole anti-fungal agents for the treatment of uncomplicated vulvovaginal candidiasis (thrush): a systematic review. *BJOG* 109:85-95.

Watson RA, Irwin Jr RJ. 2009. Chronic pelvic pain syndrome and prostatodynia. http://emedicine. medscape.com/article/437745-overview.

Weig M, Muller F-M C. 2001. Synergism of voriconazole and terbinafine against *Candida albicans* isolates from human immunodeficiency virus-infected patients with oropharyngeal candidiasis. *Antimicrobial Agents and Chemotherapy* 45:966–8.

Weinberg ED. 1999 The role of iron in protozoan and fungal infectious diseases. *Journal of Eukaryotic Microbiology* 46:231-8.

Weinberg ED. 2004. *Exposing the Hidden Dangers of Iron: What every Medical Professional Should Know About the Impact of Iron on the Disease Process.* Cumberland House Publishing, Inc., Nashville, Tennessee.

Weissenbacher T, Witkin SS, Ledger WJ, Tolbert V, Gingelmaier A, Scholz C, Weissenbacher ER, Friese K, Mylonas I. 2009. Relationship between clinical diagnosis of recurrent vulvovaginal candidiasis and detection of Candida species by culture and polymerase chain reaction. *Archives of Gynecology and Obstetrics* 279:125-9.

Weissenbacher TM, Witkin SS, Gingelmaier A, Scholz C, Friese K, Mylonas I. 2009. Relationship between recurrent vulvovaginal candidosis and immune mediators in vaginal fluid. *European Journal of Obstetrics, Gynecology, and Reproductive Biology* 144:59–63.

Westrom LV, Willen R. 1998. Vestibular nerve fiber proliferation in vulvar vestibulitis syndrome. *Obstetrics and Gynecology* 91:572-6.

White DJ, Habib AR, Vanthuyne A, Langford S, Symonds M. 2001. Combined topical flucytosine and amphotericin B for refractory vaginal *Candida glabrata* infections. *Sexually Transmitted Infections* 77:212-3.

White DJ, Vanthuyne A, Wood PM, Ayres JG. 2004. Zafirlukast for severe recurrent vulvovaginal candidiasis: An open label pilot study. *Sexually Transmitted Infections* 80:219–22.

Williams AB, Yu C, Tashima K, Burgess J, Danvers K. 2001. Evaluation of two self-care treatments for prevention of vaginal candidiasis in women with HIV. *Journal of the Association of Nurses in AIDS Care* 12:51-7.

Wilson C. 2005 Recurrent vulvovaginitis candidiasis; an overview of traditional and alternative therapies. *Advance for Nurse Practitioners* 13:24-9.

Willis K. 2019. http://theconversation.com/the-womb-isnt-sterile-healthy-babies-are-born-with-bacteria-and-fungi-in-their-guts-123123.

Wise GJ, Shteynshlyuger A. 2006. How to diagnose and treat fungal infections in chronic prostatitis. *Current Urology Reports* 7:320-8.

Witkin SS. 1985. Defective immune responses in patients with recurrent candidiasis. *Infections in Medicine* 2:40-2.

Witkin SS. 1991. Immunologic factors influencing susceptibility to recurrent candidal vaginitis. *Clinical Obstetrics & Gynecology* 34:662-8.

Witkin SS, Jeremias J, Ledger WJ. 1988. A localized vaginal allergic response in women with recurrent vaginitis. *Journal of Allergy and Clinical Immunology* 81:412-6.

Witkin SS, Jeremias J, Ledger WJ. 1989. Vaginal eosinophils and IgE antibodies to *Candida albicans* in women with recurrent vaginitis. *Journal of Medical and Veterinary Mycology* 27:57-8.

Witkin SS, Gerber S, Ledger WJ. 2002. Differential characterization of women with vulvar vestibulitis syndrome. *American Journal of Obstetrics and Gynecology* 187:589-94.

Wlodarska M, Finlay BB. 2010. Host immune response to antibiotic perturbation of the microbiota. *Mucosal Immunology* 3:100-3.

Wojdani A, Ghoneum M, Cheung GP. 1986. Measurements of humoral and cellular immunity for the diagnosis of candidiasis. *Clinical Ecology* 3:201-7.

Woodruff JD, Parmley TH. 1983. Infection of the minor vestibular gland. *Obstetrics and Gynecology* 62:609-12.

Wucherpfennig KW. 2001. Structural basis of molecular mimicry. *Journal of Autoimmunity* 16:293-302.

Yamaguchi N, Sugita R, Miki A, Takemura N, Kawabata J, Watanabe J, Sonoyama K. 2006. Gastrointestinal Candida colonisation promotes sensitisation against food antigens by affecting the mucosal barrier in mice. *Gut* 55:954-60.

Zhang X, Essmann M, Burt ET, Larsen B. 2000. Estrogen effects on *Candida albicans*: a potential virulence-regulating mechanism. *Journal of Infectious Diseases* 181:1441-6.

Zhu W, Filler SG. 2010. Interactions of *Candida albicans* with epithelial cells. *Cellular Microbiology* 12:273-82.

Zwerling MH, Owens KN, Ruth NH. 1984. "Think yeast"—the expanding spectrum of candidiasis. *Journal of the South Carolina Medical Association* 80:454-6.

Zwolinska-Wcislo M, Brzozowski T, Budak A, Kwiecien S, Sliwowski Z, Drozdowicz D, Trojanowska D, Rudnicka-Sosin L, Mach T, Konturek SJ, Pawlik WW. 2009. Effect of Candida colonization on human ulcerative colitis and the healing of inflammatory changes of the colon in the experimental model of colitis ulcerosa. *Journal of Physiology and Pharmacology* 60:107-18.

Index

NOTE: Locators in **boldface** indicate major discussions. *Figures* are indicated by f following the page number, e.g. 21f, and *tables* by t.

acute pseudomembranous candidiasis (white
form), 11–12
chronic atrophic erythematous candidiasis (red
form), 12–13
Mycamine (micafungin), 122
Mycelex (clotrimazole), 113, 114
mycelia, 7
Mycolog (steroid/antifungal cream), 90, 136
Mycostatin (nystatin), 114
mycotoxins, 20

N
National Vulvodynia Association, 42, 44
natural remedies for yeast infections, 127–28
neurologic pain, vulvodynia and, 38
neutropenia, 116, 201
neutrophils
in chronic granulomatous disease, 15
as innate defense mechanism against Candida,
22–23
pus formation, bacterial vs. yeast infections, 22
newborn infants, oral thrush in, 169
Nikkomycin Z, 123
Nilstat (nystatin), 115
Nizoral (ketoconazole)
side effects and drug interactions, 119
as systemic oral antifungal, 119
topical, in shampoo, 113
nonoxynol-9, 179
nonsteroidal anti-inflammatory drugs (NSAIDs),
149–50
Norplant implant, 181
nosocomial disseminated candidiasis, 169
nosocomial transmission of infections, 172–73
NovaDigm Vaccine (NDV-3A), 162
Noxafil (posaconazole)
disseminated fungal infections, 122, 135, 136
oral suspension, 116
NSAIDs (nonsteroidal anti-inflammatory drugs),
149–50
nutritional deficiencies
yeast infections and, 172
yeast syndrome and, 69, 102
nystatin
cost, convenience, and treatment time, 118
dosage, intestinal candidiasis, 117
efficacy, 117
enema protocol, for intestinal candidiasis, 131–32
ergosterol supplement interactions with, 118
formulation, 117
intestinal yeast overgrowth, treatment protocol,
129
for mucosal and cutaneous candidiasis, 116–18
for oral thrush, 52–53, 54
safety, 117
for yeast vaginitis, 114, 115

O
oat bran, 204
Oidium, 9, 162
opportunistic pathogens, 9
oral candidiasis (thrush)
age factors, 169
characteristics, 11
in children, 51–52
diseases mimicking, 102
prevention, 54
topical plus systemic antifungal therapy, 125
treatment, 52–53, 128–29
oral contraceptives, yeast vaginitis and, 168–69, 180
oral vaccines (sublingual immunotherapy), 161
oropharyngeal candidiasis, 125
overview of the ten-step program, **87-92**
over-the-counter (OTC) medications
self-treatment of yeast vaginitis, 32
topical antifungals, 113, 114
ovulation, yeast vaginitis and, 168

P
pain clinics, vulvar, 42–44
PCR (polymerase chain reaction), 94, 97
penicillin, 58, 166, 167
penile candidiasis. *See* Candida balanitis
penis, yeast infections of, 45
peptic ulcer treatments, 167
perianal area, 26
permeability, selective, 68
personal hygiene, candidiasis prevention and, 177
persorption, 68
pH, vaginal, 28–29, 97
phospholipase, 18–19
physical therapy, for vulvodynia, 43
physician–patient relations
medical history summary (questionnaire), 4–5t
physician referrals for yeast syndrome treatment,
83–84, 103–4
physician skepticism about yeast infections, 2–3
stay with personal physician, 5, 103, 104
pimaricin, 116
Pityrosporum (Malassezia), 13
polymerase chain reaction (PCR), 94, 97
polymorphisms, 74
polysystem chronic candidiasis (yeast syndrome), 14
posaconazole. *See* Noxafil (posaconazole)
postprandial exacerbation of symptoms, 65, 186
prebiotics
definition, 197
fiber supplements, 202
fructooligosaccharides, 202
lactulose, 202–3
promoting growth of Bifidobacterium, 91
synbiotic use with probiotics, 202–3
pregnancy
prenatal screening for neonatal yeast infection

prevention, 54
vaginal antifungal safety during, 113–14
yeast vaginitis in, 168, 169
prepubescent girls, yeast vaginitis in, 168
preventive antiyeast treatments, 167
prick (scratch) tests, 100, 154–55
probiotics
overview, 91
clinical conditions prevented by, 200
daily dosage, 198
definition, 197
efficacy for specific diseases, 198
intestinal candidiasis in children, 54–55
for intestinal disorders, 197–98
mechanisms for blocking pathogens, 200
reasons for not inserting into vagina, 207
restoring normal intestinal flora, 8, 58
safety of, 198, 199–200
tale of two yeasts, 200
for yeast vaginitis, 205–6
in yogurt, 198
progesterone therapy, yeast vaginitis and, 169
progesterone-based contraceptives, 181
prostaglandin E2, 153–54
prostatitis
Candida, 46, 47–48
chronic nonbacterial (nonspecific), 46
prostatodynia (chronic pelvic pain syndrome), 12, 46, 49–50
protocols, yeast infection, 128–37
pruritis, 2, 147
pseudohyphae, 7
pseudomembrane, in yeast vaginitis, 27
psoriasis, 13, 70
punch biopsy, vulvar, 40
pus formation, bacterial vs. yeast infections, 22

Q
Q-tip test, for vulvodynia, 40

R
raffinose and intestinal gas, 190
rash, skin, 13
RAST (radioallergosorbent test) blood tests, 154
reservoir of infection, 18, 136, 166
resistant yeast infections, 123, 135–36
rhythm method (birth control), 181
ricotta cheese, 193
ringworm, 13, 97
risk factors
antacids, 167
antibacterial antibiotics, 166–67
avoiding all yeast infection risks, 165–73
Candida transmission, 172–73
corticosteroids, 168
estrogen, 168–69
medical, 166–69

nosocomial disseminated candidiasis, 169
physiological, for candidiasis, 169
predisposing conditions, 170–72
SGLT-2 inhibitors, 167–68
susceptibility factors, identifying, 166

S
Saccharomyces boulardii, 200–202
Saccharomyces cerevisiae (baker's yeast), 8, 161, 173, 193, 201
safety of antifungals, 110
sanitary products, 176–77
scratch (prick) tests, 100, 154–55
screening tools
Candida Questionnaire and Score Sheet (Crook), 61
Yeast Questionnaire (Santelmann), 61, 62t
scrotum, and "jock itch," 46
secondary metabolites, 20
selective permeability, 68
self-tests
Candida DNA, 30
pros and cons, 30
vaginal pH, 29–30
yeast vaginitis, 29–30
Semmelweis reflex (cognitive bias), 84
sensitive but dose dependent (S-DD) yeast infections, 123–24
septa, 7
sexual practices, 38, 182
sexually transmitted infections (STIs)
relapse vs. reinfection, 183
safety tips for preventing, 183
substances in semen causing yeast vaginitis, 182
SGLT-2 (sodium–glucose co-transporter-2) inhibitors, 167–68
short-chain fatty acids (SCFA), 203, 204
sigmoidoscopy, 97
signs and symptoms, in diagnosis, 88, 93, 147
silver, colloidal, 123
simethicone (Gas-X), 190
sinusitis, 115
skin disorders
cutaneous candidiasis, 13
exfoliative, 142
skin tests
intradermal, 100, 155–56
precautions, 155
scratch (prick) tests, 100, 154–55
sources for antigens, 160
systemic reactions to antigens, 156, 160
sodium–glucose co-transporter-2 (SGLT-2) inhibitors, 9, 167–68
soluble fiber, 203, 204
spermicides, 179, 180
Sporanox (itraconazole)
C. glabrata vaginitis, 135

Printed in Great Britain
by Amazon

51434910R00156